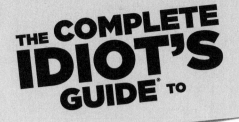

THE COMPLETE IDIOT'S GUIDE TO

Hearing Loss

by House Clinic, edited by William M. Luxford, M.D., M. Jennifer Derebery, M.D., and Karen I. Berliner, Ph.D.

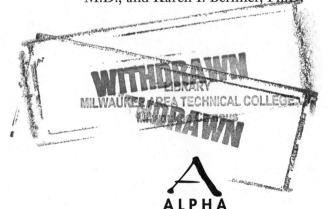
ALPHA

A member of Penguin Group (USA) Inc.

ALPHA BOOKS

Published by the Penguin Group

Penguin Group (USA) Inc., 375 Hudson Street, New York, New York 10014, USA

Penguin Group (Canada), 90 Eglinton Avenue East, Suite 700, Toronto, Ontario M4P 2Y3, Canada (a division of Pearson Penguin Canada Inc.)

Penguin Books Ltd., 80 Strand, London WC2R 0RL, England

Penguin Ireland, 25 St. Stephen's Green, Dublin 2, Ireland (a division of Penguin Books Ltd.)

Penguin Group (Australia), 250 Camberwell Road, Camberwell, Victoria 3124, Australia (a division of Pearson Australia Group Pty. Ltd.)

Penguin Books India Pvt. Ltd., 11 Community Centre, Panchsheel Park, New Delhi—110 017, India

Penguin Group (NZ), 67 Apollo Drive, Rosedale, North Shore, Auckland 1311, New Zealand (a division of Pearson New Zealand Ltd.)

Penguin Books (South Africa) (Pty.) Ltd., 24 Sturdee Avenue, Rosebank, Johannesburg 2196, South Africa

Penguin Books Ltd., Registered Offices: 80 Strand, London WC2R 0RL, England

International Standard Book Number: 978-1-59257-990-7
Library of Congress Catalog Card Number: 2009937011

12 11 10   8 7 6 5 4 3 2 1

Interpretation of the printing code: The rightmost number of the first series of numbers is the year of the book's printing; the rightmost number of the second series of numbers is the number of the book's printing. For example, a printing code of 10-1 shows that the first printing occurred in 2010.

Printed in the United States of America

Note: This publication contains the opinions and ideas of its authors. It is intended to provide helpful and informative material on the subject matter covered. It is sold with the understanding that the authors and publisher are not engaged in rendering professional services in the book. If the reader requires personal assistance or advice, a competent professional should be consulted.

The authors and publisher specifically disclaim any responsibility for any liability, loss, or risk, personal or otherwise, which is incurred as a consequence, directly or indirectly, of the use and application of any of the contents of this book.

Most Alpha books are available at special quantity discounts for bulk purchases for sales promotions, premiums, fund-raising, or educational use. Special books, or book excerpts, can also be created to fit specific needs.

For details, write: Special Markets, Alpha Books, 375 Hudson Street, New York, NY 10014.

Publisher: *Marie Butler-Knight*

Associate Publisher: *Mike Sanders*

Senior Managing Editor: *Billy Fields*

Senior Acquisitions Editor: *Paul Dinas*

Development Editor: *Julie Coffin*

Senior Production Editor: *Megan Douglass*

Copy Editor: *Nancy Wagner*

Cover Designer: *Kurt Owens*

Book Designer: *Trina Wurst*

Indexer: *Brad Herriman*

Layout: *Ayanna Lacey*

Proofreader: *John Etchison*

This book is dedicated to Howard P. House, M.D. (1908–2003), the founder of House Ear Institute and the House Clinic, and to William F. House, M.D., the father of inner ear surgery. These brothers developed so many of the surgical techniques that now help restore hearing and balance to patients worldwide. They trained ear doctors from all over the world because they believed that any new procedure could help a significant number of people only if it was widely available to them. Their motto was "So all may hear."

We also dedicate this book to the memory of Drs. James Sheehy and Antonio De la Cruz, who as members of the House Clinic dedicated considerable time and energy to the education and training of their younger colleagues and ear doctors everywhere.

Contents

Appendixes

Introduction

Bob Hope told this joke at a benefit dinner for House Ear Institute, the nonprofit research and education institution with which we are associated:

A man is talking to his doctor and says, "I don't think my wife's hearing is as good as it used to be; what should I do?" The doctor replies, "Maybe we can try a test to find out just how bad it is. When your wife's standing somewhere with her back to you, stand about 15 feet behind her and ask her a question; if she doesn't respond, keep moving closer asking the question until she hears you. Then let me know how close you had to get." The man goes home and sees his wife preparing dinner. He stands 15 feet behind her and says, "What's for dinner, honey?" He gets no response, so he moves to 10 feet behind her and asks again. Still no response, so he moves to 5 feet. Again, no answer. Finally he stands directly behind her and says, "Honey, what's for supper?" She replies, "For the fourth time, I SAID CHICKEN!!"

What is the moral of this story? Some of us may not realize just how greatly hearing loss is impacting our lives. And many people who are aware that their hearing has deteriorated don't acknowledge the problem and don't seek help.

Hearing loss is one of the most common chronic illnesses in the United States. In the year 2000, 28 million Americans—approximately 10 percent of the population—were hearing impaired. Nine million had mild hearing loss; 10 million had moderate hearing loss; 6 million had moderate to severe hearing loss; and 3 million had severe to profound hearing loss. By 2004–2005, the population with hearing loss increased to more than 31 million Americans. More than 1 million of this group are children (0–18 years); 18.4 million are grouped as working adults (18–64 years); and 11.6 million are over 65 years of age. It's predicted that within the next two decades, the number of Americans with hearing loss will swell to more than 40 million.

Approximately 30 percent of people over the age of 65 are affected by hearing impairment, with the figure rising to 35 to 40 percent in those older than 75 years. And by a 2004 survey, nearly 1 in 6 baby boomers (people from 41 to 59 years old) already had a hearing problem. It's estimated that 3 in 1,000 infants are born with serious to profound hearing loss. Take a look at these numbers—it's clearly a myth to think that hearing loss affects only "old people." In fact, the majority of those with hearing loss are younger than age 65. Do you have a hearing loss? Do you suspect you have a hearing loss? Or do you know someone with a hearing loss? Then this book is for you.

Age-related hearing loss (presbycusis) occurs gradually and, though it may go unnoticed by the individual, it's quite apparent to family and friends. Presbycusis is the most common cause of hearing loss in the United States. The aging of the baby boomers is swelling the over-60 population, increasing the number of older adults with hearing loss. Older adults with hearing loss who don't use hearing aids are more likely to report feelings of sadness, depression, anxiety, and emotional turmoil. Excessive noise is the likely culprit for the increase in the incidence of hearing impairment in the younger age groups. Damaging noise exposure may occur at rock concerts, movies, and aerobics classes. Noise-induced hearing loss can result from the use of personal music players with in-the-ear buds.

Hearing loss definitely impacts quality of life for the individual and his or her family. It has a negative impact not only on physical, emotional, and mental health but also on work and school performance. Hearing is necessary for effective communication in most work settings to create an efficient and safe environment. Compared to those with normal hearing, workers with severe to profound hearing loss as well as workers with mild to moderate hearing loss are more likely to be unemployed or underemployed, leading to significant adverse personal and social effects. Treating the hearing loss, whether mild, moderate, or severe, with medical treatment, surgery, or hearing aids, as appropriate, can improve the earning power of the worker. Not treating the loss can lead to lost wages, lost promotions, lost opportunities, and, as a result, lower income in retirement.

Hearing loss can also markedly affect the life of a child. Children with severe to profound hearing loss are more likely to receive further testing and treatment, while children with milder losses are often not identified or treated. However, even a mild hearing loss can have a significant negative effect on speech development, educational achievement, and formation of social skills. Don't minimize the potential impact that any degree of hearing loss can have on your child.

A complete otologic (ear) examination is necessary to determine the type of hearing impairment, its probable cause, and recommended treatment. Hearing is the natural and normal way to understand speech. If your hearing can be improved by medical or surgical means or through the use of a hearing aid, you should take advantage of any opportunity. The vast majority of Americans with hearing loss, probably 95 percent, could be helped with hearing aids, and most of the other 5 percent can likely find improvement through medical or surgical treatment. This book will educate you on the many causes of hearing loss and what can be done to improve hearing.

How to Use This Book

The Complete Idiot's Guide to Hearing Loss is divided into five parts, each covering an aspect of hearing or hearing loss to help you understand how you hear and what goes wrong when you can't hear.

Part 1, The Basics, describes the four basic parts of the ear: the external ear, the middle ear, the inner ear, and the brain. We describe how waves in the air become sound in the brain. And we tell you about the various categories of hearing loss based on the part of the hearing system that is affected. We'll help you answer the question, "Do I have a hearing loss?" and introduce the types of health-care professionals you might need to see regarding your hearing.

Part 2, External and Middle Ear Hearing Loss, deals with the most common external and middle ear causes of hearing loss. We explain issues such as earwax, foreign objects in the ear, and "swimmer's ear." You'll learn how important the Eustachian tube is and how fluid buildup in the middle ear can lead to hearing loss as we discuss the symptoms and treatments for these and other causes of middle ear hearing loss.

Part 3, Inner Ear Hearing Loss, focuses on the many problems that can affect the inner ear and cause hearing loss. Aging and noise are at the top of the list. We provide tips and advice for preventing inner ear problems as well as what you can do to make the best of it when it does occur.

Part 4, Other Issues of Hearing Loss, covers issues such as how allergy can affect all parts of the ear and the very common problem of tinnitus. Hearing problems in children and the treatment of problems in children get special attention because of the importance of detecting and treating hearing loss as early as possible.

Part 5, Help for Hearing Loss, deals with different types of help available beyond treatments for specific diseases. One of the major types of help is the use of a hearing aid, so we explain how hearing aids work; we cover the different styles and their special features; and we give you helpful hints for learning to use a hearing aid.

We also talk about assistive listening devices designed to help with the problems of hearing loss. When other treatment options fail to help severe or profound deafness, several surgically implanted devices are available. We explore the surgical procedures and the expected outcomes of surgery.

How do hearing-impaired people and their family and friends cope with hearing loss? You'll find out how best to communicate, whether you have a hearing loss or are talking to someone who does.

And finally, many of the chapters end with a section titled "True Stories." These are stories or anecdotes about actual patients from our clinic records, but of course, the names and perhaps some facts have been changed to protect patient privacy. We believe these stories can help you understand more about the causes of and treatments for hearing loss.

In addition, you'll find the following:

Appendix A, Glossary, defines some of the words we use that may not be part of your regular vocabulary.

Appendix B, Resources, provides contact information for organizations related to hearing and hearing loss, print references, and companies from which to obtain assistive listening devices.

Appendix C, Noise Levels of Common Sounds, gives examples of the loudness levels of everyday sounds and how much exposure you can have before potential damage to hearing occurs.

Appendix D, Low-Sodium, Low-Caffeine Diet, provides examples of salt and caffeine levels in common food items for those with hearing loss related to inner ear fluid imbalances or anyone else who is interested.

Appendix E, Hearing Loss and Learning Needs, details the impact of different degrees of hearing loss on a child's speech and language development, the social impact of that level of loss, and some of the educational accommodations and services that might be necessary.

Appendix F, Comparison of Digital Hearing Aids, provides a list of technological features available in hearing aids and which features can be found at different levels of technology and cost.

Extras

Throughout your reading, you'll find sidebars that offer interesting facts, warnings, and helpful hints related to the ears and hearing.

DEFINITION

These boxes provide key words and phrases to help you understand the ear, hearing, and hearing loss.

HAVE YOU HEARD?

Look here for interesting facts or amusing information about the ear and hearing.

LISTEN UP

In these boxes, you find warnings to help prevent hearing loss or injury to the ear.

SOUND ADVICE

Check these boxes for useful information and things you should know to help you deal with hearing loss or to communicate better as—or with—a hearing-impaired person.

Acknowledgments

Although three of us "edited" this book, the content comes from and couldn't have been done without all of the physicians of House Clinic. The otologists (ear doctors) of House Clinic are:

Derald E. Brackmann, M.D.

Antonio De la Cruz, M.D. (1944–July 31, 2009)

John W. House, M.D.

William M. Luxford, M.D.

M. Jennifer Derebery, M.D.

William H. Slattery, III, M.D.

Rick A. Friedman, M.D., Ph.D.

Jose N. Fayad, M.D.

Eric P. Wilkinson, M.D.

(Fred H. Linthicum, Jr., M.D.—retired; currently, Director Temporal Bone Histopathology Lab of House Ear Institute)

Much of the basic material for many of the chapters came from a series of patient booklets prepared by House Clinic on a wide variety of ear and hearing problems and made available to the clinic's patients. Material for specific chapters was also contributed by Margaret Winter, M.S., Clinical Coordinator of House Ear Institute's Children's Auditory Research and Education (CARE) Center; Allen Senne, Au.D., Director of Audiology for House Clinic; the 2008 and 2009 Clinical Fellows—Joseph Ursick, M.D., Alexander G. Bien, M.D., John Goddard, M.D., and Felipe Santos, M.D.; Maria T. Vargas, Au.D., of House Ear Institute; and Rebecca Cihocki, Au.D., of House Clinic.

Much information about hearing and hearing loss is available online. We gleaned considerable information from the websites of House Ear Institute, House Clinic, Better Hearing Institute, the American Academy of Otolaryngology—Head & Neck Surgery (AAO-HNS), the American Speech-Language-Hearing Association (ASHA), and National Institute on Deafness and Other Communication Disorders (NIDCD), among others.

Of course, we all want to thank our spouses for putting up with the time commitments required in the writing of this book. And we must not forget the thousands of patients who visit our clinic and provide the basis for our experience and clinical and research expertise.

Trademarks

All terms mentioned in this book that are known to be or are suspected of being trademarks or service marks have been appropriately capitalized. Alpha Books and Penguin Group (USA) Inc. cannot attest to the accuracy of this information. Use of a term in this book should not be regarded as affecting the validity of any trademark or service mark.

The Basics

1

Before we can discuss any specific cause of hearing loss, you, the reader, need to know how we hear and how we determine the amount and type of hearing loss. In Part 1, we describe the four basic parts of the ear: the external ear, the middle ear, the inner ear, and, of course, the brain, and we explain how the ear works and the various categories of hearing loss based on the part of the hearing system that is affected.

Do you ever wonder if you have a hearing loss? Or maybe you're concerned about a family member. We describe the general symptoms of hearing loss, the types of health-care professionals you might need to see regarding your hearing, and the tests you'll need to have to determine the degree and cause of any hearing loss.

How the Ear Works and How We Hear

In This Chapter

- The basic anatomy of the ear—names and purposes of important parts
- The way pressure waves in the air become sound in the brain
- The characteristics and measurements of sound
- The types of hearing loss

The human ear is extremely complicated, and hearing is commonly considered the most complex of the human senses as scientists are still investigating the smallest details of how the ear works. The ear's main purpose is to transform pressure waves from the air into electrical signals that the brain can interpret as sound. The human ear can perceive a broad range of tones and loudness levels, can help an individual determine the direction from which a sound comes, and can pick out a particular voice from all background sounds. How does it do all of these things?

In this chapter, we give you a basic overview of the anatomy and function of the human ear. We describe the major divisions of the ear that make up the auditory system: the external ear, the middle ear, the inner ear, and the brain. We describe how pressure waves in the air become sound in the brain and explain the measurement units that define the pitch and loudness of a sound. As hearing loss can occur from problems with any part of the hearing system, from external ear to the brain, we briefly define the various categories of hearing loss based on the affected part of the hearing system. In Parts 2, 3, and 4, we discuss specific causes of hearing loss that can affect each part of the auditory system.

We introduce many new words in this chapter (see Appendix A for definitions). We realize it may seem pretty technical and complicated, but we want to give you a very complete picture so you can fully understand any kind of hearing loss situation that you or a loved one may experience. With careful reading in the technical parts and with the help of Appendix A, we feel sure this book will help you recognize, face, comprehend, and/or live with hearing loss, whether yours or someone else's.

Parts of the Ear

The ear is commonly divided into three parts that represent both a physical division as well as a division by function: the external, middle, and inner ear. We refer to the brain as a fourth part because hearing does not occur without this central component. So let's take a look at each of these parts, including the names of many of the different structures of each part.

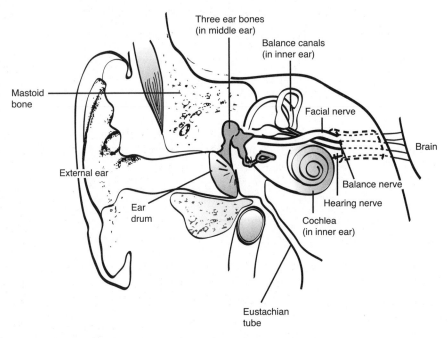

Diagram showing many of the basic structures of the auditory system.

External Ear

The external part of the ear that we all see and think of as the ear is the pinna, which comes from the Latin word *pinna*, meaning "wing" or "feather," and is sometimes called the auricle. We call the normally curled outer rim of the pinna the helix. The bowl-shaped depression in the center of the ear is the concha, and the triangle-shaped piece in front of the ear canal, nearest to the cheek, is the tragus. These various curvatures and outcroppings are made of skin draped over a cartilage framework. The ear lobe, or lobule, is mainly skin and fatty tissue with no cartilage underneath. These external parts serve as a funnel to gather sound waves and transmit them to the ear canal and on to the eardrum. Both the pinna and canal continue to grow during childhood. When the external ear does not form correctly during fetal development, it may be smaller than normal or lacking some parts (a condition called microtia) or it can be missing entirely (a condition called anotia).

The rest of the external, middle, and inner ear structures are contained within the temporal bone, a pyramid-shaped bone that forms part of the base of the skull on each side. The hard, or petrous, part of the temporal bone contains the inner ear structures involved with hearing and balance. The mastoid bone houses the honeycomblike system of air cells that connect to the middle ear behind the eardrum.

HAVE YOU HEARD?

The petrous portion of the temporal bone is the hardest bone in the human body!

The ear canal, or external auditory canal, is the tubelike structure located between the pinna and the eardrum and is about an inch long. The skin toward the outside of the canal contains cerumen glands, which make earwax, and hair. A branch of a major nerve from the brain supplies sensation to part of the ear canal. When you stimulate it by using a cotton swab or putting a finger in the ear, it can cause a tickle in the throat or even a cough because it may be stimulating other branches of the same nerve. This experience is known as referred pain. Many people say they get an "ice cream headache" (or brain freeze) after eating or drinking something cold. This is also a referred pain experience. The cold food or beverage is freezing a nerve to the palate, but the pain occurs in the eye and forehead!

Just as some people are born with an absence or malformation of the pinna, others are born with similar problems with the ear canal. When it's closed completely and the eardrum is not visible, this is known as aural atresia. Aural atresia is often associated with microtia.

In front of the ear canal, the jawbone forms its connection to the base of the skull, a structure you've most likely heard of—the temporomandibular joint (TMJ). Sometimes the front wall of the ear canal is missing a part of the bone, and the jaw joint protrudes into the ear canal. This appears as a mass beneath the skin of the ear canal that enlarges when the jaw is closed and gets smaller when the jaw opens. Yes, your jaw might actually stick into your ear!

SOUND ADVICE

Inflammation of the TMJ is a common nonear-related cause of perceived ear pain. Also, you might sometimes notice a clicking sound when you open your mouth or chew. This can occur from overaggressive chewing, grinding your teeth (during the day or while sleeping), or trying to pop your ears by excessive yawning. The best treatment is refraining from chewing hard foods or gum, using anti-inflammatory medications such as ibuprofen, and applying warm compresses. If the pain due to TMJ inflammation doesn't respond to those simple treatments, your dentist may recommend a bite block during sleep or perhaps surgery.

Behind the ear canal is the mastoid bone, normally filled with dozens of tiny air pockets known as air cells. Below the ear canal lies the base of the skull.

The eardrum, or tympanic membrane, is a light gray to tan colored see-through piece of skinlike tissue that is the border between the external and middle ear. The eardrum has two main functions. Of course, it's involved in sound transmission. When sound waves from the environment strike the eardrum, they cause a vibration that is carried on to the middle ear bones. Also, the eardrum protects the middle ear from exposure to water and micro-organisms (bacteria and fungi) that can cause infection.

HAVE YOU HEARD?

The skin of the eardrum flakes off and is replaced just like skin elsewhere on the body. The old skin moves outward from the eardrum at a rate of about a millimeter (0.04 inches) a day and eventually falls out with the earwax.

Middle Ear

The middle ear is the space between the eardrum and the inner ear. Lined with mucosa, or a mucous membrane, it contains a number of important structures as the ossicular chain, the three bones of hearing, or ossicles, are located here. The malleus, or hammer, the first bone of hearing, is attached to and can be seen through the eardrum. The incus, or anvil, the second bone, transmits vibrations from the malleus to the stapes, or stirrup, the third bone of hearing. The stapes has two components. The arch, or superstructure, connects with the incus. The stapes footplate sits in what's called the oval window—a membrane-covered opening into the inner ear. Vibration of the stapes is transmitted by movement of the oval window membrane to the fluids of the inner ear hearing organ. A second opening into the inner ear, the round window, allows the vibration carried to the inner ear by the stapes to escape back to the middle ear space so no pressure builds up in the fluids of the inner ear. A thin membrane also covers the round window to prevent leakage of inner ear fluid.

HAVE YOU HEARD?

The stapes is the smallest bone in the human body, measuring just a few millimeters in height. The muscle that attaches to the stapes, the stapedius muscle, is the smallest muscle in the human body. The stapedius muscle receives its nervous input from the facial nerve!

Two muscles inside the middle ear play a protective role. The tensor tympani muscle attaches to the malleus, and the stapedius muscle attaches to the stapes. One function of the stapedius muscle is to protect the inner ear from loud sounds that can cause large, damaging vibrations. When a loud sound is presented to the ear, the hearing nerve picks up the signal and notifies a relay center, or nucleus, in the brainstem. This nucleus transmits the signal to another and, eventually, the signal is sent back to the stapedius muscle, which causes a reflexive, or automatic, contraction of that muscle. Involuntary contraction or spasm of either of the two middle ear muscles can cause an intermittent fluttering sound, something most people occasionally hear. These two middle ear muscles also act to stabilize the ossicular chain and can alter the sound frequencies entering the inner ear.

The Eustachian tube is a cylindrical cartilage framework surrounded by fat and muscle tissue that connects the back of the nose to the middle ear cavity. Yes, your nose and your ear are directly connected! For the eardrum to vibrate efficiently in response to a sound wave, the air pressure of the middle ear must be roughly equal to that of the outside environment. The Eustachian tube functions as a pressure-release valve to maintain this balance. Although the tube is normally closed to prevent secretions from the nose from entering the ear, it opens in response to yawning, swallowing, or forcefully blowing the nose. These actions ventilate the middle ear space and prevent negative pressure from building up behind the eardrum. (See Chapter 4 for hearing problems due to Eustachian tube dysfunction.)

Several nerves run through the middle ear, the most important of which is the facial nerve (cranial nerve VII). This nerve runs next to the hearing and balance nerve (cranial nerve VIII) between the brain and inner ear. The first structure it passes through on its way to the face is the internal auditory canal (IAC), a bony tunnel in the temporal bone through which the facial, hearing, and balance nerves travel. At the end of the IAC, the facial nerve sends off a nerve branch that eventually causes tearing and nasal mucus production on the same side of the face. The facial nerve then winds its way through the middle ear and eventually exits the skull base to supply the muscles of facial movement.

The chorda tympani nerve branches off from the facial nerve and travels through the middle ear on its way to innervate taste buds at the front of the tongue on the same side of the face. Because the facial nerve is so intimately involved in the temporal bone areas, diseases of the ear or surgical procedures used to treat some types of hearing loss may affect it and its branches; both ear disease or ear surgery can affect facial movement and taste. A branch of the ninth cranial nerve involved in stimulating the salivary glands also travels along the bony inner wall of the middle ear.

The floor of the middle ear includes the bony covering of the jugular bulb, the beginning of the large jugular vein that drains blood from the brain through the neck on its way to the heart. Sometimes, the bony covering of the jugular bulb is absent. In such a case, a bluish mass is visible behind the eardrum. In some people, the jugular bulb is located higher than the floor of the middle ear and can actually interfere with the normal movement of the round window membrane, which can lead to a hearing loss.

Inner Ear

The petrous temporal bone contains the inner ear structures involved with hearing and balance.

HAVE YOU HEARD?

The inner ear is adult size at birth. In fact, studies show that a baby is probably able to hear some sound even before it's born. A person's cochlea is completely formed by week 26 of gestation. Some studies have shown evidence that babies in the womb can respond to loud sound at 30 weeks of age.

The hearing portion of the inner ear, or cochlea, is composed of three fluid-filled ducts within a spiral or snail-shaped bony shell (see the following figure). The central cochlear duct, or scala media, contains a fluid called endolymph that is rich in potassium. On either side of the scala media are two other ducts, the scala tympani and scala vestibuli. They are connected at the end of the spiral and are filled with a fluid called perilymph, which is rich in sodium. The scala tympani and scala vestibuli are each separated from the scala media by a thin membrane, scala tympani by the basilar membrane and scala vestibuli by Reissner's membrane.

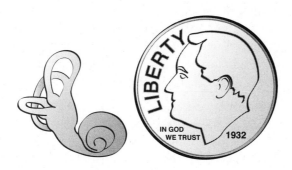

Picture of the entire inner ear system shown for actual size next to a dime.

Within the scala media is the organ of corti, the inner ear hearing organ. This structure contains sensory cells, or hair cells, that transform sound vibrations from the middle ear bones into electrical signals. They're called hair cells because they are composed of a body with tiny filaments called stereocilia coming from their upper surface—the filaments are the "hairs." The cell bodies rest on the basilar membrane. The hairs touch another membrane called the tectorial membrane. There are two types of hair cells: inner hair cells and outer hair cells. The inner hair cells are responsible for most of the auditory input to the brain. The outer hair cells help to fine-tune the auditory signal. Each inner hair cell is attached to several tiny nerve endings that eventually unite to form the hearing, or cochlear, nerve.

The inner ear also contains the organ of balance. Cranial nerve VIII, the hearing nerve, is also called the vestibulocochlear nerve. Part of this cranial nerve transmits sound, and part transmits balance, or vestibular, information to the brain. The organ of balance consists of three half-circular, interconnected tubes called the semicircular canals, as well as other components. Because this book is about hearing loss, we don't discuss the balance mechanism in any detail, but now you'll understand why so many causes of hearing loss also cause dizziness or balance problems. The presence of the symptom of dizziness and its severity are sometimes clues to the cause of the hearing loss.

Brain

Once the hair cells create their auditory message, they send it to the brain via the cochlear nerve. The cochlear nerve carries its message to the brainstem, where nerve fibers pass through several relay stations or nuclei. The first relay station is the cochlear nucleus. Some nerve fibers pass to the cochlear nucleus on the same side; others actually cross to the opposite side. Within these relay stations, nerve fibers interact with one another, eventually sending the auditory information up the brainstem to the midbrain relay centers and then to the auditory cortex located in the temporal lobe of the brain. You'll find more about some of these structures and their roles in hearing loss or in restoration of hearing in later chapters.

Normal Hearing: How We Hear

To understand hearing loss and all the ways it might occur, we first need to understand how we hear. As we already mentioned, the ear is a very complex organ, and hearing is a complicated series of events.

From Pressure Wave to Sound

Sounds we hear are actually invisible pressure waves created by vibrating objects. These waves require both a source of vibration (for example, your vocal cords) and also a medium through which to transmit the vibration (for example, air or water). The medium is a set of interconnected particles that vibrate in turn and keep the wave moving. These particles vibrate back and forth at a given rate, known as frequency. The frequency of a wave is the number of times a particle vibrates back and forth in a certain amount of time. For hearing, frequency is measured in units called Hertz (Hz), the number of vibrations, or cycles, per second.

HAVE YOU HEARD?

Sound waves require a medium through which to travel. This medium must be composed of particles close enough to each other to transmit a vibration. Any medium composed of one or more of the three states of matter (solid, liquid, or gas) can conduct a sound wave. But outer space is a near perfect vacuum and contains very few gas particles. They are too far apart to pass vibrations to one another. Because of this, space cannot propagate sound waves and is therefore silent.

The human ear can hear sound frequencies ranging from 20 Hz all the way to 20,000 Hz. The frequencies most important in human speech are from 500 Hz to 3000 Hz. Middle C on a piano keyboard is roughly 256 Hz. Anything above the range of frequencies we can hear is known as ultrasound. Dogs and cats detect sounds of very high frequencies—up to 85,000 Hz. This ability is the basis of the dog whistle, as the sound it makes is a high frequency dogs can hear but humans can't. Bats detect frequencies up to 120,000 Hz, and dolphins, up to 200,000 Hz. The human sensation of sound frequency is known as pitch. High-pitched sounds correspond to high-frequency waves; low-pitched sounds to low-frequency waves.

The intensity, or loudness, of a sound is determined by how much energy is applied to a medium in a given amount of time. The amount each particle moves in response to the applied energy is known as the particle's (or wave's) amplitude. Using the example of a guitar string, a gentle strum of the string imparts less energy on the string, causing a smaller displacement of air particles (in other words, less amplitude) and therefore a quieter sound. A strong plucking of the guitar string imparts much more energy, leading to a larger amplitude wave and a louder sound.

The task of the human ear is to transform a pressure wave, usually in the air, into an electrical signal the brain can understand. Briefly, sound (in the form of a pressure wave) enters the ear and strikes the eardrum, causing a vibration. Then the three bones of hearing carry the vibration to the inner ear. The vibration causes the fluid in the inner ear to move, stimulating the hair cells to generate an electric impulse that travels along the nerve of hearing to the brain. And every part of the system must function properly for normal hearing to occur. You should keep in mind that sound is a pressure wave in a medium until it encounters an ear and is changed in form, but from now on, we will refer to such waves as sound waves or just sound.

 HAVE YOU HEARD?

A philosophical question has had people arguing for centuries. "If a tree falls in the forest and there is no one around to hear it, does it make a sound?" Let's assume that "no one" means no critters of any sort. The answer may depend on the definition of sound you choose to use. You can think of sound in the scientific sense—as vibrations created in the air or some other medium. Or you can say that sound is the interpretation of these vibrations by the brain after the pressure waves have been converted to an electrical signal by an ear. This latter definition is how most of us think of sound. We are not going to offer an opinion about the correct answer to this age-old question. An Internet search on the question yielded more than 700,000 hits!

The pinna acts as a funnel to focus sound waves toward the eardrum, and in doing this, amplifies the sound signal. The other external and middle ear structures also amplify sound waves. The ear canal acts as a resonating tube. The eardrum and the ossicles are most efficient at transmitting sounds with frequencies between 500 Hz and 3000 Hz. Is it any coincidence that most speech sounds fall between these frequencies?

The middle ear (and specifically the ossicular chain) has the important task of transforming sound energy from the medium (again, usually the air) into a liquid medium inside the cochlea. The structure and function of the middle ear ensures that sound energy is not lost as this transformation is made. First, the vibrating surface of the eardrum is much larger than that of the oval window. This results in a 17:1 increase in sound energy.

Second, because the malleus is longer than the incus, the force the stapes receives from the incus is 1.3 times that received by the malleus from the eardrum. In other words, as the vibrations pass through the middle ear system, they are increased. These two mechanisms result in a 22:1 increase in energy as sound passes from the eardrum to the stapes footplate, which is part of the reason the human ear is so sensitive to such a wide range of sound intensity.

When the stapes vibrates, the vibration is transmitted to the fluid in the scala vestibuli of the cochlea by movement of the oval window membrane. The fluid wave causes movement of the membranes separating the scala media from the two other compartments. Movement of the basilar membrane causes the stereocilia (remember those "hairs"?) of the hair cells to bend in relation to the membrane they touch. This bending causes first potassium from the endolymph fluid and then calcium to leak into the hair cell, leading to the release of a chemical messenger or neurotransmitter. The neurotransmitter stimulates the hearing nerve, which then conveys the auditory information to the brainstem. From there, the signal is transmitted to higher centers in the brain where it is transformed into meaningful information.

The hair cells along the basilar membrane are organized with respect to the frequency of sound to which they are most sensitive. The hair cells in the base of the cochlea near the oval and round windows are more sensitive to high-frequency sounds. The hair cells toward the top or apex of the cochlear spiral are responsible for coding low-frequency sounds. This is referred to as the tonotopic principle.

How Loudness Is Measured

Physicists measure sound in units known as watts per meter squared (W/m^2). However, measuring sounds that humans can hear in this way is impractical. The human ear is sensitive to a very wide range of sound intensity. In fact, the faintest sound the human ear can hear would move air particles by one billionth of a centimeter (a centimeter is less than half an inch). On the other end of the spectrum, the ear is able to hear sounds of very high intensity, such as jet airplane engines. Because the range of intensities that the human ear can hear is so large, scientists created a new scale for measuring sound intensity—the decibel (abbreviated dB) scale.

For those of you interested in mathematics, the decibel scale is a logarithmic scale of sound intensity. The threshold of hearing for most people, 1×10^{-12} W/m^2, has been assigned the number 0 dB. A loudness level of 0 dB does not mean no sound is occurring. Rather, it represents the lowest sound level the majority of humans can detect. Some people have thresholds for hearing of –5 dB or even –10 dB (see Chapter 2). The human ear is just able to distinguish differences in sound intensities of one decibel. The decibel scale is based on multiples of 10. If a sound increases from 0 to 10 decibels, it's 10 times more intense. However, because the decibel scale is logarithmic and not linear, a sound that increases from 0 dB to 20 dB is 100 times more intense.

Complex Hearing Functions

In addition to detecting pitch and loudness, people can usually determine from what direction a sound is coming. We tend to take this ability for granted, yet it's actually a very complex function of the auditory system. Having two ears is part of what makes localization of sound possible. Depending on the direction from which the sound is coming, it arrives at one ear slightly before the other. This timing difference provides a cue to the direction or angle of the sound source. There may also be a difference in sound level or loudness entering the ears, which can also serve as a clue to direction. What about when the sound is coming from directly in front or in back of us? Moving the head can add more information. We often cock our head to one side or turn it slightly when trying to determine the location of a sound. We won't attempt to cover this complicated topic in detail, but you should now understand how a hearing loss in one ear might affect your ability to tell from what direction a sound is coming.

Another complex function of our auditory system is that we are able to focus on one sound out of many. We can still hear and understand conversation even when there are other noises and other speakers in the background. Hearing scientists as well as cognitive psychologists who study attention and information processing have studied this ability.

HAVE YOU HEARD?

We still don't completely understand how the human brain manages to pick out and follow a single conversation from competing similar background noises, a phenomenon we call the cocktail party effect. We can listen to and understand what one person says; yet if someone across the room calls out our name suddenly, we also notice that sound and respond to it immediately.

The ability to localize sound and the ability to hear in noise are not completely independent abilities. Binaural (two-ear) directional hearing plays a role in our ability to communicate in noise. Any degree of hearing impairment, therefore, can affect both of these abilities and make communication more difficult.

Types of Hearing Loss

We categorize hearing loss into three main types: conductive, sensorineural, or mixed (a combination of the other two). In conductive hearing loss, sound waves are not able to reach the inner ear hearing structures at normal levels. In sensorineural hearing loss, the sound conduction mechanism can be normal, but the inner ear hearing organ or hearing nerve is not functioning properly. These different types of hearing loss can be due to problems with the external, middle, and inner ears, as well as with the brain.

External and Middle Ear Hearing Loss

Hearing loss due to problems with the external ear is usually conductive (see Chapter 3). The most common cause of hearing loss worldwide is earwax plugging the ear canal, as the wax plug interferes with sound waves trying to reach the eardrum. Similarly, narrowing of the ear canal due to inflammation, bony growths, or from aural atresia causes a conductive hearing loss.

Problems with the eardrum can interfere with the fidelity of sound transmission (see Chapters 4 and 5). A thickened, scarred, or torn eardrum can't vibrate normally, so this leads to a conductive hearing loss because sound loses energy as it passes through the eardrum. Fluid or blood behind the eardrum from infection (see Chapters 4 and 5), trauma (Chapter 6), or allergies (Chapter 12) can also interfere with the normal vibration of the tympanic membrane and lead to a conductive hearing loss.

Any abnormality of the middle ear bones can cause conductive hearing loss (see Chapters 5 and 6). If the hearing bones are fixed in position, are lacking a strong connection to one another, or are malformed, they can't properly transmit vibrations from the eardrum to the inner ear. Chronic infections and diseases of the middle ear bones can affect their ability to move properly. Tumors and cysts can also grow within the middle ear space and cause erosion of the ossicles.

If a hearing loss is purely conductive and the inner ear and hearing nerve are working well, it's usually possible to improve hearing by surgically fixing the problem with the external or middle ear.

Inner Ear Hearing Loss

Hearing loss due to damage to inner ear structures is typically sensorineural. This term refers to a loss occurring either in the cochlea (sensory) or the hearing nerve itself (neural) or both. There are many causes of inner ear hearing loss, the most common being age-related loss or presbycusis (see Chapter 7). Other causes include toxins (mercury, some intravenous antibiotics), loud noise exposure, trauma (fracture through the cochlea), viral or bacterial inner ear infections, developmental abnormalities of the inner ear, and tumors (Chapters 8 through 11).

Each of these causes affects the inner ear in different ways, but many of them lead directly to hair cell loss. While outer and middle ear causes of conductive hearing loss can often be improved with surgery, inner ear hearing loss is usually irreversible. Once hair cells have been damaged or lose their function, there is no way to repair or replace them.

HAVE YOU HEARD?

Humans are not able to regrow lost hair cells, but some other species can. Fish, amphibians, and birds can grow new hair cells to replace damaged ones, but so far, mammals can't regenerate hair cells on their own. According to the National Institutes of Health (NIH), scientists have been able to grow new hair cells in laboratory animals using gene therapy and stem cell research, in some cases restoring some hearing to deafened mammals. Such promising results have led researchers to wonder if we might be able to regenerate hair cells in people one day.

The primary treatment for people with some, but not total, sensorineural hearing loss is a hearing aid (see Chapter 16). These devices provide a higher volume of sound to the inner ear to make up for the loss of hair cells. If someone becomes deaf in both ears, a cochlear implant can restore some hearing (see Chapter 18). This device is surgically implanted in the inner ear and replaces the function of the cochlea by electrically stimulating the hearing nerve.

Mixed Hearing Loss

Mixed hearing loss is simply a combination of conductive and sensorineural hearing loss and is usually caused by a middle ear problem that also affects the inner ear. For example, chronic ear infections can cause erosion of the ossicles—a conductive loss. But over time, the infection and inflammation can cause damage to the inner ear, leading to a sensorineural hearing loss as well. Inner ear malformations can also cause mixed loss.

Central (Brain) Hearing Problems

As we've said, the auditory system does not end at the level of the inner ear or hearing nerve. There are several further connections in the brainstem, midbrain, and temporal lobe of the brain. Damage at any of these higher levels of the auditory pathway may cause different problems than conductive and inner ear sensorineural hearing loss. Because it's at these higher levels that sounds become meaningful to the listener, a central cause of hearing loss might still allow an individual to hear tones, but yet have trouble understanding speech.

The Least You Need to Know

- The ear is a complex structure that includes external, middle, and inner portions.
- The middle ear bones, called ossicles, are the malleus (hammer), the incus (anvil), and the stapes (stirrup).
- The frequency or pitch of a sound is measured in Hertz (HZ); the intensity or loudness of a sound is measured in decibels (dB).
- When sound waves strike the eardrum, they cause a vibration that is carried to the middle ear bones, so anything that blocks the sound waves in the external ear or the transfer of the vibrations through the middle ear bones causes a conductive hearing loss.
- The hearing portion of the inner ear is the cochlea, and damage to its sensory cells (hair cells) or nerve fibers causes sensorineural hearing loss.

Do I Have a Hearing Loss?

In This Chapter

- Knowing the symptoms of hearing loss
- The health professionals who deal with hearing loss
- Personal information the doctor needs to know to diagnose the cause of your hearing loss
- Hearing tests that help determine the degree and type of hearing loss
- Other tests that determine the cause of your hearing loss

The person who has a hearing loss doesn't always realize it. In fact, for many adults, other family members often first recognize the hearing loss problem. Because a person may be able to hear and understand family conversation some of the time, yet misinterpret or totally ignore a speaker at other times, family members may decide the person (often the husband or father) has "selective hearing." I know—it seems as if we're picking on the man of the family, but in our experience, men are less likely to recognize or acknowledge having a hearing problem than are women!

Hearing loss—certainly if it's severe to profound and even if it's mild to moderate— can have a big impact on a person's ability to communicate and can be frustrating for both the individual and for family members. It can be devastating for a young child whose early onset of hearing loss may delay or significantly impair his or her ability to communicate. We discuss the impact of hearing loss in more detail in Chapters 14 (children) and 20 (adults). But first, one must recognize a hearing loss—either in one-self or in a family member, see the appropriate health-care professional, and undergo testing to determine the exact cause of the hearing loss. In this chapter, we tell you what symptoms might lead you to suspect you have a hearing loss, whom to see about it, and what type of examination and tests you might need to have.

General Symptoms

You might think it should be obvious to people that they have a hearing loss. Certainly people do notice a sudden onset of a significant hearing loss. But often, hearing loss is only mild or moderate or sneaks up on you, only gradually getting worse. In the following list of common warning signs for hearing loss, in either an adult or a child, are some signs you might notice in yourself. Other warning signs you might notice in a family member or a friend—or they might notice them in you. You should have your hearing checked if you believe you've experienced more than a few of these signs of hearing loss.

First, we list signs related to understanding speech. A person with a hearing loss might …

- Think everyone is mumbling.

- Often miss certain words, confuse words, or misunderstand conversations.

- Give inappropriate responses (due to not understanding the question).

- Seem to understand better when intently watching the faces of speakers.

- Say "What?" or "Huh?" frequently or ask the speaker to repeat.

- Have trouble understanding on the telephone and/or switch ears frequently when on the phone.

- Have more difficulty understanding speech in a group or when there is background noise such as in a restaurant or at a party.

- Tend to turn one ear toward a speaker to hear better.

- Hesitate to respond or not respond to soft and moderate-level speech (or environmental sounds), even when there are no other distractions.

- Sit closer to the TV or speaker when the volume is acceptable to others, or increase the volume to levels uncomfortable for others.

If someone is speaking too loudly for the situation, it's often a sign that the person may have a hearing loss. Or if someone seems to always try to control the conversation, he or she might have a hearing loss. By controlling the conversation and knowing the topic, the person may not feel the need to admit having a hearing problem. When older adults seem to misunderstand or not respond, we often assume it's because they're senile or confused. But sometimes they just haven't heard us correctly!

Besides difficulties related to understanding conversation, there are other warning signs of hearing loss. An individual with a hearing loss might …

- Feel tired or stressed from trying to hear.

- Fail to startle at loud or sudden sounds.

- Have difficulty locating the source of a sound.

- Receive questions from family members, friends, or colleagues about whether there might be a hearing problem.

- Experience delays or differences in speech and language development, attention or behavioral difficulties, or a decline in academic performance (when a child has the hearing loss).

- Have a history of work-related noise exposure.

- Miss important sounds such as the telephone, doorbell, alarm clock, smoke alarm, or approaching motor vehicles.

- Have difficulty hearing environmental sounds such as birds, barking dogs, or other common background sounds.

A number of other symptoms are commonly associated with hearing loss. These include fullness or a feeling of pressure in the ear; pain or ache in the ear; bleeding or drainage from the ears; ringing in the ears, called *tinnitus*; dizziness or balance problems; weakness or paralysis of the facial muscles; or a decrease in feeling in the face. These other symptoms are an important part of determining the cause of one's hearing loss.

 DEFINITION

Tinnitus is a sound in one or both ears, such as a buzzing, ringing, hissing, or whistling, that occurs even when there is no external sound present. Tinnitus, often referred to as head noise, is a common symptom in many diseases of the ear but may also occur on its own without apparent cause.

What Professional Should I See?

If you think you have a hearing problem or have been told by your family physician that you may have a problem, you may wonder what kind of a doctor or medical specialist to see about it. A number of specialists—including health care providers in the fields of otolaryngology, otology, neurotology, audiology, and radiology—diagnose and treat problems involving the ear and hearing. Following are some specifics on each specialty:

- **otolaryngology**   Also referred to as ear, nose, and throat, or ENT, this is the field of medicine broadly concerned with the ear and other head and neck structures.

- **otology**   Dealing with diagnosis and management of disorders of the ear and balance system and related structures of the head and neck, an otologist is a board-certified otolaryngologist who has specialized in treating ear disease.

- **neurotology**   Working in diagnosis and treatment of the hearing nerve, balance nerve, and facial nerve, a neurotologist is an otologist who has special training in performing surgery for treatment of ear disease.

- **audiology**   With the measuring of hearing and hearing aid consultation, an audiologist performs special tests to determine the amount of hearing loss and best type of hearing aid.

- **radiology**   Using X-ray, computerized axial tomography (CT or CAT), magnetic resonance imaging (MRI), and other radiological tests, a radiologist "reads" and interprets the test results to help diagnose problems.

Otolaryngologists are physicians (with M.D. degrees) who have specialized residency and internship training in the medical conditions of the ear, nose, and throat. Those who specialize in the ear and hearing—otologists and neurotologists—complete additional fellowship training. An otologist is knowledgeable in the basic sciences of hearing, balance, nerve function, infectious disease, and anatomy of the head and neck. Their diagnostic, medical, and surgical skills include treatment of hearing loss and tinnitus; dizziness; infectious and inflammatory diseases of the ear; facial nerve disorders; congenital malformations of the ear; and tumors of the ear, hearing nerve, and skull base. As part of a team with neurosurgeons, neurotologists also manage diseases and disorders of the cranial nerves and skull base.

Audiologists have a Master's or doctoral degree in audiology and have completed a postgraduate fellowship in clinical practice to become licensed. The initials CCC-A following an audiologist's name and degree indicate that he or she has a Certificate of Clinical Competence in Audiology. The American Speech-Language-Hearing Association (ASHA) sponsors this certification program.

In addition to these medical- or graduate degree-level professionals, other individuals specialize in the fitting of hearing aids and are often called hearing aid specialists or hearing instrument specialists. The education requirements for this category of hearing health-care providers varies by state, although most states require them to pass an exam before being issued a license. A hearing aid dispenser (someone who selects the proper hearing aid for you, fits it to you, and sells it to you) may be an audiologist or a hearing aid specialist.

HAVE YOU HEARD?

Otolaryngology is the oldest medical specialty in the United States.

Your family physician or pediatrician can refer you to the proper hearing health-care professional. If ear disease is suspected, you or your child will most likely need to see an otolaryngologist (ENT) or otologist and an audiologist. Depending on the results of his or her evaluation, an ENT may then send you to an otologist or neurotologist for more specific diagnosis and treatment.

The Office Examination

Regardless of which specialist you choose to see or are sent to see, the opening routine will be much the same. The doctor will ask many, seemingly far-ranging questions about your work, your lifestyle, and your health as it's necessary to get a complete picture before a physical examination and any diagnoses are made. After taking a history of your ear symptoms and your medical history, the doctor will examine your ears and other areas of the head and neck.

Here we describe the types of questions that the doctor will ask and tell you why they are important to diagnosing the cause of a hearing loss. We get you to think about the characteristics of your hearing loss so you can be prepared to answer the doctor's questions. And we tell you what the doctor looks for in the physical examination of the ear and related structures such as the nose and sinuses.

Medical History

The first question the doctor will probably ask, especially if you are an adult male (there we go again), is whether you're in the office because you feel you have a hearing problem or because you've been "dragged in" by your spouse, children, friends, or co-workers who feel you have a hearing problem. Treatment may actually be influenced by whether you feel you need help or you feel someone has forced you to seek this consultation.

In the case of a child, various reasons may foster a visit to a hearing specialist. These include failure to pass the newborn screening test, a delay in speech and language development, or a change in responses in the home or classroom (see Chapter 14).

The doctor will take a careful history, asking about the onset of the hearing loss and symptoms, how long the symptoms last when they occur and how often they occur, what activities seem to make the symptoms better or worse, and how the symptoms responded to any treatments you may have already had. Are the symptoms on one side only, or do they involve both ears? Did the symptoms appear gradually, or was there a sudden change in hearing? Is there hearing loss in the family, either immediate or distant? The doctor will also ask about your medical history, which is relevant for reasons such as these:

- Hearing is affected by the aging process, probably through a change in circulation (see Chapter 7).

- Medical conditions such as diabetes, hypertension, or thyroid abnormalities can add to hearing impairment.

- Certain medications can be harmful to the hearing system (ototoxicity). Many of these are given for life-threatening illnesses, such as severe infections and cancer.

The medical history also tries to assess how you perform in the work setting, with family, and in social situations in relation to your hearing and balance problems. Most sensorineural hearing losses that occur, either through age or noise, involve the higher frequencies of speech. As noted in Chapter 1, vowels are primarily in the low-frequency portion of the speech range; consonants are primarily in the high-frequency portion. So in most settings, someone with a high-frequency hearing loss is able to hear the vowels and be aware that someone is talking, but because the consonants are not clearly heard, does not understand what is said (see also Chapter 19). This difficulty is made worse when there's a lot of background sound such as at a family gathering, restaurant, classroom, and so on. It's also more of a problem when one is trying to hear women's voices or the voices of young children, which are usually higher pitched.

Your doctor will undoubtedly question you about your possible noise exposure. Noise, either in one sudden exposure to a very loud sound (acoustic trauma) or through long-term repeated exposures to sounds at an intensity and duration beyond safe limits, can cause hearing loss (see Chapter 8). There are three primary sources of noise exposure: work, military service, and hobbies, so the doctor may ask you to describe each of these to help determine your possible exposure to unsafe sound levels.

Ear Exam

The doctor will work from the outside in, examining first the outer ear, the pinna, looking for any abnormalities in shape, flexibility, or tenderness. Then, working inward, the doctor will use an *otoscope*, a handheld instrument, or a microscope to examine the external ear canal and the eardrum or tympanic membrane.

DEFINITION

An **otoscope** is a special instrument doctors use for examining the external ear canal and eardrum, which consists essentially of a magnifying lens and a light.

Earwax is natural and meant to be present in the ear canal. Occasionally, there can be too little wax from overzealous cleaning of the canal with cotton-tipped applicators, or there can be an excess amount of wax pushed deep into the canal up against the eardrum, again because of the use of cotton-tipped applicators (see Chapter 3). In older men, sometimes too much hair at the opening of the ear canal blocks the entrance and traps wax in the ear canal, so the doctor will sometimes trim these hairs to see into the ear canal and remove any trapped wax. During this stage of the examination, the doctor will note whether there is drainage from the ear or any inflammation or infection of the ear canal.

When examining the eardrum, the doctor will look for perforations (holes) or abnormalities in its shape and notice whether it's bulging outward due to too much positive pressure or perhaps pulled inward due to poor Eustachian tube function (see Chap-ter 4). The eardrum is usually a blue-gray color. Occasionally, scarring of the eardrum can make a portion of it appear more whitish. The doctor is alert to these color differences as well as to evidence of drainage or findings consistent with an infection of the middle ear. Occasionally, an ear doctor will use a special type of otoscope called a pneumatic otoscope to examine movement of the eardrum.

The doctor may briefly inspect the nose and sinus area as a wide range of conditions or circumstances may be affecting hearing or causing hearing loss. Sinus disease can create Eustachian tube problems, which can lead to middle ear infections and ear symptoms with hearing loss (Chapter 4). The physician will also examine the mouth, tongue, and teeth because, occasionally, lesions in the back of the throat can cause the sensation of ear pain even though the problem is not really with the ear. Symptoms that occur at a site away from the cause are called referred symptoms. Similarly, ear symptoms can be referred from temporomandibular joint (TMJ) dysfunction.

The doctor will also examine the neck for any enlarged lymph nodes that might be a response to ear infections. Occasionally, arthritis of the neck can create a sense of unsteadiness that might send a person to an ear specialist. The facial nerve motor function allows you to pucker your lips, smile, wiggle your nose, close your eyes, and lift your eyebrows. The doctor will look for any unevenness or difference between the right and left sides of the face. Any abnormal findings such as drainage, swelling behind the ear, or facial nerve weakness indicate that other studies should be ordered.

As part of the physical exam, doctors often carry out "tuning fork" tests. Tuning forks come in different frequencies, but the two frequencies routinely used are 512 Hz and 1,024 Hz. Although several tests involve the use of tuning forks, the two most important tests are called the Rinne and the Weber tests. Both tests help determine whether a hearing loss might be conductive or sensorineural in nature. To perform the tests, the doctor starts the tuning fork vibrating by striking it against something and then holds it in different positions around or touching your head.

HAVE YOU HEARD?

A British musician is said to have invented tuning forks in 1711. A tuning fork consists of a steel stem with two prongs and produces a musical tone of definite, constant pitch, or frequency, when struck. They serve as a standard for tuning musical instruments. Prior to the availability of modern hearing tests, tuning forks were used for testing hearing, and they are still used as an initial test of whether a hearing loss is conductive or sensorineural in nature.

Hearing Tests

The purpose of the basic hearing, or audiometric, test is to determine the following:

- Whether a person has a hearing loss.
- At what frequencies (low, middle, or high tones) the loss occurs.
- To what degree (mild, moderate, severe, or profound) the loss is.
- Whether the loss is one-sided or on both sides.
- Whether the loss is conductive, sensorineural, or a mixed loss.

The basic test package also helps determine how well a person can process speech sounds (speech discrimination), which provides important information about how well one might be able to use hearing aids, as well as information that could suggest that a serious problem is the cause of the hearing loss. The set of basic tests also determines whether there are problems of the middle ear, which can create hearing loss. In addition to tests of one's ability to hear pure tones of different frequencies and to discriminate speech sounds, other frequently and infrequently used tests might be used to help evaluate hearing, but the doctor will decide which tests are necessary.

Pure-Tone Hearing Test

The pure-tone hearing test determines your ability to hear sounds at different frequencies and your thresholds for these sounds—the faintest sound that your ear can consistently perceive. The testing tones of low and high frequencies are presented at various levels of loudness in a sound-treated or soundproof room. To test air conduction thresholds, earphones that either cover the ear completely or insert in the ear canal are used so each ear can be tested separately. To test bone conduction, a special vibrator device is placed on the bone behind the ear. (Infants and young children may require special test procedures, which are discussed in Chapter 14.)

Often, it's necessary to introduce a loud noise into the other ear, the one not being tested. This distraction, called a masking sound, is necessary to ensure that the test tones are being heard only in the ear under evaluation. Each frequency is tested separately to determine your threshold for that frequency. The record of your pure-tone hearing test results, called an audiogram, shows the intensity level, in decibels (dB), that you are able to hear, usually for all frequencies from 250 Hz to 8,000 Hz.

Degree of hearing loss is often categorized as shown in the following table.

Categories of Hearing Loss Based on Pure-Tone Threshold Test Results

Threshold	Hearing Loss	Description
0–25 dB	Normal hearing	
26–40 dB	Mild	Unable to hear soft sounds; difficulty hearing speech in noisy environments
41–55 dB	Moderate	Unable to hear soft and moderately loud sounds; considerable difficulty understanding speech, especially with background noise
56–70 dB	Moderately severe	Can barely hear loud speech, with considerable difficulty understanding when any noise is present
71–90 dB	Severe	Can hear only loud sounds; effective speech communication without use of hearing aids is unlikely
>90 dB	Profound	Can hear only extremely loud sounds; speech communication without a hearing aid is impossible; might need a cochlear implant to provide any detection of speech or other sounds

The following figure shows an example of an audiogram where one ear has normal hearing and one has a mild hearing loss.

Speech Discrimination Test

The ability to hear and understand speech is different from the ability simply to detect sounds. In this test two different samples of speech are presented through earphones or through a loudspeaker in a sound-treated room. One series of words is presented at different degrees of loudness, which tests the speech recognition threshold (SRT)—the softest level at which a person can correctly recognize half the words. A second group of words is presented at a comfortable listening level. This word recognition test determines one's ability to understand single-syllable words presented at a level loud enough for a person to hear them. It's not a test for "hearing" (awareness of speech), but a test of how well one can process, or discriminate, and understand speech.

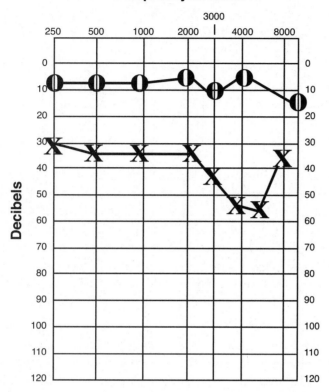

Audiogram shows normal hearing in the right ear (circles) and mild hearing loss in the left ear (Xs).

HAVE YOU HEARD?

Understanding speech is a two-step process when it comes to hearing. First, the speech sounds must be loud enough for you to detect their presence. This depends on your thresholds for hearing different frequencies. Second, the sounds you hear must be properly processed so you can understand what you've heard. Difficulty understanding conversation can result from either or both of two problems. The first is lack of audibility. If you can't hear what is said, you have nothing to process and won't understand the conversation. The second is a problem of processing—the inability to discriminate. You can detect that speech is occurring but can't seem to understand the words. Some causes of hearing loss affect only your ability to detect speech sounds. Other causes might affect your ability to discriminate, even when the sound is loud enough to hear. Both your pure-tone and speech thresholds and your speech discrimination ability are important clues to determining the cause of your hearing loss.

One other aspect of hearing is the ability to understand speech in the presence of noise, so you may be given a speech in noise test. One such test, the hearing in noise test (HINT), measures your ability to repeat sentences you hear presented in noise and compares your results to those of normal-hearing listeners. The ability to understand speech in noise is not related to your audiogram. Often, people who have normal audiograms (normal thresholds for all tested frequencies) report significant difficulties in understanding speech in noise.

Middle Ear Function Tests

To help diagnose the cause of your hearing problem, it's important to know how well your middle ear is functioning. Impedance audiometry and acoustic reflex testing evaluate the sound-transmitting properties of the middle ear bones (the ossicles) and hearing nerve, the function of the Eustachian tube and middle ear muscles, and the middle ear pressure. A small earplug containing a special measuring device is inserted into the ear canal, and a low-pitched humming sound is delivered to the ear, accompanied occasionally by small pressure changes (similar to those caused by altitude changes). From this test, the doctor or audiologist acquires information about the ear without requiring any response from you.

The tympanogram measures the mobility of the eardrum. Decreased mobility—that is, stiffness of the drum—may be a result of fluid in the middle ear space or scarring of the fibrous layer of the middle ear. Increased movement, or hypermobility, of the drum may be a result of previous infections or medical treatments that have weakened the fibrous layer, causing the drum to sag. The acoustic reflex test is used primarily to determine whether there is fixation of the third bone of hearing, the stapes bone, from a condition called otosclerosis (see Chapter 6). In very young children or in others whose ear canals are so narrow that the eardrum can't be seen, impedance testing can help determine whether there might be a perforation in the eardrum.

Inner Ear Tests

When the outer hair cells in the cochlea are stimulated, they not only send information onward toward the brain but also transmit a response backward through the ossicles and eardrum into the external ear canal. The otoacoustic emission (OAE) test takes advantage of this fact. When a brief sound burst is used to bring out a response from the inner ear, a soft probe tip placed in the external ear canal records these responses. This test requires only a quiet setting and a cooperative patient—the patient doesn't have to do anything but sit still—and takes only a few minutes to perform. This type of test is also used for newborn hearing screening (Chapter 14). The OAE test is particularly good in assessing patients with ototoxicity—drug-related damage to hearing—or acoustic trauma—exposure to very loud sound, where damage to the outer hair cells may have occurred.

A computerized hearing test called auditory brainstem response (ABR) audiometry can help determine the site of an inner ear or brainstem hearing disorder. It's also used to evaluate degree of hearing loss in people who can't respond to standard hearing tests. This would include, for example, infants and young children or those with disabilities that prevent them from making a physical or verbal response to let the tester know that they've heard a sound. Small discs placed on the skin of the ear and scalp record electrical responses in the brain resulting from sound stimulation. A computer then analyzes this information to determine the location and type of hearing disturbance. In infants and young children, sedation may be necessary during this test.

Electrocochleography is another test that can help determine the location of an inner ear hearing defect, and is performed in the office under local anesthesia. An electrode is inserted through the eardrum to record electrically the response of the inner ear and hearing nerve to sound stimulation. This information is computer-analyzed.

Other Diagnostic Tests

Research during the past decade has greatly increased our medical and surgical knowledge of the ear and related structures, and this improved technology aids doctors in making accurate diagnoses. For many causes of hearing loss, relatively few tests are necessary for a diagnosis. But sometimes a large number of tests, even requiring multiple visits, are necessary to establish an accurate diagnosis, which is essential before proper medical or surgical treatment can begin. Some additional tests are done in the otologist's office while others, such as X-ray tests, may require going to a different facility for the necessary specialized equipment.

Tests of the Balance Mechanism

As explained in Chapter 1, the inner ear and the eighth cranial nerve also include the balance or vestibular system. Because of this, many ear diseases affect balance and can cause dizziness, imbalance, or vertigo. So tests of the balance system may be necessary to determine the cause of your hearing loss.

The electronystagmography (ENG) test measures eye movement with electrodes that are taped on the skin around the eyes. Videonystagmography (VNG) uses goggles that cover the face and contain a video camera to record eye movements. For either test, the patient sits in a reclining position, and cool and warm water are alternately put into each ear canal for 30 seconds. The resulting responses of the balance mechanism, which are expressed through the eye movements, are automatically recorded.

Posturography uses a computer to help record input to the balance system from the four components of balance: ears, eyes, muscle-joint sense (proprioception), and brain. If you have this test, you'll be asked to stand on a platform in different ways, for example, with your eyes open, your eyes closed, on one foot, with one foot in front of the other, and so on. Your movement patterns on the platform are sent to the computer and analyzed to help determine the nature and source of any balance problems.

X-Ray Studies

These days, it's likely that you or someone you know has had a CT or CAT scan (computerized axial tomography) or an MRI (magnetic resonance imaging) of some part of the body. A CT uses a computer to analyze the body's absorption of small quantities of X-rays. An MRI uses no X-rays but rather measures the magnetic field given off by the targeted part of the body after exposure to a strong magnet. To help diagnose the cause of a hearing problem, you might have a CT or MRI of the head. The result of the scan is a photograph of the contents of the skull showing any major abnormalities in or around the structures of the temporal bone. To the radiologist who interprets these tests, abnormalities within the skull appear different from normal brain tissue. These tests are usually performed at an outpatient facility.

Nerve Tests

Because the hearing and balance nerve is closely associated with other nerves within the brain, disorders of one may affect another. So to make a diagnosis, it's sometimes necessary to have a complete neurological examination. Your doctor may want to evaluate the tearing mechanism of the eye to get additional information regarding the site of nerve disorders within the temporal bone. A nerve excitability test compares the response of the facial muscles to electrical stimulation. Each facial nerve is stimulated with small electrical currents, and the degree of muscle movement on the right and left is compared. Electroneuronography is a computerized test of facial muscle movement in response to electrical stimulation of the facial nerve. Recording electrodes are applied to the face to detect the muscle contractions, which are then recorded by computer.

Metabolic and Allergy Tests

Hearing loss can sometimes be associated with metabolic or allergic problems, so you may be asked to have a thyroid profile blood test to determine the function of the thyroid gland. Also, inability to metabolize sugar in a normal manner can result in hearing or balance problems, so you may need to have a glucose tolerance test, which evaluates the body's ability to use sugar. Blood samples are drawn to determine the sugar content after fasting for 12 hours and then over a 5-hour period after drinking a sugar solution. And several ear problems appear to be related to immune abnormalities, or autoimmune diseases, so you may also have an immune profile test to determine whether the immune system is functioning properly.

Allergy tests of the skin, blood, and foods may be performed to determine sensitivities to inhalants (things you breathe in such as pollen, dust, and mold) and foods. Chapter 12 discusses the role of allergy in hearing loss and describes these tests.

After the Diagnosis

After the history and physical exam, the hearing tests, and any other required tests, the otolaryngologist (ENT), otologist, or neurotologist will tell you the likely cause of your hearing loss and make recommendations for treatment. Depending on the degree and cause of the hearing loss, the doctor might recommend no treatment, medical treatment, surgery, use of a hearing aid or cochlear implant, or use of special assistive devices. In the following chapters, we'll describe the many different causes of hearing loss and the many possible treatments.

The Least You Need to Know

- People don't always recognize or admit to a hearing loss.
- Knowing the signs of hearing loss can help you detect it in yourself and in others.
- If you think you have a hearing problem or if your family physician has told you you may have a problem, see a hearing health-care professional.
- Your ear doctor needs to know all your symptoms, your medical history, and your history of exposure to noise.
- Hearing tests of both pure-tones and speech discrimination are necessary for accurate diagnosis.
- Tests of balance function, facial function, CT or MRI, or allergy may be necessary to diagnose the cause of a hearing loss.

External and Middle Ear Hearing Loss

2

Now you know *how* we hear, so in this part we talk about how and why we *don't* hear by exploring the most common external and middle ear causes of hearing loss. You'll read about earwax, "swimmer's ear," abnormal anatomy, chronic infection, disease of the middle ear bones (otosclerosis), and the effects of accidental injuries and abnormalities present at birth.

If you're a parent, you may be all too familiar with the Eustachian tube and the problems it can lead to, such as fluid in the ear and ear infections. If it's been the object of many doctor visits with your child, then here we give you the whole story about what is happening, what could happen, and what you should do about it. It's also the Eustachian tube that can cause you ear pain when flying or diving. Learn what to do to prevent such problems.

External Ear Causes of Hearing Loss

In This Chapter

- All about earwax
- Things that shouldn't be in your ear
- Proper cleaning of the ears
- The symptoms and consequences of external ear infections
- Abnormal anatomy of the external ear

As a review of Chapter 1, the external ear is composed of the pinna or the auricle, the ear canal, and the outer layer of the tympanic membrane, the eardrum. The external ear (sometimes called the outer ear) helps transmit sound to the middle ear, acting as a resonator. The ear canal also protects the middle ear from the outside environment. Part of the ear canal is lined by a fragile, paper-thin skin that is closely attached to the bone and so is easily damaged. It contains nerve endings from a number of different cranial nerves. Because of this, pain from external ear problems is often severe enough to interfere with sleep.

Both common and rare conditions of the external ear can affect hearing. In this chapter, we address some external ear problems that can lead to hearing loss and the treatment of those problems. We also discuss a number of "no-no's," even though many people frequently do these things. Because the ear, even the external part, is so delicate and complicated, your efforts to keep your ears clean could even be risking your ability to hear!

Earwax

The ear canal is shaped somewhat like an hourglass—starting wide outside, narrowing in the middle, and then widening again. The skin of the outer part of the canal has special glands that produce earwax or cerumen, which traps dust and foreign objects to keep them from reaching the eardrum. The presence of wax is not a sign of poor hygiene! Wax is healthy in normal amounts, and the absence of earwax can result in dry, itchy ears. Cerumen has many beneficial roles in the ear canal:

- It lubricates the ear canal.
- It repels water.
- It traps debris.
- It appears to have antimicrobial properties.

Earwax varies in color from a light golden brown to a dark red brown or even a black color. Some people have very dry wax while others have wet wax.

HAVE YOU HEARD?

In 2006, the gene responsible for determining whether one has the dry or wet type of earwax was discovered (called ABCC11). The dry variation of the gene, the more common type in Chinese and Korean populations, is thought to have originated in northeast Asia and spread to other populations around the world.

Normally the body is quite efficient at moving earwax out of the canal along with dead, flaky skin cells that are a normal part of skin turnover. In fact, the ear canals are self-cleaning; earwax and skin cells slowly move from the eardrum outward to the ear opening where it usually dries and falls out. Chewing and jaw motion help propel this outward movement. When this process is disrupted or the ear is not efficient at clearing, the wax builds up and can lead to an impaction. This occurs more commonly in people, both children and adults, who have either a very small opening to the ear canal or have narrow ear canals. Signs of a wax impaction include pain, fullness or a plugged feeling, difficulty fitting a hearing aid, impaired function or "whistling" from a hearing aid, hearing loss (which may be progressive), tinnitus, coughing, and infection of the ear canal with itching, odor, or discharge.

When everything is working properly, the ear canals don't need to be cleaned. Earwax is formed in the outer part of the ear canal. So if you have wax blockage against the eardrum, it's probably because you've been putting such things as cotton-tipped applicators, bobby pins, ballpoint pens, or twisted napkin corners into your ear canal in an attempt to clean it. These objects only push the wax in deeper, causing an impaction! It may be an old saying, but it has some value: never put anything smaller than your elbow in your ear!

If enough earwax does accumulate to cause symptoms, you need to clean the canals. First, try washing the external ear with a cloth, but remember, don't insert anything into the ear canal. Home treatments used to soften wax can often help earwax impaction. You can try putting a few drops of mineral oil, baby oil, glycerin, or commercial drops into the ear. Detergent drops, such as hydrogen peroxide or carbamide peroxide, might also aid in wax removal.

Follow the drops with an irrigation of the ear canal. To do this, mix equal amounts of white vinegar and tap water in a cup. Suck some of this mixture up into either an eyedropper or a small syringe. Tilt your head to the side—with the involved ear up—and fill the ear canal with the fluid mixture. Refill the dropper or syringe, place the tip in the ear canal, and squeeze the bulb—or move the plunger—rapidly to stir up the fluid filling the canal. Then tip the irrigated ear down to allow the fluid and debris to fall out of the ear.

If the wax is really hard, you can use a stool softener (for example, Colace) to soften the wax. Be sure to get the liquid form of Colace, which is available without a prescription. Using a dropper, put the liquid into your ear; wait 10 minutes or so; and then irrigate the ear canal as described in the previous paragraph.

You can also try commercially available irrigation kits, whose common solutions include water and saline. Whether a commercial or homemade solution, warm it to body temperature, or you might experience dizziness when you put it into the ear canal.

Do not irrigate your ears if you have diabetes, a perforated eardrum, a tube in the eardrum (see Chapter 4), or a weak immune system. If you have one of these conditions, an ear doctor should remove your earwax manually using suction and special instruments. Manual removal is also the best option if your ear canal is very narrow. If the home treatments don't work or if so much wax has accumulated that it blocks the ear canal (and hearing), your doctor may irrigate or vacuum it out. Occasionally, an ear doctor will need to remove earwax using a microscope for visualization.

If there's a possibility that you have a hole (perforation or puncture) in the eardrum, you must consult a physician before trying any over-the-counter remedies. Putting ear drops or other products in the ear with the presence of an eardrum perforation may cause pain or an infection. Even irrigating with water in the presence of such a hole could start an infection. The American Academy of Otolaryngology Head and Neck Surgery recommends that persons prone to repeated wax impaction or who use hearing aids should see their doctor every 6 to 12 months for a checkup and routine preventive cleaning.

Foreign Objects in the Ear Canal

Many objects can and do become stuck in the ear canal, including erasers, beans, batteries, and even cockroaches! Foreign objects (often called foreign bodies) in the ear canal are a surprisingly common problem in adults as well as children. Children and toddlers are curious and tend to stick things in their ears. And insects that like dark warm places have been known to crawl into the ear, usually when people are asleep. Sleeping on the floor or outdoors increases the chance of this happening.

Fortunately, most people can tell if something's in their ear because the ear canal—where most objects get stuck—and the eardrum are very sensitive. The most common symptom of a foreign object in the ear canal is pain, but if the object blocks most of the canal, hearing may be decreased. Irritation can cause nausea and vomiting, and bleeding is also common, especially if the object is sharp. Or you may cause bleeding by trying to remove the foreign body by sticking something else into your ear. A live insect in the ear is particularly distressing as its movements can cause a buzzing sound and be quite uncomfortable. Occasionally, a foreign body in the ear will go undetected and cause an infection. In this situation, you may notice ongoing infectious drainage from the ear.

An object in the ear canal may itself cause damage, or the damage may occur as a result of attempts to remove the object. Injuries may include cuts, hematomas or bruising, eardrum perforations, and burns (for example, from a leaking battery). The resulting trauma to the ear canal makes the skin more susceptible to infection. Objects left in the canal can lead to recurring infection, scarring, and hearing loss.

Most objects can be removed without damaging the ear canal or eardrum. Damage is more likely when multiple attempts are needed to get rid of the object. You can do several things at home to help remove a foreign object from your ear. First, turn the affected ear downward and gently wiggle the pinna. This changes the shape of the ear canal, so you may be able to move the object enough for it to fall out. If you have the misfortune of having a live insect in your ear, you'll be eager to get the bug to stop moving—it's pretty uncomfortable. Putting a few drops of mineral or other oil into your ear should suffocate the bug and allow you to calm down enough to get to the doctor. If you're going to the doctor to get something removed, don't eat or drink anything for about 8 hours before the visit. Sometimes sedation is required for safe removal, and sedation is safer if you haven't swallowed anything for 8 to 12 hours before the procedure.

LISTEN UP

If you have a foreign body in the ear that won't come out, you need to see a qualified medical professional. Urgent removal is called for if the object is a button battery as chemicals can leak out and cause a burn. Food or plant material, such as beans, should be removed immediately because they swell when moistened and can damage the ear canal or eardrum.

An ear doctor will commonly use a microscope and special instruments to remove a foreign object, but ER doctors are less likely to have these tools available. Instead, the ER doctor may apply gentle suction to the ear canal to pull the object out or use small forceps or medical instruments that have a loop or hook at the end. If the object is metallic, the doctor might use a long magnetized instrument to pull the object from the ear. Another common method is to perform warm water irrigation. The water is squirted in and moves past the object. When the eardrum turns it back, the object often washes out. If the foreign object is a live insect, anesthetic solutions can put the insect to sleep before the doctor removes it.

As a preventive measure, teach your children never to put anything into their ears. If you suspect a child has put something into his or her ear, it's very important to ask about it in a nonjudgmental, nonthreatening manner. When children think they'll be punished, they're more likely to deny having done a deed. This can delay the discovery and safe removal of a foreign object and allow complications to occur.

Swimmer's Ear and Irritations of the Ear Canal

Swimmer's ear, or otitis externa, is an inflammation and irritation or infection of the external ear canal. The infection, which is usually bacterial but may be fungal, typically begins as a result of irritation to the ear canal from an underlying skin condition such as eczema (a skin disorder that causes itching) or scratching of the ear or other trauma. When water gets trapped in the ear, it allows bacteria to spread. Because of this, otitis externa commonly affects swimmers, divers, or others who spend time in the water—hence the term swimmer's ear. It affects mostly children and teenagers but can also affect people with eczema or excess earwax. Acute *otitis externa* (lasting less than four weeks) occurs in approximately 4 of every 1,000 people annually in the United States, and the chronic form (lasting more than four weeks or occurring more than four times in a year) affects 3 to 5 percent of the population.

Causes of Swimmer's Ear

Bathing, showering, increased humidity, and living in warm moist climates all create conditions conducive to moisture being trapped in the ear canal. In this moisture, the bacteria that are normally present can multiply, causing infection and irritation. Some conditions or situations that increase the risk of developing swimmer's ear include the following:

- Swimming, bathing, or seeking recreation in polluted water, whether it be a natural body of water, a swimming pool, or a hot tub.

- Excessive cleaning of the ear canal with cotton swabs (the most common cause of otitis externa).

- Cuts or abrasions in the skin of the ear canal from attempts to remove earwax or foreign objects or from other trauma.

- Skin conditions, such as eczema or seborrhea, that may be aggravated by greasy foods, carbohydrates, and chocolate.

- Getting hair spray or hair dye chemicals in the ear canal. Avoid this by blocking the ears with cotton balls when using these products.

Symptoms of Swimmer's Ear

The most common symptoms of swimmer's ear are an itchy ear and mild to severe pain that gets worse when you tug on the pinna or push on the tragus—the little triangular piece just in front of the ear canal. Itching is especially problematic because it can lead to a cycle of scratching, further irritation, and infection. Other symptoms include a feeling that the ear is blocked or full; drainage from the ear; fever; decreased hearing; pain that radiates to the neck, face, or side of the head; swollen lymph nodes in the neck; and redness and swelling of the skin around the ear. Your pinna may even seem to be pushed forward or away from the head.

SOUND ADVICE

Once the skin of the ear canal is inflamed, external otitis can rapidly become worse either from scratching the ear canal or from allowing water to remain in the ear canal for any length of time. As much as it might itch, try not to scratch, don't stick any kind of implement or cotton swab into the ear canal, and don't squirt water into the ear thinking it will relieve the itching or pain.

Multiple episodes or recurrent infections of the external ear canal or inflammation from causes such as dermatitis can lead to scarring of the inner third of the ear canal, which can actually create a plug in the ear canal. If left untreated, hearing loss can occur or become worse. However, when the infection clears up, hearing usually returns to normal.

Sometimes ear infections can spread into the bony floor of the external ear canal, resulting in a condition called malignant *otitis externa*. In spite of that scary word *malignant*, this is not a cancer, but it is very painful and dangerous. If untreated, it can spread to the base of the skull, brain, or cranial nerves and can become life-threatening. Diabetics and older adults are more at risk, as are people who have weakened immune systems, so diabetic and immunocompromised individuals having symptoms of *otitis externa* should see a doctor right away.

Treatment of Swimmer's Ear

For mild *otitis externa*, refraining from swimming or washing your hair for a few days, as well as keeping all implements out of the ear, will usually take care of the problem. But if the infection is moderate to severe or if the climate is humid enough to keep the ear moist, the condition may not improve on its own. Treatment for the early stages of swimmer's ear includes careful cleaning of the ear canal by a physician and using eardrops to inhibit bacterial growth.

Mild acid solutions such as boric or acetic acid are sometimes effective for early infections. If you're certain you don't have a perforated eardrum, you can make your own eardrops using rubbing alcohol or a mixture of half alcohol and half white wine vinegar. These eardrops will evaporate excess water and keep your ears dry. For more severe infections, your doctor may prescribe antibiotic ear drops. Sometimes the ear canal is actually swollen shut, and in this situation, an otolaryngologist may place a sponge or wick in the ear canal so the antibiotic drops can reach the affected areas. If you have tubes in your eardrum, use nonototoxic (not dangerous to your hearing) topical antibiotic ear drops. The doctor may also prescribe pain medication and oral antibiotics if the infection goes beyond the skin of the ear canal.

Follow-up appointments are very important to monitor progress of the infection, to repeat ear cleaning, and to replace the ear wick as needed. If routine treatment from your primary care doctor is not effective, an otolaryngologist has specialized equipment and expertise to clean the ear canal and treat swimmer's ear. With proper treatment, most infections should heal in 7 to 10 days.

Fungal infections—called otomycosis—are less common than bacterial infections but produce many of the same symptoms. Otomycosis is treated with antifungal medications that may be drops, powder, or ointment.

If the infections result in damage to the ear canal, surgery is indicated for treatment of the conductive hearing loss that may result from the scarring that plugs the ear canal.

SOUND ADVICE

A dry ear is less likely to become infected, so it's important to keep the ears free of moisture during swimming or bathing. Use earplugs when swimming. After swimming or bathing, use a dry towel to dry the outer ear and use a hair dryer held about one foot away from the ear on a lukewarm setting to dry the ear canal. Have your ears cleaned periodically by an ear doctor if you have itchy, flaky, or scaly ears or extensive earwax. Avoid scratching your ears. Placing a petroleum jelly–coated cotton ball just at the opening of the ear canal (not into the ear canal) while showering can prevent moisture from accumulating. But use a new one every time!

Although acute external otitis generally resolves in a few days with topical washes and antibiotics, complete return of hearing and cerumen gland function may take a few more days. Once healed completely, the ear canal is again self-cleaning. Until it recovers fully, it may be more prone to repeat infection from further physical or chemical insult.

Other Problems of the External Ear

Exostoses are bony outgrowths of the external auditory canal that typically line both the front and back of the canal and can cause extensive narrowing of the canal. Exostoses occur more often in people exposed to cold water and wind, such as surfers and divers, so it's sometimes called surfer's ear. Exostoses usually don't cause any symptoms at first, but as they grow, they begin to fill the external auditory canal and therefore trap water in the canal, which leads to infections. Because of the altered shape of the ear canal, these infections can be more difficult to treat. If you have exostoses and get recurring infections, you might be a candidate for surgical removal of the exostoses. Rarely, exostoses will cause a conductive hearing loss because they serve as a bony earplug, and in these cases, surgery can help eliminate the hearing loss. If you engage in activities that might predispose you to exostoses, consider wearing earplugs.

A variety of dermatologic skin conditions can also affect the external ear. Most of these don't directly cause hearing loss, but many can lead to infections that may result in hearing loss. As we've mentioned, one of these is eczema, which typically affects people with allergies, especially food allergies, or asthma (see also Chapter 12). Other skin conditions include psoriasis, seborrhea, and contact dermatitis, an allergy-based condition (see Chapter 12).

Abnormal Anatomy

Developmental abnormalities can affect the normal structure of the pinna and the ear canal. The causes of these abnormal formations may be genetic, teratogenic (toxic substances), infectious, or environmental. Some abnormalities result only in cosmetic problems, but others affect hearing function or predispose an individual to infection or other ear problems.

Narrowing of the ear canal, called atresia, ranges from a slight narrowing to complete absence of the external ear canal. There may also be changes in the shape of the pinna (called microtia) and malformations of the middle ear structures, including missing hearing bones (see Chapter 6). Atresia of the external ear requires evaluation by a multidisciplinary team including an otolaryngologist, audiologist, and radiologist. An absent ear canal leads to a conductive hearing loss even if the inner ear and nerve function are normal. In addition to hearing loss, a narrow canal can predispose one to infections or, in more severe cases, cysts of the middle ear called cholesteatomas (see Chapter 4). The external ear canal can be surgically reconstructed to improve hearing, or bone conduction hearing aids may be an option (see Chapter 16). Both solutions are useful for hearing only if the middle ear and inner ear hearing structures are intact or, in the case of the middle ear, can be reconstructed.

Preauricular tags are appendages of skin, with fat and/or cartilage. The tags themselves are not a problem, but in some newborns they can be associated with other congenital abnormalities, including congenital hearing loss. Preauricular pits are small holes occurring just above the tragus (in front of the opening to the ear canal). These pits can become infected and should be surgically removed if they repeatedly are infected. These pits, which tend to run in families, can be part of a range of congenital abnormalities that may include sensorineural hearing loss.

True Stories

In this section, we tell you some stories about patients we've seen who had problems related to the external ear. Because of what you now know from this chapter, you may even be able to guess what the problem or treatment is before you finish a story.

Surf's Up

A doctor at an urgent care facility recently referred Travis, a surfer for most of his 47 years, to an ENT physician for severe left ear pain. In spite of the ear drops and oral antibiotics Travis had received through the urgent care facility, his pain persisted. He noticed hearing loss and fullness, also in the left ear. The right side felt fine. But he did say that after surfing, he felt as if water was trapped in both ears.

The ENT doctor found a very swollen left ear canal, closed both by bone (exostoses) and by soft tissue swelling from infection (acute external otitis). The right ear also was involved with exostoses but had no infection. The medications were continued, and, in a few days, the infection improved and his ear pain went away. However, his sense of fullness persisted. When an audiogram showed a mild conductive hearing loss, Travis elected to undergo surgery to remove the exostoses. Following surgery, his hearing improved, and the feeling of fullness disappeared. He now wears earplugs in the right ear when he surfs to avoid having the same problem there.

Something's in the Wrong Place

Rebecca, age 18, noted some pain in her right ear following a camping trip with her senior high school class. She had no drainage and no history of ear problems. Although her pain was mild, it persisted and was irritating, so she went to an ear doctor who discovered that she was transporting an ant in her ear! The ant must have crawled into the ear canal at night while Rebecca was in her sleeping bag. By the time she got to the doctor's office, the ant was no longer alive, so the doctor used a small forceps to pick it out of her ear. No infection was present, and ear drops were not prescribed.

Little Matthew, age three, was helping in the kitchen when he decided to store a fresh lima bean in his ear. When he began to show signs of ear discomfort, his grandmother suspected he'd put something in his ear. When Matthew's parents got home, they tried to flush the bean out. Unfortunately, this caused it to swell up, making the pain worse. The next day they took Matthew to the ER. The ENT doctor who was on call looked under the microscope and found a lima bean swollen to twice its normal size. Using fine instruments and a suction device, the doctor removed the bean.

A Tip

Harvey was a dapper older gentleman, always properly turned out. Besides the usual shower and washing his hair, he spent extra time trimming his beard, cleaning his glasses, and drying his ears with cotton swabs. Not only did the moisture in the ear canals bother him, but also his mother had always lectured him that gentlemen did not have dirty ears. One day following his morning ritual, he noticed an immediate loss of hearing in his left ear. He didn't have any pain; he just couldn't hear on that side. Worried that something serious had happened, he immediately went to the doctor who saw that Harvey's ear was blocked with wax. The nurse at the office tried unsuccessfully to irrigate his ear and wash the wax out. His hearing didn't improve, so he obtained a referral to an ear doctor who used a microscope, instruments, and suction to clean the impacted wax from his ear. This time, he left with his hearing restored. His only prescription was to no longer use cotton swabs. He actually discovered that instructions on the cotton swab box said not to use them in the ears.

Don't Delay Treatment

Betty, not one to complain, had a week of constant drainage from her left ear. Finally, her daughter gave her ear drops she had left over from a prior infection, but the pain persisted. In addition, her diabetes became increasingly difficult to control with insulin. Ultimately she went to an ENT doctor, who diagnosed *otitis externa*. Her diabetes made the situation potentially dangerous, so after she had her ear canal cleaned, Betty had to be hospitalized to receive IV antibiotics to clear up her infection.

The Least You Need to Know

- Earwax, or cerumen, is a naturally occurring protector of the ear canal and is healthy in normal amounts.
- Never stick cotton swabs or sharp objects in your ears; doing so is likely to cause earwax impaction or damage the skin of the ear canal.
- If you have a foreign object in your ear that you can't easily remove, see an ear doctor.
- To prevent swimmer's ear (*otitis externa*), keep your ears dry and avoid scratching them; if prone to this condition, wear earplugs in the water.
- If you have itchy, flaky, or scaly ears or extensive earwax, have an ear doctor periodically clean your ears.

Problems of the Eustachian Tube

In This Chapter

- The Eustachian tube
- Abnormal Eustachian tube function
- Causes and treatments of fluid in the middle ear
- Preventing ear problems when flying or diving

You might not have heard of the Eustachian tube by name before, but you've at least thought about it. It's the thing involved when you feel as if you have to "pop" your ears. Dysfunction of the Eustachian tube can result in ear fullness along with associated discomfort, popping or crackling sounds, pressure, and diminished hearing. People often describe the fullness that arises from this dysfunction as feeling as if their head were in an empty barrel or inside a tunnel.

The Eustachian tube is a 1½-inch-long, narrow channel connecting the nasopharynx (area connecting the back of the nose to the throat) with the middle ear space. It lies deep within the head, is made of cartilage and bone, and is surrounded by muscles and other soft tissues. Each ear, right and left, has one. The Eustachian tube is named for an Italian anatomist, Bartolomeo Eustachi, who lived in the sixteenth century. Eustachi described many anatomic findings, but he's best known for his discovery of this tube that now bears his name.

In this chapter, we describe the function of the Eustachian tube and explain how blockage or dysfunction of this tube can lead to hearing loss and how problems are treated, especially fluid in the middle ear. We also give some specific helpful hints regarding the pressure equalization function of the Eustachian tube when atmospheric pressure changes, such as when we fly or go diving.

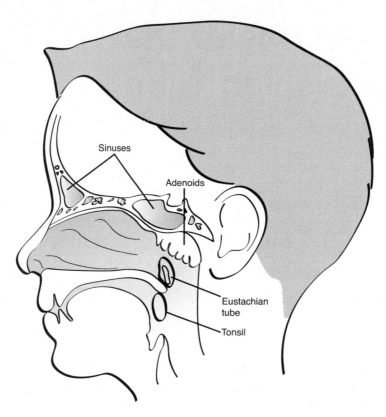

This drawing shows the location of the opening of the Eustachian tube in the nasopharynx at the back of the nose in relation to other structures.

Function of the Eustachian Tube

The Eustachian tube acts as a pressure-equalizing valve for the middle ear, which is usually filled with air. Normally closed, the tube opens for a period of less than a second when we swallow, yawn, or sneeze. This opening allows air to pass into the middle ear space from the back of the nose, which is necessary because the lining of the middle ear constantly absorbs the air, which must be replaced. When there's a change in pressure, as with altitude changes, the Eustachian tube allows pressure between the middle ear and the atmosphere to equalize.

The Eustachian tube, in its closed state, also prevents mucus and secretions from the back of the nose from rising into the middle ear, which would likely cause infection. In spite of this protective function, infections can arise from the nose and travel into the middle ear through the Eustachian tube. This happens more often in children than in adults. The Eustachian tube also allows secretions from the middle ear to drain into the back of the nose. A problem that interferes with the Eustachian tube performing any of these functions properly can lead to hearing loss and other ear symptoms.

Blockage of the Eustachian tube opening (at either end—within the nose or within the ear) leads to a negative middle ear pressure (a vacuum) because air can't enter the middle ear space from the back of the nose. This eventually causes the eardrum to be sucked inward, a process called retraction. A retracted eardrum may lead to ear pain, a feeling of fullness or pressure, head noise—tinnitus, and hearing loss.

LISTEN UP

Your ear doctor may use the word *retraction* when describing the findings of an examination of your eardrum. A retracted eardrum can make you more susceptible to recurrent infections, so it needs close monitoring and, sometimes, surgery.

Over time, continued blockage of the Eustachian tube, with the associated negative middle ear pressure, can lead to fluid being drawn out of the tissue lining the middle ear. This leads to a condition called otitis media with effusion (OME) or fluid in the middle ear. If the fluid in the middle ear becomes infected, it's called acute otitis media. OME is the most common cause of hearing loss in children today. Children are more susceptible to this condition because their Eustachian tubes are not fully developed. In comparison with adults, a child's Eustachian tube is shorter and has a less angled orientation, so it is less effective at maintaining equal pressure between the middle ear and the back of the nose.

Also, children are more likely to get upper respiratory infections, such as colds or flu, which can lead to blockage of the Eustachian tube and fluid buildup in the middle ear through swelling and mucus production. The Eustachian tube reaches its adult size and orientation by age seven, but improper function of this tube can and does continue into adulthood in some people.

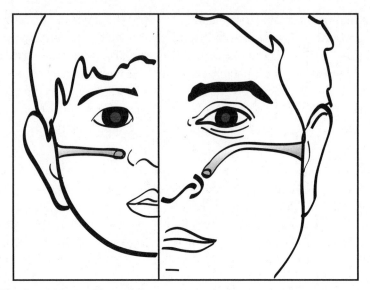

An illustration of the difference in size and shape of the Eustachian tube between adults and children.

Fluid in the Middle Ear

Otitis media with effusion may be acute, subacute, or chronic. Acute episodes generally are those that occur for one to four weeks; subacute episodes last one to three months; and chronic disorders last for more than three months. If infection occurs, it's acute otitis media—commonly called "an ear infection." Most parents of toddlers are familiar with this condition; 75 percent of children experience at least one episode by their third birthday and nearly half will have had three or more ear infections by then. After the acute infection is treated, fluid may remain even though it is no longer infected.

OME is diagnosed by looking at the eardrum through an otoscope. The eardrum may be retracted or appear "full." When the ear is normal, the ossicles show as a particular pattern on the eardrum, but when fluid is present in the middle ear, this pattern may not be visible. A special attachment to the otoscope blows a slight puff of air into the ear, which should cause movement of the eardrum. When there is fluid behind the eardrum, this movement may be less than normal or absent. When infection is present (acute otitis media), the eardrum may appear red and swollen. If fluid or pus is draining from the ear, the doctor can collect a sample and test it to determine what organism might be causing the infection.

Causes of Fluid in the Middle Ear

OME may result from any of several conditions that interfere with the periodic opening and closing of the Eustachian tube. The causes may be congenital (present at birth), related to infection or allergy, or a result of blockage of the nasal opening of the tube by enlarged adenoids or other tissue. The adenoids are specialized tissue located in the middle of the back of the nose between the openings of the two Eustachian tubes. This tissue typically decreases in size by adulthood but can block the back of the nose and hold bacteria in children. Such blockage may lead to mouth breathing, snoring, fatigue, and recurrent nasal and ear infections. (Many things can lead to a blocked tube, but it's a common misconception that getting water in a baby's ears is one of these things.)

Known risk factors for the development of OME include prematurity and low birth weight, young age, a positive family history, altered immune system function, abnormal facial features such as cleft palate, neuromuscular disease, Down syndrome, and various environmental factors such as day care attendance, crowded living conditions, low socioeconomic conditions, exposure to tobacco and pollutants, pacifier use in toddlers, sleeping on the stomach, and prolonged bottle-feeding. If otitis media runs in a child's family, that child is five times more likely to be susceptible to the disease.

Acute otitis media is usually the result of blockage of the Eustachian tube from an upper respiratory infection, sinus infection, or an attack of nasal allergy. In the presence of bacteria, the fluid buildup may also become infected. When infection does not develop, the fluid remains until the Eustachian tube again begins to function normally. Then the fluid is absorbed or drains down the tube into the throat.

HAVE YOU HEARD?

The lining membrane, or mucous membrane, of the middle ear and Eustachian tube is connected with, and is the same as, the membrane of the nose, sinuses, and throat. Infection of these areas results in mucous membrane swelling, which in turn may result in Eustachian tube obstruction. In short, a stuffy nose can lead to stuffy ears.

Chronic OME (fluid present in the middle ear for more than three months) may result from continued and persistent Eustachian tube blockage or from thickening of the fluids so they can't be absorbed or drained through the Eustachian tube. This chronic condition usually produces a hearing impairment of as much as 10 to 30 decibels. There can be ear pain, especially with a cold. But children with OME, unlike an acute ear infection, are often not sick, and the condition can go unnoticed. Parents may notice that the child wants the TV volume too loud, or a teacher may see that the child is not paying attention in class. Fortunately, OME can last for many years without producing any permanent damage to the structures of the middle ear, but the presence of fluid in the middle ear does make it very susceptible to recurrent episodes of acute otitis media. These recurrent infections may result in middle ear damage. And for children, the hearing loss can have substantial consequences (see Chapter 14).

LISTEN UP

As you know, the middle ear is composed of the eardrum and the three ear bones or ossicles. Recurrent infections can lead to damage of any of these structures, which can lead to a hearing loss. If you have ear pain and/or ear discharge along with changes in hearing, see an ear specialist. Also, children with cleft palate or other craniofacial abnormalities, such as those that occur in children with Down syndrome, should have their ears evaluated regularly because they are predisposed to having fluid within the middle ear and therefore susceptible to hearing loss.

Allergic reactions in the nose and throat result in mucous membrane swelling, and this swelling may also affect the Eustachian tube. This reaction may be acute, as in a hay fever–type reaction, or may be chronic, as in many varieties of chronic sinusitis or ongoing inflammation of the sinuses.

Treatment of Acute Fluid and Ear Infections

Treatment of OME is medical and usually directed toward treatment of the upper respiratory infection or allergy attacks. Treatment may include antibiotics, antihistamines (anti-allergy drugs), decongestants (drugs to decrease mucous membrane swelling), and nasal sprays. We discuss allergy and its treatment in Chapter 12. When the diagnosis is an ear infection, antibiotic treatment usually takes care of the problem and normal middle ear function occurs within three to four weeks.

If antibiotics don't do the job, a surgical procedure may be required for acute otitis media. Tympanocentesis involves piercing the eardrum with a needle and suctioning out fluid for diagnostic examination. The hole created by this procedure is small enough so that it usually heals within one or two days. In a myringotomy, a small surgical cut is made in the eardrum, and the fluid is removed from the middle ear space. After myringotomy, the ear may drain pus and blood for up to a week. The eardrum then heals and hearing usually returns to normal within three to four weeks. During this healing period, varying degrees of ear pressure, popping, clicking, and fluctuation of hearing may occur, occasionally with shooting pains in the ear. Myringotomy with ventilation tube insertion is performed to maintain the opening to the middle ear for longer-term drainage, access for medication, and ventilation of the middle ear space. Ventilation tubes are usually made of plastic or silicone and are also called tympanostomy tubes or pressure equalization (PE) tubes.

Children less than two years old frequently develop acute otitis media and have ear pain without significant hearing loss. In fact, 70 percent of all children experience one or more attacks of acute otitis media by age two. Antibiotic treatment is sufficient in most cases. Recurrent episodes of acute otitis media are best treated with myringotomy and ventilation tube placement.

Treatment of Chronic Fluid

Resolution of an acute infection occasionally leaves uninfected fluid in the middle ear. When this fluid remains for more than three months, it's called chronic otitis media with effusion. Like acute OME, treatment of chronic OME may be either medical or surgical. Someone with chronic OME may also have other chronic problems. For example, as a cold or flu subsides, it may leave a persistent sinus infection in addition to the fluid within the middle ear. Pus from the sinuses and nose can then drain over the Eustachian tube opening in the back of the nose, resulting in Eustachian tube blockage and dysfunction. Antibiotic treatment may be necessary to help clear the sinus infection. Besides chronic sinus infection, chronic OME can signal the presence of other medical problems. This is particularly important to consider in children. General health factors are important to a child's resistance to infection. A deficiency in some of the blood immune proteins, or antibodies, may predispose the child to recurrent infections and prolonged colds. Though rare, immune problems should be suspected if recurrent or persistent infections or colds occur following appropriate treatment. Periodic injections of gamma globulin might be helpful in some of these cases.

Allergy is often a major factor in the development or persistence of OME. Inflammation of the mucous membranes lining the nose, sinus cavities, and Eustachian tube can result from exposure to various allergens, leading eventually to middle ear problems. Mild cases are often treated with antihistamine drugs. More persistent cases might require allergic evaluation and treatment, including allergy shots (see Chapter 12).

Eustachian tube insufflation may also be helpful. This means blowing air through the nose into the obstructed Eustachian tube and middle ear to help relieve congestion and reestablish middle ear ventilation. This is typically done by a *Valsalva maneuver* or by *Politzerization*.

DEFINITION

A **Valsalva maneuver** is a means for getting air from the back of the nose into the Eustachian tube. It's accomplished by carefully blowing air into the middle ear while holding the nose, often called "popping the ear."

Politzerization is a way to blow air into the Eustachian tube by using a special instrument called a middle ear inflator.

To perform the Valsalva maneuver, take a deep breath in through the mouth. With lips sealed, blow gently out through the nose. While doing so, pinch your nose closed (both nostrils) for several seconds, release, then pinch again, and release, for a total of 10 to 15 seconds. Closing off the nose forces air from the nose into the middle ear through the Eustachian tube. Don't do this if you have a cold or nasal discharge, because it can lead to the spread of an infection into the middle ear. And don't blow your head to the moon; be gentle!

Politzerization is accomplished by blowing air with a special syringe, called a middle ear inflator, into one nostril while blocking the other and swallowing at the same time. This forces the air into the Eustachian tube and middle ear. Also, don't do this if you have a cold.

You can also insufflate the Eustachian tube by using a special instrument called the Ear Popper. This commercially available, battery-powered device delivers a constant flow of air to the nasal cavity, and you must hold the device firmly against the nostril opening. When you press a button, a stream of air enters the nose. While the air is flowing, you swallow frequently to try to open the Eustachian tube and allow the air into the middle ear. The Ear Popper may be purchased from your local pharmacy and is often covered by insurance.

Surgical treatment of chronic OME may be necessary to reestablish ventilation of the middle ear, keep the hearing at a normal level, and prevent recurrent infection that might damage the eardrum and middle ear bones. The same procedures described for acute OME may be used, including myringotomy with insertion of a ventilation tube and, in some cases, adenoidectomy.

In adults, myringotomy and ventilation tube insertion is usually performed in the office under local anesthesia. In children, it's often done in a hospital setting but on an outpatient basis. The adenoids can be removed at the same time if they are enlarged. The ventilation tube temporarily takes the place of the Eustachian tube in equalizing middle ear pressure. This plastic tube usually remains in place for three to nine months until the Eustachian tube blockage subsides. When the tube falls out, the eardrum heals, and the Eustachian tube resumes its normal pressure equalizing function. In rare cases, the eardrum does not heal following dislodgement of the tube; but if this happens, the perforation can be repaired later.

Most often when the ventilation tube dislodges, there is no further middle ear ventilation problem. If OME recurs, it may be necessary to insert a new tube, and in some difficult cases, a longer-lasting type of tube may be inserted. Removal of this type of tube may require a second procedure in a hospital outpatient setting.

A person can perform most normal activities when a ventilation tube is in place. Opinions do vary, but some physicians believe that when a tube is in place, no water should be allowed to enter the ear canal or middle ear as this could lead to an infection. Other physicians feel that only contaminated water, such as water from ponds, lakes, streams, or oceans, needs to be avoided. Your physician may recommend an earplug for use when showering, shampooing, or swimming.

Children who suffer from chronic OME are usually older than two years and rarely have pain. However, these children often have measurable hearing loss and frequently have delayed language development and difficulty in school. Specialized hearing tests can be performed to determine the degree of hearing loss. Myringotomy with ventilation tube placement is often extremely helpful in such children. When the fluid within the middle ear is drained, hearing rapidly improves. Removal of enlarged adenoids may provide some additional benefit in children with chronic OME. Tonsillectomy is not done for ear problems but most often for problems related to snoring, airway obstruction, or recurrent throat infections.

Polyps in the nose can also lead to partial or complete blockage of the Eustachian tube, leading to problems of fluid buildup in the middle ear. Smoking has been shown to impair the function of the mucous membranes, which can lead to problems with the Eustachian tube as well. Avoidance of smoking is an important concept for the entire body, and the ear is no exception to this rule.

Persistent Fluid Formation

Chronic serous mastoiditis and idiopathic hemotympanum are uncommon conditions that have the same symptoms as chronic OME. They differ in that the middle ear fluid continues to form, either draining out the ventilation tube or blocking it completely so that the tube dislodges shortly after surgery. This persistent fluid formation is due to changes in the mucous membrane of the middle ear and mastoid. In both of these conditions, mastoid surgery may be necessary to control the problem and reestablish a normal middle ear mechanism.

LISTEN UP

Hemotympanum is the presence of blood within the middle ear space. Most cases of hemotympanum are due to trauma to the bone around the ear, which results in leakage of blood into the middle ear. Anyone who suffers a blow to the head should be evaluated by a physician to rule out a serious problem.

Other Eustachian Tube Problems

Abnormal patency or openness of the Eustachian tube, also known as a patulous Eustachian tube, is a condition in which the Eustachian tube remains open for prolonged periods. This abnormality may produce many distressing symptoms: ear fullness and blockage, a hollow feeling in the ear, hearing one's own breathing, and voice reverberation. It does not typically produce true hearing impairment.

The exact cause of an abnormally patent Eustachian tube is often difficult to determine. In many instances, it develops following a loss in weight, such as occurs following stomach surgery or treatment with chemotherapy. It can develop during pregnancy or while taking oral contraceptives or other hormones. In other cases, patulous Eustachian tube may develop because the Eustachian tube is narrow and stiff and does not open and close properly.

Treatment of this harmless but bothersome condition is often difficult. A number of different medications have been used and may be successful in alleviating the symptoms. Myringotomy with insertion of a ventilation tube is often effective. Some physicians perform surgery through the nose or through the ear to try to block the Eustachian tube. But the outcome of these surgeries varies considerably as the procedure is not always successful and may need to be repeated.

Palatal myoclonus is a rare condition in which muscles of the palate (the back of the roof of the mouth) twitch rhythmically many times a minute. The cause of this harmless muscle spasm is unknown. With this condition, you might experience a rhythmic clicking or snapping sound in the ear as the Eustachian tube opens and closes. Sedatives or tranquilizers often are effective in controlling the symptom, but in many cases, no treatment is needed. Occasionally, the snapping sound in the ear is caused by simultaneous spasm of the two muscles attached to the middle ear bones. Cutting one or both of these muscles usually relieves the symptoms. The operation is performed on outpatients under local anesthesia through the ear canal, and patients are able to return to usual activities in a few days.

A person can have the same ear symptoms we've been describing for Eustachian tube dysfunction (fullness, pressure, or pain) despite the ear and the Eustachian tube both being completely normal. In these situations, pain is referred to the ear from other body parts as a result of the complex interaction of the many nerves of the head and neck. Also, heartburn can occasionally lead to pain in the ear through irritation of the back of the throat.

HAVE YOU HEARD?

Doctors sometimes refer to the 10 Ts of referred ear pain: temporomandibular joint, tonsils, throat, thyroid, teeth, Eustachian tube, trachea, tongue, tics, and tendons. Problems with any of these other areas of the body may cause ear pain even though nothing is actually wrong in the ear.

When You Fly

People with Eustachian tube problems may experience difficulty equalizing middle ear pressure when flying. When an aircraft takes off and ascends, the atmospheric pressure drops, which means there is a relative increase in middle ear pressure. During the descent, the opposite occurs: there is an increase in atmospheric pressure, with a relative decrease in the middle ear pressure. In either of these situations, if the Eustachian tube is not working properly, discomfort may develop within the ear—it is often worse during aircraft descent. Try these general things to prevent Eustachian tube-related symptoms when flying:

- Chew gum, suck on candy, or yawn vigorously during the descent to stimulate swallowing and equalize pressure in the middle ear. Drinking a glass of water or eating a snack can help toddlers.

- Parents should wake children at the start of the descent. We swallow less when asleep, so children often wake up crying when the plane begins to descend due to the uncomfortable buildup of pressure in their ears.

- Place a pacifier or bottle in an infant's mouth during take off and landing to encourage swallowing. Nursing mothers can help their infants by nursing during takeoff and landing.

To avoid middle ear problems, do not fly if you have an acute upper respiratory problem (cold, allergy attack, or sinus infection). If you must fly with such a problem or if you have a chronic Eustachian tube problem, you can help avoid ear difficulty by taking the following steps:

1. Obtain Sudafed tablets and a plastic squeeze bottle of mild (0.25% phenylephrine HCL) Neo-Synephrine nasal spray from your drug store (no prescription is necessary).

2. Following the container directions, begin taking Sudafed tablets the day before your air flight. Continue the medication for 24 hours after the flight if you have experienced any ear difficulty.

3. Following the container directions, use the nasal spray shortly before boarding the aircraft. If your ears plug up upon ascent, hold your nose and swallow. This will help suck excess air pressure out of the middle ear.

4. Forty-five minutes before the aircraft is due to land again, use the nasal spray every 5 minutes for 15 minutes. Chew gum to stimulate swallowing.

Should your ears plug up despite this, hold your nose and blow forcibly to try to blow air up the Eustachian tube into the middle ear (that's the Valsalva maneuver).

If you must fly with an acute upper respiratory infection, do not perform the Valsalva maneuver in step 4. None of these recommendations or precautions is necessary if you have a middle ear ventilation tube in your eardrum.

In both adults and children, the failure to properly clear the ears could lead to a more serious condition. Decongestants can help minimize the impact of changing cabin pressure on tiny ears of a congested baby while flying. However, parents must have the proper prescriptive and dosage advice from a pediatrician in these situations.

One other way to avoid or alleviate problems while flying is to use EarPlanes, which are silicone ear plugs with a ceramic pressure regulator that allow eardrums to adjust to changes in altitude pressure at a slower and more natural rate. Sized for both children and adults, EarPlanes cost less than $10 at drug stores, mass retailers, and air terminal shops.

When You Dive

Special problems, not unlike the problems that may arise while flying, can arise in the middle ear during underwater diving. During diving (SCUBA or other), the external ear is immersed in water, which by definition is an incompressible liquid. Because changes in pressure on the eardrum occur more quickly during diving than while flying, there is danger of hearing loss, imbalance, eardrum rupture, and dizziness.

Ear pain occurs during a diver's descent. Increased water pressure on the external surface of the eardrum is sometimes referred to as ear squeeze. The initial change in pressure that occurs in going from the surface to just a few feet underwater can be enough to lead to ear squeeze, causing problems for the diver. To counterbalance this pressure, the air pressure must increase on the inner surface of the eardrum. To do this, the Eustachian tube will open and allow the pressure behind the eardrum to equalize with the outside pressure of the seawater in the ear canal. But if the Eustachian tube can't open as the seawater pressure in the ear canal increases, the eardrum is forced inward, inflaming the eardrum and causing pain. If the pain is ignored and the diver goes deeper, the pressure will continue to increase and the eardrum may burst or rupture. Cold seawater will then rush into the middle ear, causing nausea, vomiting, and dizziness.

If you plan to do some deep-water diving, practice pressurization of the middle ear first—to test your Eustachian tubes for patency and to perform middle ear pressurization before beginning actual descent. Doing so can cushion the ears against trauma. If, when you do dive, you feel fullness or pain, stop the dive and attempt to clear your ears. If this fails, you must end the dive. Always complete the decompression steps, if necessary, when returning to the surface. If the eardrum ruptures, a diver may become disoriented or vomit, which can lead to panic, and panic may lead to ascending too rapidly. You and your diving partner should always carefully observe and assist each other during the ascent.

True Stories

In this chapter, we talked about a wide variety of problems that can arise due to dysfunction of the Eustachian tube. Here are a few patient stories from our medical records to help you better understand the diagnosis and treatment of some of these problems.

A Common Problem

The parents of four-year-old Clarissa brought her to the clinic and reported that she had had four or five ear infections in the past year that were treated with oral antibiotics. They also related that Clarissa snored and did a lot of mouth breathing. On examination, the doctor found that Clarissa had a persistently open mouth and some mucus in the front of the nose. The exam also showed evidence of fluid behind both eardrums, with reduced movement of each drum. A hearing test showed a conductive hearing loss in both ears. In the past, Clarissa had taken a nasal steroid spray with no relief. She was diagnosed with chronic otitis media with effusion and enlarged adenoids. After the parents learned about the risks, benefits, and alternatives to placement of ear tubes with adenoidectomy, Clarissa had successful placement of the tubes and removal of her adenoids. The tubes fell out after 11 months and Clarissa's hearing has returned to normal. She has not had another episode of otitis media, and her snoring has decreased.

Yes, Adults Can Get Otitis Media

Following a recent cold, 24-year-old Marisa went to her ENT doctor with complaints of fullness, popping, and crackling noises and the feeling that she couldn't hear as well in her right ear. She had never had ear problems before and said her hearing had been fine up until the recent cold. Now the cold symptoms were gone, and she was back at work but continued to have ear problems. On examination, the doctor detected fluid behind the eardrum and the eardrum had reduced movement. A hearing test revealed a very slight conductive loss in the affected ear. The rest of the head and neck exam was normal and the opposite ear was also normal. Diagnosed with otitis media, Marisa was counseled on treatment options, including continued observation versus myringotomy. Marisa, tired of her symptoms, elected to have a myringotomy performed. Immediately after the procedure, Marisa's symptoms were better, and she has had no further problems.

Weight Loss and the Ears

Linda, a 42-year-old woman with a recent history of 130-pound weight loss following gastric bypass surgery, presented with a new ear complaint. She reported hearing her own voice much more audibly than before and having a muffled sound in both ears. When she lowered her head between her knees, the muffled sound went away. On examination, the doctor noted that the eardrum moved in rhythm with the patient's breathing. No other abnormalities were noted. A hearing test was performed and revealed no evidence of hearing loss. Linda was diagnosed with patulous Eustachian tube. Her doctor counseled her about the nature of this condition and its treatment and prescribed his favored treatment, a saturated solution of potassium iodide (10 drops in a glass of orange juice taken twice a day). She was scheduled for a routine follow-up visit. Three months later, Linda felt things were better, though not perfect. However, she was content and did not feel further intervention was needed.

Clear to Dive

A 19-year-old college student, Brian, presented with complaints of ear pain, bleeding, and decreased hearing. Having recently participated in a SCUBA diving course, Brian noted that these symptoms started following a dive. He did have a history of ear infections in childhood and had had several sets of ear tubes, even into his elementary school years. Brian also reported having some nasal allergies for which he took a nasal steroid and an oral antihistamine on a regular basis. During the initial descent of the recent dive, he noted he was unable to clear his ears. As he dove deeper, he assumed his ears would clear at any moment, but they didn't, and he felt a sudden onset of pressure and pain in his right ear. He also experienced some mild nausea when this occurred, so he slowly came back to the surface with his dive partner. Upon examination of the ear in the clinic, a small amount of dried blood was noted in the ear canal.

The doctor could see a perforation of the tympanic membrane and some moist debris within the middle ear space. Brian began applying topical antibiotics and was told to avoid further diving as well as to prevent water from entering the ear canal. A dysfunctional Eustachian tube was the likely cause of the inability to clear the ears during the dive. The perforation has now healed and Brian is ready to try diving again. But he knows to stop his descent if his ears do not clear as they should.

The Least You Need to Know

- The Eustachian tube acts as a pressure-equalizing valve for the middle ear.
- Dysfunction of the Eustachian tube can result in ear fullness or pressure, pain, popping or crackling sounds, and hearing loss.
- Otitis media with effusion (fluid in the middle ear) can occur at any age but is more common in children than in adults.
- To help equalize middle ear pressure when flying, hold the nose and swallow on ascent and hold the nose and blow gently on descent.

Chronic Infection in the Middle Ear

In This Chapter

- Symptoms and consequences of an ongoing infection in the middle ear
- Caring for an ear with infection
- Medical and surgical treatments for long-lasting infection
- Risks and complications of surgery

Any disease affecting the eardrum or the three small bones may cause a conductive hearing loss by interfering with the transmission of sound to the inner ear. Such a hearing impairment may be due to a perforation in the eardrum, partial or total destruction of one or all of the three little ear bones or ossicles, or scar tissue. A chronic infection of the middle ear can cause any or all three of these problems, leading to hearing loss. In Chapter 4, we discussed acute otitis media, short-lived ear infections, usually lasting no more than a month. But when infection remains in the middle ear for more than a month, it's called chronic otitis media (COM).

If you have chronic otitis media, it's important for you to know the potential risks and complications of the treatment, as well as the anticipated benefits. So in this chapter, we describe common symptoms of chronic otitis media, give basic advice on how to care for an infected ear, and discuss the surgical repair of the damage caused by COM.

The Diseased Middle Ear

In Chapter 4, we talked about the possibility that a middle ear infection can cause a perforation in the eardrum and that with acute otitis media, this perforation usually heals on its own. But when *chronic otitis media* is present, it's less likely that a perforation can heal.

DEFINITION

Chronic otitis media (COM) is a long-lasting infection of the middle ear that often produces a perforation in the eardrum and can lead to damage of the ossicles (middle ear bones) or tissue membrane of the middle ear, resulting in hearing loss.

In addition to a perforated eardrum, COM may lead to other conditions or complications. One such complication is tympanosclerosis—scarring or calcification in the middle fibrous layers of the eardrum and in the middle ear. Remember, the eardrum is made up of four layers: an outer layer of skin, an inner layer of mucosa, and two middle layers of fibrous tissue. Tympanosclerosis stiffens the eardrum, often affecting its movement. If the tympanosclerosis spreads to involve the ossicles, hearing loss will occur. Your doctor can tell when you have tympanosclerosis because the appearance of the eardrum changes from its normal blue-gray to white.

Chronic otitis media and perforation of the eardrum can also lead to formation of cholesteatoma—a collection of skin cells and connective tissue that forms a cyst in the middle ear. This results from the movement of skin from the ear canal wall down through the hole in the eardrum into the middle ear space. Cholesteatoma is not a cancer or even a benign tumor. It's a collection of skin trapped in an area where the skin does not belong. Cholesteatomas have the capacity for continued growth, causing erosion of surrounding bone by direct pressure or by chemical breakdown of the bone, and can damage the ossicles to produce hearing loss.

Cholesteatoma in the middle ear can cause drainage as well as conductive hearing loss by involving the ossicles. If it involves the inner ear, it can also cause a permanent sensorineural hearing loss and dizziness. The dizziness is caused because the cholesteatoma can erode through one of the semicircular canals of the inner ear balance system (the labyrinth).

A fistula test can determine whether cholesteatoma has affected the inner ear balance system. The medical term *fistula* means an abnormal connection between organs or structures—a hole, of sorts. A cholesteatoma can create an opening through the bone to the membrane portion of the balance system. For a fistula test, the doctor uses an instrument called a pneumatic otoscope. But you can do a fistula test by placing a finger into the opening of the external ear canal and gently pushing in and out. This causes a column of air to move against the eardrum, which transfers that pressure through the middle ear space to the exposed membrane of the labyrinth. The movement creates a sense of vertigo or dizziness only when the balance system is exposed because of a hole in the bone.

Symptoms of Chronic Ear Infection

Infections of the middle ear can cause hearing impairment and discharge from the ear. Occasionally, symptoms of more advanced chronic ear disease are present, such as pain, dizziness, or facial weakness. Symptoms depend upon whether the condition is active or inactive, whether or not the mastoid bone is involved, and whether or not there is a hole in the eardrum. A careful evaluation of the symptoms and findings allows the physician to determine the need for medical or surgical treatment; the urgency, if any; and the possible outcomes of treatment.

Ear Drainage

Drainage from the ear is the most common symptom of middle ear infections. An odorless mucous type of discharge is usually an indication of middle ear mucosal disease or Eustachian tube dysfunction—often temporary. The discharge tends to be intermittent, clearing rapidly with proper care of the ear. But a foul-smelling discharge that may be bloody and is either constant or frequently recurring usually indicates significant middle ear (COM) and mastoid disease (a complication of COM that can include cholesteatoma or inflammation of the mucosa in the mastoid area). Purulent discharge, or pus, is an indication of infection. Bacterial infection of the mucous membrane of the middle ear is usually brief and clears rapidly with treatment. Purulent discharge that doesn't subside with treatment is an indication of a resistant organism, irreversible mucous membrane disease, cholesteatoma, or all of these.

Hearing Loss

The extent of hearing loss in chronic otitis media depends primarily on the degree of disruption of the three middle ear bones, not on how much disease is present. A conductive hearing loss of 20 dB or less usually indicates that the ossicles are intact. Disruption or fixation of the ossicles usually results in a hearing loss of 30 dB or more. Cholesteatoma can cause significant disruption of the ossicles.

It's not unusual to have normal hearing in an ear with a perforation near the top of the eardrum with a cholesteatoma in the attic area of the middle ear. The normal hearing may be misleading. In reality, the cholesteatoma may not only have broken the chain of the three middle ear bones, but in essence replaced it, so that the sound transmission travels through the mass of the cholesteatoma to the inner ear.

A progressing conductive hearing loss when there is no active infection tells us that the middle ear bones may be becoming fixed and can't move properly. In such a case, tympanosclerosis may be causing the fixation of any of the three ossicles and hearing aids or surgery may be required to improve hearing.

HAVE YOU HEARD?

Another condition, otosclerosis, can cause fixation of the footplate of the stapes—the third middle ear bone. Hearing loss due to otosclerosis is discussed in Chapter 6.

Pain

Pain is not a frequent complaint in people with COM unless they also have an infection of the external ear canal (see Chapter 3), which can be quite painful. Occasionally, however, the patient with COM and cholesteatoma will complain of a dull pain that can be severe enough to disturb sleep. This pain indicates that the cholesteatoma is expanding, causing pressure against the tissue that separates the brain from the mastoid space. Occasionally, an abscess, or infection, may form in that space that can lead to pain. In this situation, you should not delay treatment.

A feeling of pressure in the ear is not uncommon in cholesteatoma. Often, this pressure builds when the ear stops discharging and is relieved when drainage begins again. This feeling of pressure is not usually an urgent symptom.

Other Symptoms

We frequently see minor degrees of vertigo with chronic otitis media. But if you have significant vertigo, especially if it has just started, and an infection of the middle ear, this could mean that there is inflammation of the labyrinth (called labyrinthitis) or that a cholesteatoma has caused a fistula in one of the three semi-circular canals as we mentioned earlier. The erosion of the semicircular canal can often be seen on a CT scan. Don't delay surgical treatment here, as a delay in treatment can result in complications such as a permanent sensorineural hearing loss.

LISTEN UP

Facial nerve weakness in patients with COM is rare but does develop in less than 1 percent of people with cholesteatoma from infections of the middle ear. Treatment should be undertaken without delay to be able to relieve the pressure on the facial nerve.

Care of the Infected Ear

If you have a perforation of your eardrum, don't allow water to get into your ear canal. When showering or washing your hair, use an earplug, or place cotton or lamb's wool in the external ear canal and cover it with a layer of petroleum jelly. When bathing a young child with a perforation, don't allow the child's head to become submerged. The dirty bathwater entering the middle ear space through the perforation is a common source for drainage.

Experts differ in their opinions about whether patients with perforations should swim. Most allow swimming in the family pool. Fewer allow swimming in a public pool. Some allow swimming in lakes or rivers, but swimming in the ocean is not recommended. Earplugs, even custom-made ear molds, can keep most, but not all, water out of the ears. If drainage from the middle ear does occur, stop the swimming activity.

SOUND ADVICE

To prevent any infection in your nose from spreading to the ear through the Eustachian tube, avoid blowing your nose if you have COM. Instead, draw backward and expectorate (yes, spit out) any nasal secretion. If it's absolutely necessary to blow your nose, don't block or close one nostril while blowing the other.

If you have ear drainage, keep the ear canal clean by using a small cotton-tipped applicator. Using the hand opposite the ear to be cleaned, reach across the back of the head and pull the top of the ear up and back (in other words, the right hand reaches across the back of the head and pulls the left ear up and back). This straightens out the ear canal and makes it easier to introduce the cotton-tipped applicator. Gently insert the applicator into the ear canal and blot the ear. Repeat this procedure with a fresh cotton applicator until the ear is dry. Do not place the applicator deep into the ear canal, and don't ever leave an applicator in the ear canal while doing something else. Trauma to the eardrum can and has occurred from inappropriate use of cotton-tipped applicators (see Chapter 3).

Evaluation for Treatment

Based on your symptoms and findings, your ear doctor may want to perform tests, including tests of hearing and balance and radiographic studies (see Chapter 2).

Hearing tests are performed routinely when assessing patients with COM. The decision to perform surgery is not made only on the basis of the hearing impairment; however, the hearing evaluation will be helpful in advising you about what outcome to expect from surgery.

Imaging studies (CT or MRI scans) are not necessarily needed, even in patients with COM who are scheduled for surgery. The doctor will more likely request an imaging study when there's a complication of the disease (such as labyrinthine fistula or facial nerve weakness) or extensive involvement of the ear. If imaging is needed, a CT scan of the temporal bone is performed, which provides excellent details of bony erosion of the middle ear or mastoid that might affect the inner ear balance system or facial nerve. The CT can also show whether the ossicles have been damaged. MRI scans are rarely done for COM but can help determine whether there's any brain involvement by the cholesteatoma if symptoms suggest the need.

Medical Treatment

Three important factors underlie chronic or intermittent infection in chronic otitis media: moisture, diseased tissue, and opportunistic organisms—meaning bacteria. These factors form the basis for treatment approaches. You can eliminate moisture by keeping the ear dry and using proper techniques for cleaning the ear, as described earlier in this chapter. The physician can remove damaged or diseased tissue (see the following section on surgical treatment). And you can control opportunistic organisms by the application of antibiotic ear drops or powder. Medication is often prescribed for patients with ear drainage. Because of the potential for these ear drop medications to cause more inner ear hearing loss (ototoxicity, see Chapter 9), many medications formerly used are no longer prescribed. Today, a select list of ear and occasionally eye drops treat ear drainage. Yes, you did read correctly; in a few instances, eye drops are prescribed for use in the ear to treat ear drainage.

SOUND ADVICE

The easiest way to apply, or instill, medication ear drops is to lie on your side with the draining ear up. Place the appropriate number of drops into the draining ear. Remain lying down for about 5 minutes; then stand and place a small piece of cotton loosely in the lower portion of the outer ear. The cotton will catch any drops or drainage, but you don't want to block the ear canal. It's important to allow as much air as possible to get into the ear canal to help the ear heal. Change the cotton as needed throughout the day.

Powder, frequently effective when ear drops are not, is available only through a pharmacist. Occasionally, the doctor may suggest use of vinegar or Betadine irrigations to clean the infected ear. You should carefully clean the ear prior to the use of drops or powder. Oral antibiotics aren't usually prescribed but can be helpful in some people with perforations and irritated, diseased mucosa.

HAVE YOU HEARD?

Because a cholesteatoma is a collection of dead skin, it has no blood supply. This means that antibiotics taken by mouth and absorbed into the bloodstream from the stomach and intestines have no effect on an infected cholesteatoma.

Surgical Treatment

For many years prior to the 1950s, surgical treatment for chronic otitis media was used primarily to control infection and prevent serious complications. But developments in surgical techniques have made it possible to reconstruct the diseased or damaged hearing mechanism in most cases. So now, you may have surgery for any one or all of the following: elimination of infection, closure of a perforation, and improvement in hearing. These objectives are accomplished by the following procedures:

- Myringoplasty—Repairing a perforation in the eardrum.
- Mastoidectomy—Removing diseased tissue such as cholesteatoma from the mastoid.
- Tympanoplasty—Repairing or replacing the middle ear bones.

Let's briefly look at each of these types of surgery, though each surgeon uses his or her own preferred specific techniques.

Repairing a Perforation in the Eardrum

Myringoplasty is performed to repair a perforation in the eardrum when there is no middle ear infection or disease of the ear bones. This procedure, which seals the middle ear and may improve the hearing, is usually performed under local anesthesia through the ear canal. Ear tissue is used to repair the defect in the eardrum. This tissue might be from the covering of the chewing muscle behind the ear (fascia), from the covering of ear cartilage (perichondrium), or even from some synthetic materials. Sometimes a combination of tissue materials is used. The procedure is usually done in a hospital outpatient setting, and the patient can return to work in a week. Healing is complete in most cases within six weeks, and any hearing improvement is usually noticeable during this recovery period.

Surgery to Remove Middle Ear Diseased Tissue

When destruction by cholesteatoma or infection is widespread in the mastoid, surgical elimination of the infection may be difficult. Surgery—in this case, a mastoidectomy—is performed through an incision behind the ear. The primary objective is to eliminate infection and regain a dry, safe environment in the ear. When cholesteatoma is present, it's usually not possible to eliminate infection and restore hearing in one operation. In the first operation, which requires a general anesthetic as a hospital outpatient, the infection is eliminated and the eardrum rebuilt. The patient should be able to return to work in one to two weeks. During the later, second stage surgery (see the following paragraphs), the surgeon inspects the ear spaces for any residual disease and, if possible, reconstructs the hearing mechanism.

More complex surgical procedures may be needed to stop discharge or completely remove all diseased tissue, so a modified radical mastoidectomy is performed to remove all disease in the mastoid area but leave any eardrum and parts of the ossicles in order to preserve some hearing. By contrast, in a radical mastoidectomy, these tissues may be removed as necessary to eradicate the infection without consideration of hearing improvement. A mastoid obliteration operation is performed to get rid of any mastoid infection and to fill in a previously created mastoid cavity, an open space where mastoid bone was removed to get rid of infection.

Replacing Middle Ear Bones

An ear infection may cause not only a perforation of the eardrum but also damage to the middle ear tissue and ossicles. Fixation that causes a significant hearing loss involving the first or second bone of hearing can be taken care of at the same time the eardrum perforation is repaired. If, however, fixation involves the third bone, the stapes, surgery usually is performed in two stages. The first stage is to repair the hole in the eardrum, eliminate disease, and create a dry, healed ear. At the second surgery, artificial ossicles can be placed in an attempt to restore better hearing.

Tympanoplasty is the operation performed to eliminate any infection and to repair both the sound-transmitting mechanism and any perforation of the eardrum. There are a number of different types of tympanoplasty procedures, depending on the extent and location of disease. When repair of the eardrum is not necessary, the operation is usually performed as a hospital outpatient under local anesthesia through the ear canal or through an incision made behind the ear. Most types of tympanoplasty procedures are performed through an incision behind the ear, under local or general anesthesia, usually in a hospital outpatient setting. The perforation is repaired with ear tissue, and sound transmission to the inner ear is restored by repositioning or replacing diseased ear bones. The patient can return to work in 7 to 10 days. Healing is usually complete in eight weeks, but hearing improvement may not be noted for a few months.

Several circumstances require tympanoplasty to be performed in two stages. These circumstances include the following:

- Cases in which there are extensive, inflammation-caused changes in the middle ear mucosa.

- Cases in which the complete removal of cholesteatoma is uncertain.

- Cases in which the third bone of hearing, the stapes, is fixed by tympanosclerosis.

In a two-stage situation, the surgeon first repairs the eardrum and 9 to 12 months later, in a planned second stage, reconstructs the sound-transmitting mechanism. At the first surgery, a piece of stiff plastic is placed in the middle ear to allow tissues to heal but to prevent scar tissue from forming in the middle ear space. Although use of a planned second stage for hearing reconstruction is common practice, some experts prefer to do both eardrum and sound mechanism repair at one surgery.

Whether it's at the first or second surgery, a variety of methods is used to repair a damaged ossicular chain, the three middle ear bones. Sometimes it's possible to reposition the patient's own ear bones. In a few cases, synthetic bone cement is used to reattach a partially broken second bone of hearing to an undamaged third bone. But commonly, a surgeon uses a synthetic material to recreate the chain of bones, reconnecting the eardrum and the inner ear. If the third bone is undamaged, a partial ossicular replacement prosthesis (PORP) is used. When only a part of the stapes (the footplate part of the "stirrup") remains usable, a total ossicular replacement prosthesis (TORP) is used. The most recent synthetic material used for PORPs and TORPs is titanium.

HAVE YOU HEARD?

Titanium is not magnetic and will not set off a metal detector at airports or interfere with MRI scans.

After a planned second stage hearing reconstruction operation, the patient may return to work in four to seven days. Healing is usually complete in six weeks and hearing improvement is frequently noted at that time.

What to Expect Following Surgery

Some symptoms, which we mention in other chapters as well, may follow any ear operation: pulsation; popping, clicking, and other sounds in the ear; and a feeling of fullness. Occasional sharp, shooting pains in the ear are not unusual, and often, you may feel as if you have liquid in the ear. Taste disturbance and mouth dryness are not uncommon for a few weeks following surgery, and in some people, this disturbance is long-lasting. Tinnitus, frequently present before surgery, is almost always present temporarily after surgery. It can persist for one to two months and then decrease as hearing improves.

Temporary loss of skin sensation in and around the ear is also common following surgery. This numbness may involve the entire outer ear and could last for six months or more. As the jaw joint is in intimate contact with the ear canal, some soreness or stiffness in jaw movement is very common after ear surgery but usually goes away within one to two months. A bloody or watery discharge from the ear can occur during the healing period, so change the cotton placed in the outer ear as necessary. In general, however, the less done to the ear the better. A yellow discharge suggests infection and is an indication to call for an appointment to see your doctor.

After surgery, it's common to have pain involving the head at the site of surgery and neck pain or stiffness. The source of the chewing muscle, which is just above the ear, is affected in two ways: (1) incisions made at the time of surgery often involve the muscle, and (2) fascia, the covering of the muscle, is used to repair the eardrum perforation. Head pain can occur when talking or chewing, but eating a softer diet for a few days after surgery helps. As the surgical incisions also often involve the muscles of the neck, you could have some pain when turning your head. Taking over-the-counter pain medication on a regular basis for two to three days after surgery usually treats the problem of head and neck pain.

Rarely is a hearing improvement noted immediately following surgery, and it may even be worse temporarily due to swelling of the ear tissues and surgical packing in the ear canal. Patients might notice an improvement six to eight weeks after surgery, but maximum improvement may require four to six months of healing.

SOUND ADVICE

Following middle ear surgery, your doctor will tell you not to blow your nose or "pop" your ears until your ear has healed. So what do you do? You can draw any accumulated secretions in the nose back into the throat and spit it out. If it's necessary to sneeze, do so with your mouth open, but be polite and cover your mouth with a tissue or your shirt sleeve!

Don't get water in your ear until your doctor advises that the ear has healed. When showering or washing your hair, place cotton in your outer ear opening and cover it with petroleum jelly. If a surgical incision was made in the skin behind your ear, keep that area dry for several days.

Air travel is okay as soon as two days following surgery.

Risks and Complications of Surgery

Fortunately, major complications are rare following surgery for correction of chronic ear infection. However, complications that *can* occur include the following:

- Ear infection with drainage, swelling, and pain may persist following surgery or, on rare occasions, may develop following surgery due to poor healing of the ear tissue. Additional surgery might be necessary to control the infection.

- In about 3 percent of ear operations, permanent hearing loss occurs due to the extent of the disease or complications in the healing process; nothing further can be done in these instances. Rarely, a total loss of hearing occurs in the operated ear.

- Dizziness may occur immediately following surgery due to swelling in the ear and irritation of the inner ear structures. Some unsteadiness may persist for a week postoperatively, but on rare occasions, dizziness is prolonged. About 10 percent of patients with COM and cholesteatoma have a labyrinthine fistula (abnormal opening into the balance canal). When this problem exists, dizziness may last for six months or more.

- Because the facial nerve travels through the ear bone in close association with the middle ear bones, eardrum, and mastoid, a rare postoperative complication of ear surgery is temporary paralysis of one side of the face. This may occur as the result of an abnormality or a swelling of the nerve and usually subsides on its own. On very rare occasions, the nerve may be injured at the time of surgery or removed to eradicate disease. When this occurs, a skin sensation nerve is removed from the upper part of the neck to replace the facial nerve. Paralysis of the face under these circumstances might last six months to a year, and there would be a permanent residual weakness. Eye complications, requiring treatment by a specialist, could develop.

- A hematoma, a collection of clotted blood under the skin, develops in a small percentage of cases, prolonging hospitalization and healing. Re-operation to remove the clot may be necessary if this complication occurs.

- A cerebrospinal fluid leak (leak of fluid surrounding the brain) is a very rare complication following mastoidectomy. Re-operation may be necessary to stop the leak.

True Stories

As in other chapters, here we tell you some stories from our case files. People of all ages can have problems resulting from chronic infection in the middle ear or require one of the surgical procedures described in this chapter. Here are just a few examples.

Born with It

Emily is six years old. Her pediatrician referred her to the otologist for evaluation of a whitish mass noted behind her right eardrum in the middle ear space. The mass was seen on her routine checkup although she had no complaints of pain and no history of ear drainage or hearing loss. In fact, she had no history of any prior ear infections.

The otologist used a microscope with a video feed that allowed the parents and Emily to see her eardrum and the whitish mass. The left ear was normal. The history and these findings led to a diagnosis of congenital cholesteatoma. Even though Emily had no history of any disease and her hearing was normal, the doctor reviewed with Emily's parents the potential risks and complications of allowing the cholesteatoma to remain in the middle ear space. It would continue to grow slowly, and, in time, would cause hearing loss and potential problems to the inner ear with dizziness and perhaps even facial nerve paralysis.

Because the potential that these complications would occur without surgery was greater than the risks of surgery, Emily's parents elected to proceed with a right tympanoplasty with possible mastoidectomy. Emily was admitted to the hospital as an outpatient, and her surgery was performed under general anesthesia. The surgeon completely removed the cholesteatoma, a small, pearl-like structure localized to the middle ear space. The eardrum was not involved, so a graft was not needed. The chain of middle ear bones was not involved and was left intact. Emily's ear healed well, and when a hearing test was performed 12 weeks after surgery, her hearing level was the same as before surgery.

Headed for a Hole

Mark is a 19-year-old college student. During a soccer game with the crosstown rival, while he was jostling for position to head the ball into the goal, the ball scored a direct hit on his left ear. He immediately felt ear pain and fullness but had no dizziness, so he continued to play until a teammate saw a trickle of blood coming from his left ear canal. The bleeding stopped and Mark soon forgot about the whole incident. But a few days after going swimming at the beach, he noticed some drainage from the ear. When Mark's family physician recommended that he see an ear doctor, the examination revealed a moderate-size perforation in the left eardrum. A hearing test revealed a mild conductive hearing loss.

Mark was given antibiotic ear drops and told to keep his ear dry, but the infection persisted. When he returned in several weeks to see if the eardrum perforation had spontaneously healed, it had not. When after three months the eardrum perforation was still there, surgery was suggested to close the hole in the eardrum. Mark was admitted to the hospital as an outpatient. Under local anesthesia, a myringoplasty was performed through the external ear canal, using a fascia graft to close the perforation. Eight weeks after surgery, the eardrum had healed completely, and Mark's hearing had also improved.

Staged Right

Karen is 39 years old. She was referred for treatment of persistent drainage from her right ear. The referring doctor had performed a tympanoplasty five years before, repairing a perforation in the eardrum. In addition to the draining ear, Karen noticed some unsteadiness and a progressive hearing loss. She had no facial weakness, but she did have tingling of the right side of her face. On examination, the otologist found a perforation in the portion of the eardrum over the position where the second and third bones of hearing would normally be. The findings were consistent with cholesteatoma. A CT scan revealed erosion of mastoid bone by soft tissue. The bone covering a portion of the facial nerve also was missing. The ossicles were either partially or totally involved by the cholesteatoma, which filled the middle ear space.

Arrangements were made for Karen to undergo a right tympanoplasty with mastoidectomy as an outpatient under general anesthesia. The procedure was staged; hearing would be restored at a later date. The surgeon placed stiff plastic in the middle ear and used fascia to repair the eardrum. By four months, the eardrum graft had healed, and Karen was able to swim over the summer. But her hearing loss remained because there was no connection from the eardrum to her inner ear. Nine months after her first-stage procedure, she underwent a second-stage tympanoplasty with mastoidectomy. No residual cholesteatoma was found, and a total ossicular replacement prosthesis was used to repair her hearing connection. Postoperatively, she maintained her dry healed ear and had hearing improvement.

The Least You Need to Know

- A chronic infection of the middle ear (chronic otitis media) can cause a hole in the eardrum or formation of cholesteatoma, a skin-filled cyst, and can lead to damage of the middle ear, producing hearing loss.
- Drainage from the ear and hearing loss are the most common symptoms of chronic ear infection.
- If you have a perforation of your eardrum or have had surgery to repair a hole, don't allow water to get into your ear canal until the ear doctor says it's okay.
- Surgery may be necessary to repair a hole in the eardrum, remove cholesteatoma, or repair or replace the middle ear bones.
- Hearing may be worse temporarily following surgery, with improvement six to eight weeks later; maximum improvement may take four to six months.

Other Middle Ear Hearing Problems

In This Chapter

- Disease of the middle ear bones (otosclerosis) as a cause of hearing loss
- Symptoms, cause, and diagnosis of otosclerosis
- Surgical replacement of the stapes bone as treatment for otosclerosis
- Other causes of middle ear hearing loss, such as accidental injury or changes in pressure
- Middle and inner ear abnormalities present at birth that can cause hearing loss

In Chapters 4 and 5, we discussed otitis media and chronic infections that occur in the middle ear and cause hearing loss and told you that chronic infections could erode or damage the ossicles, the middle ear bones. Other types of disease and injury can also impair the function of the middle ear bones and cause conductive hearing loss. One of the most common causes of conductive hearing loss is a disease of the middle ear called otosclerosis. In this chapter, we discuss this disease and its treatment in detail. In addition, accidental injuries to the middle ear and abnormalities present from birth may cause hearing loss.

Otosclerosis: a Disease of the Middle Ear Bones

Otosclerosis is the medical term for a disease that causes stiffening, or hardening, of the third middle ear bone, the stapes. It comes from the Greek *skleros*, meaning "hard" and *osis*, meaning "condition." Throw in the *oto* for "ear," and you have, literally, a hard condition of the ear! Because of this hardening, the stapes becomes fixed in place, and sound transmission from the middle ear to the inner ear is impaired. Remember, it's the movement of the stapes bone that sets the inner ear fluids in motion, starting the process to stimulate the hearing nerve.

DEFINITION

Otosclerosis is a disease of the ear in which abnormal growth of bone, called remodeling, causes eventual stiffening or hardening of the stapes bone in place, interfering with its movement and leading to a progressive loss of hearing.

Otosclerosis is one of the most common types of acquired hearing loss, affecting about 15 million people in the United States alone. Most common among whites, some estimate that otosclerosis affects 10 percent of the adult Caucasian population. It's less common among people of Japanese and South American descent and is rare in African Americans. It affects twice as many women as men, and this is thought to be because of hormonal influences. Pregnant women with otosclerosis sometimes experience a rapid drop in hearing.

Symptoms of Otosclerosis

Gradual hearing loss is the most common symptom of otosclerosis. Typically, hearing loss develops over many months or years and slowly gets worse. It usually (in 85 percent of occurrences) affects both ears, but the loss might start at different times in each ear, and each ear can have different degrees of loss. The first signs of otosclerosis may begin any time between the ages of 15 and 45 but usually start in the early 20s. Even if you don't notice hearing loss until your 40s, this is long before the signs of typical "old-age" hearing loss begins. If you have otosclerosis, you might not notice a hearing loss until it reaches 25 to 30 dB on the audiogram. Difficulty understanding speech during a conversation may be the first sign that you have hearing loss.

HAVE YOU HEARD?

In the early stages of otosclerosis, you might actually find it easier to hear in a noisy environment. The observation that some people with middle ear hearing loss seem to hear conversation better in noise, a phenomenon called paracusis, was first described in 1680! In most cases, the person does not actually hear better in noise, he or she just does not require as great an increase in the strength of the speech signal as a normal-hearing person, and so the disability in the presence of noise will appear to be less in comparison.

Another sign that you, or someone around you, may have otosclerosis is that you may start to speak more softly. A person with a conductive hearing loss like that caused by otosclerosis hears his or her own voice louder than other people do. The natural reaction to this is to speak more softly. Other symptoms of otosclerosis may include tinnitus and, rarely, dizziness or balance complaints.

Cause of Otosclerosis

What causes otosclerosis? Bone in other parts of the body undergoes a constant turnover; that is, normal, healthy bone is absorbed and replaced with new bone, a process that does not normally occur in the ear. However, in otosclerosis, the normally very hard bone of the stapes and inner ear actually breaks down and is replaced by spongy bone with lots of blood vessels in it (another name for otosclerosis at this stage is otospongiosis). This spongy bone is eventually replaced by a type of denser, thicker bone (otosclerotic bone). Usually, this newly formed, denser new bone affects the base, or footplate, of the stapes first. The very thin ligament that connects the stapes to the inner ear becomes stiff and can't move, and this prevents the stapes from moving as it normally does to transmit sound to the inner ear. This fixation of the stapes produces a conductive hearing loss.

LISTEN UP

Occasionally, the area of stiffening, or otosclerotic focus, can spread to the inner ear, a condition called cochlear otosclerosis. If this occurs, what started out as a primarily conductive hearing loss can actually produce a significant sensorineural hearing loss as well. Although the conductive component can be treated, the sensorineural part can't. On occasion, the otosclerosis may spread to the balance canals and cause episodes of unsteadiness.

How or why did you develop otosclerosis? In about 60 percent of cases, otosclerosis is of genetic origin. As it's well known that otosclerosis runs in families, your doctor may ask you whether anyone else in your family has had a similar type of hearing loss. The inheritance pattern, or the way otosclerosis is passed from generation to generation, is believed to be autosomal dominant. This means that a person needs to have only one copy of the otosclerosis gene, as it were, to show the condition. If you have one parent with otosclerosis, you have a 25 percent chance of getting the gene. If both parents have it, the risk goes up to 50 percent. However, simply because you have the gene for otosclerosis doesn't mean you will develop a hearing loss. And if you do, it might not be the same degree of loss that others in your family have. The degree of hearing loss can be influenced by environmental factors, including things that make you more susceptible such as the measles virus.

Diagnosing Otosclerosis

The diagnosis of otosclerosis is based upon the findings on your audiogram and physical examination. Your ear doctor will carefully examine your ear to rule out other causes of conductive hearing loss. If there's active disease, meaning the presence of the spongy bone before it becomes hardened, there may be a reddish-blue color behind the eardrum. This color results from the increased number of blood vessels that are present in this newly formed spongy bone. If the disease is already in the later, hardened, bone stage, your ear can appear normal.

The audiologist will do a pure-tone test for both air conduction and bone conduction. When there's no conductive hearing loss, the results should be the same whether the sound is introduced through the air or through the bone (using a vibrator placed on the skull behind your ear). When they're not the same, the difference between them is known as the air-bone gap. In the beginning stages of otosclerosis, your audiogram will show a conductive hearing loss (an air-bone gap) that's primarily in the lower frequencies. As your stapes bone becomes stiffer and more fixed, the size of the air-bone gap will get larger, and the conductive hearing loss will spread to higher frequencies.

One hearing test finding, called the Carhart notch, is unique to otosclerosis. The Carhart notch is a dip in the sensorineural hearing as shown on the audiogram when there really is no sensorineural hearing loss. This false loss, which is greatest at 2,000 Hz and can be as much as 15 dB, often will disappear after surgical correction of otosclerosis.

In addition to the standard audiogram, your doctor will do some other special tests, including tuning fork tests (see Chapter 2). One test helps localize which ear is affected by the disease as the affected ear will cause you to hear the sound vibrations from the tuning fork louder on that side. In another test, your doctor will place the tuning fork on the mastoid bone immediately behind your ear and then hold the tuning fork a few inches directly to the side of your ear. This test helps determine whether you're hearing better through bone or through air. Normally, you should hear the tuning fork sound vibrations better through the air, but if your otosclerosis is bad enough, you'll hear the sound vibrations better when the tuning fork is held against the mastoid bone.

You may also have middle ear function tests such as tympanometry and acoustic reflex testing (see Chapter 2). In otosclerosis, the movement of the eardrum should be normal, or when the otosclerosis becomes advanced, you may have decreased movement of the eardrum. This is in contrast to the type of tympanogram that occurs if there's fluid in the middle ear. Also, an abnormal or absent stapedial reflex can often be one of the earliest signs of otosclerosis, sometimes even before a conductive hearing loss is apparent.

You shouldn't need a CT or MRI scan to diagnose otosclerosis. Occasionally, the doctor may order a CT scan if you have a large sensorineural component to your hearing loss and might have inner ear involvement of your otosclerosis. This can show up on a CT scan as an area of low-density bone surrounding the normally very dense, hard bone of the inner ear.

Treatment

If you've been diagnosed with otosclerosis, what are the treatment options to improve your hearing? Basically, you have four: do nothing, simply observe and monitor your hearing loss; treat your otosclerosis medically; wear a hearing aid; or undergo surgical correction.

Observation: If only one ear is affected and even that affected ear has only a mild conductive hearing loss, it might not be too bothersome, and you might choose to do nothing at present. Otosclerosis is not going to affect other parts of your body, but if left alone, it will usually progress and cause a continued decline in hearing over time. You should have a yearly audiogram if you choose simply to observe your otosclerosis. Eventually, you may decide on further treatment.

Medical Treatment: No local treatment to the ear itself or any medication will improve the hearing of people with otosclerosis. In some cases, though, medication might be helpful in preventing or slowing the further loss of hearing. Medication use is thought to slow the breakdown of bone that occurs in otosclerosis and promote the formation of healthy bone. However, widely varying results have occurred with the use of these medications.

One medication used to stabilize and potentially slow the progression of hearing loss is sodium fluoride. This medication comes as fluorical, which is actually a combination of fluoride and calcium. Treatment with fluorical is not recommended for people with kidney problems, rheumatoid arthritis, pregnant or lactating women, children, or anyone allergic to fluoride. The most common side effect from taking fluoride is an upset stomach. Even if you choose fluoride as your sole treatment, you should still have your hearing monitored yearly to track any progression of hearing loss.

Another class of medications, called the bisphosphonates, are sometimes used to try to slow the progression of otosclerosis. This type of medication has traditionally been used to treat osteoporosis. A common example of this medication is Fosamax™. Bisphosphonates are thought to slow the progression of the disease similar to fluoride, by slowing the absorption and remodeling of normal bone that occurs in otosclerosis.

Wear a Hearing Aid: Most people with otosclerosis still have good hearing nerve function; they have only a conductive loss (the otosclerosis has not spread to the inner ear). This means that they are usually excellent candidates for a hearing aid (see Chapter 16). Although using a hearing aid avoids the risks associated with surgery (see the following paragraphs), there are still disadvantages. These disadvantages include the cost of the aid and its maintenance, poorer sound quality than usually results from surgery, cosmetic issues, comfort, and being able to hear only when the hearing aids are in place (and turned on!).

Surgical Treatment: Most people with otosclerosis are candidates for surgery. Keep in mind, though, that surgery for otosclerosis is an elective procedure. This means that, while surgery can correct your hearing loss, it doesn't have to be done nor does it come without risks. The surgical procedure performed to correct otosclerosis is called a *stapedectomy*.

DEFINITION

Stapedectomy is the surgical procedure to remove all or part of the stapes bone of the middle ear and replace it with an artificial device. It is most commonly performed for otosclerosis.

Stapedectomy is performed through the ear canal, usually under local anesthesia. At times, an incision may be made above the ear to remove muscle tissue for use in the operation. Under high-power magnification, the eardrum is lifted, and the stapes is partially or completely removed by using surgical instruments, a drill, or in some cases, a laser. A prosthesis—an artificial device—is inserted to replace the stapes, and the eardrum membrane is then replaced in its normal position. The stapes prosthesis allows sound vibrations to pass from the eardrum to the inner ear fluids. The hearing improvement obtained is usually permanent, and the patient can return to work in 7 to 10 days, depending upon his or her work requirements. The doctor may suggest refraining from nose blowing, swimming, or other activities that can get water in the operated ear until about two weeks after the surgery.

SOUND ADVICE

Stapes prostheses can be made of many different materials. Many years ago, they were often made of stainless steel wire. But most prostheses today are made from titanium or other nonreactive metal or Teflon. Today, it's perfectly safe for you to have an MRI scan after you have had stapes surgery.

Risks of Surgery

Some of the risks associated with surgical correction of otosclerosis are relatively minor, while others can be more severe. One of the minor complications is a perforation of the eardrum, which can usually be repaired at the time of the stapedectomy operation. However, there is the risk of persistent perforation and even infection. Another potential complication of surgery is some altered sensation of taste in the immediate time period after surgery. As you recall from Chapter 1, the chorda tympani nerve supplies taste sensation to the front part of the tongue. This nerve must often be moved out of the way during surgery to obtain a good view of the stapes bone. Even if this tiny nerve is only stretched, you might experience an altered sensation of taste—sometimes described as metallic—after surgery. This distortion of taste usually disappears after several months, even if the nerve is completely cut. In very rare cases, some taste alterations can be long-lasting.

In rare cases, the facial nerve can be injured during stapedectomy surgery. This is a particular risk if your facial nerve partially covers the footplate of your stapes (this occurs in less than 0.5 percent of people). If the facial nerve is covering more than half the footplate, the surgeon will usually stop the procedure. There are several other rarely occurring risks, such as vertigo and tinnitus. If these symptoms occur, they usually go away with time. Of course, if you have tinnitus before surgery, there's no guarantee that it will improve after surgery—and it could get worse.

Sometimes (in 5 to 10 percent of cases), many years after the surgery, a repeat or revision surgery may be necessary. Some things that can cause this include displacement of the prosthesis, erosion of bone where the prosthesis is hooked onto the incus, and regrowth of the otosclerosis over the remainder of the footplate of the stapes.

Finally, the most serious risk of surgery to correct otosclerosis is permanent hearing loss. The risk is less than 1 to 2 percent that you could have a permanent, total hearing loss after surgery. But if it happens, this hearing loss can't be helped by use of a hearing aid or further surgery. Sometimes permanent hearing loss after a stapedectomy occurs immediately, but it may not occur for months. We don't really know what causes this kind of hearing loss to happen. Because of this possibility, if you have otosclerosis in both ears, the ear with the greatest hearing loss is operated first.

Accidental Injuries

Life is full of mishaps, and some of these can affect our hearing. A foreign body in the external ear canal can cause a conductive hearing loss (see Chapter 3). On the more severe end of the spectrum are those causes of conductive hearing loss due to traumatic injuries. Middle ear trauma most often comes from blast injuries and insertion of foreign objects into the ear. One type of injury is when an object penetrates the external ear canal and punctures the eardrum. Usually this perforation will heal without special treatment, but occasionally the punctured eardrum is just the tip of the iceberg. In some cases, the object that perforated the eardrum also causes a disruption of the ossicles. This can range from partial disruption of one ossicle to complete separation of the malleus (the first middle ear bone) from the eardrum and the stapes from the inner ear. The forceful displacement of the stapes into the inner ear can cause a sensorineural hearing loss in addition to a conductive hearing loss—a mixed hearing loss.

LISTEN UP

Most penetrating injuries are self-inflicted and occur when people use a cotton-tipped swab, paperclip, hairpin, rat-tail comb, or even a coat hanger in an attempt to scratch an itch in the ear canal or remove earwax. Don't do that! Twigs or small tree branches can also produce ear injury. Thermal injuries can occur when molten slag enters the ear during welding. Blast injuries, produced by a rapid positive pressure wave through the external auditory canal, occur when you get too close to the detonation of an explosive device, such as fireworks. Compressed air, auto airbags deploying, lightning, or even a slap to the ear can cause a nonexplosive blast injury. One of the most common causes of perforated eardrums in the United States is waterskiing. If you fall and hit the water, pressure in the ear canal may rise enough to cause a perforated eardrum.

Another cause of traumatic conductive hearing loss is temporal bone trauma. When high-velocity forces are applied to the skull, for instance in a car accident or blow to the head, the hard temporal bone (remember, the temporal bone is the hardest bone in the human body!) can fracture. The fracture may run directly through the middle ear and can cause a disruption of the ossicles. While it's more common for a fracture of the temporal bone to cause a conductive hearing loss, occasionally the fracture will be oriented in such a way that it damages the inner ear and causes a sensorineural hearing loss. The conductive hearing loss caused by a temporal bone fracture can often be restored. However, if a fracture causes a sensorineural hearing loss, hearing can't be restored.

Injury from Changes in Pressure

Injuries to the ear from changes in pressure occur when the ear is subjected to extremes from either increases or decreases in pressure. Activities that can cause injury to the ear due to changes in pressure include diving and airplane flights (see Chapter 4). Less commonly recognized activities that cause changes in ear pressure include not only explosions and other accidental "blast" events but also heavy lifting or childbirth.

Scuba diving can expose the ear to pressure changes. Even normal earwax in the external ear canal can become a dangerous object when subjected to the high pressures experienced in underwater diving. The pressure many feet underwater can cause the earwax to become stuck at the narrow portion of the ear canal or can push it against the eardrum. As you know, the Eustachian tube helps equalize pressure in the ear. When you dive, the air in the middle ear shrinks because of the pressure exerted on it by the weight of the water all around you. If the air pressure inside the middle ear is not equalized with the pressure all around you (remember the Valsalva maneuver?), then the eardrum can be sucked in to such an extent that fluid or blood accumulates in the middle ear. Or the retraction of the eardrum can be so severe and/or sudden that the eardrum actually ruptures. Rupture of the eardrum can also happen when you ascend too quickly from a dive. In this case, the air inside the middle ear expands. If your Eustachian tube is not functioning properly to equalize the pressure, your eardrum can rupture. Any sudden injury to the ear due to pressure changes is called barotrauma.

LISTEN UP

Being in as little as 4 feet of seawater can be enough to cause some harmful pressure effects on the ear. Do *not* wear ear plugs while diving unless they have a vent hole in them. Otherwise, air can become trapped between the ear plug and the eardrum and, with increasing depth, this air can become squished, causing pain and hearing loss.

The treatment of middle ear barotrauma centers around the use of oral decongestants, nasal decongestants, and proper treatment (myringoplasty) of a tympanic membrane perforation (see Chapter 5). Do not dive again until your ear is healed and you can again equalize the pressure in your ears.

Pressure-induced injury in the middle ear can specifically affect the inner ear. Increased pressure can cause rupture of one or both of the thin, small membranes that lead to the inner ear—the oval and round windows, leading to escape of the perilymph fluid of the inner ear. This injury is called a perilymph fistula. The symptoms of a perilymph fistula can include vertigo, tinnitus, and sensorineural hearing loss. Initial treatment of a perilymph fistula includes bed rest, elevation of the head of the bed, stool softeners (so as not to strain), and refraining from coughing and sneezing. If symptoms persist, surgery can be performed to try to seal the leaking membrane. Temporal bone fracture can also cause a perilymph fistula. The oval and round window membranes are considered part of the middle ear. A rupture in either specifically causes inner ear symptoms, but like other middle ear problems, surgical repair may be possible. If sensorineural hearing loss has occurred, it can't be improved, but further loss of hearing can be stopped.

Congenital Abnormalities

Congenital abnormalities of the ear are those malformations present at birth, but do not confuse congenital with genetic. While some of these abnormalities may be genetic, not all such abnormalities are inherited. As you know, abnormalities of the external ear can affect not only the appearance of the ear but also its ability to transmit sound to the middle and inner ears (Chapter 3). So let's take a look at some of the congenital abnormalities of the middle ear that can affect one's hearing.

Most middle ear congenital abnormalities involve the three middle ear bones, the ossicles. The entire ossicular chain can be involved or only one or two of the three ear bones may be abnormal. Either way, the end result is usually a conductive hearing loss.

Congenital anomalies involving only the stapes account for 40 percent of all congenital problems that have to do with the ear bones. One congenital condition very similar to otosclerosis is called congenital stapes fixation. If you recall, in otosclerosis the stapes is stiff or fixed and doesn't move effectively to transmit sound to the inner ear. Stapes fixation is the most common isolated problem with the ear bones, but other abnormalities of the stapes don't involve the footplate of the stapes as congenital stapes fixation does. These abnormalities include malformations of different parts of the stapes that may still allow it to function relatively well in conducting sound. Or the stapes may actually be formed normally but is attached to other structures by a bony bridge that prevents it from moving. In most cases, the stapes bone can be freed up or replaced with a prosthesis (similar to otosclerosis surgery) to provide improved hearing.

In the same way that the stapes can be abnormal so, too, can the malleus and incus be. Malformations of the malleus and incus often occur together because these two bones are formed from the same parts of the developing embryo. The most common abnormality of the malleus is fusion of the top or head of the malleus to the bone surrounding it. Obviously, in this situation the malleus can't move as it should. In a similar way, the top or body of the incus can become fused with surrounding bone, preventing its proper movement. If for any of these reasons one or more of the middle ear bones can't move properly, hearing will be affected. Just as with stapes abnormalities, very small prosthetic replacements for ear bones can be used to replace a malformed malleus or incus to improve hearing.

True Stories

These clinical case reports of diagnosis and treatment demonstrate a few of the middle ear causes of hearing loss discussed in this chapter. See if you can guess the diagnosis before we tell you.

Women's Choices

Mary, a 42-year-old teacher, was having difficulty understanding speech in her classroom, especially when her students had high-pitched voices. She also had problems hearing conversation in staff meetings, and at home she needed to increase the TV volume. She remembered that both her grandmother and an aunt had hearing problems, so she decided to have her hearing checked. Sure enough, her evaluation showed hearing loss in both ears. The loss was a conductive hearing loss, worse in the right ear. Diagnosed with otosclerosis, she opted to have a stapedectomy on the right ear. After her surgery, Mary immediately experienced improvement in hearing and reported that when driving home, she could hear every bump and noise on the road and many background noises. When she returned to the classroom, Mary was able to hear students in the back of the room without difficulty! Because the surgery on the right ear had gone so well, she recently returned and had an equally successful stapedectomy on her left ear.

Lori, 45 years old, came to the office complaining of hearing loss in her left ear. She said her mother had had an operation on her ear in the 1960s that improved her hearing. On examination, Lori was found to have normal eardrums, but her hearing test showed a conductive hearing loss on the left. Knowing Lori's family history, the ear doctor diagnosed otosclerosis in the left ear. She was counseled about her options, including observation, a hearing aid, or a stapedectomy surgery. Lori decided that for now, while her right ear was still good, she would try a hearing aid. She was fit with an aid and has been using it successfully. Recently, though, because her right ear has started to show some hearing loss, Lori is considering undergoing a stapedectomy in her poorer hearing ear.

Yes, We Can Fix That

Vincent, now four years old, was born with bilateral severe narrowing of his external auditory canals (congenital atresia). He was diagnosed at an early age with bilateral conductive hearing loss and had been fitted at the age of one month with a bone conduction hearing aid. On examination, the pinna looked good on both sides. Radiologic evaluation showed an absent eardrum as well as the extremely narrow ear canals. His middle ear bones were malformed, but the mastoid area was present and the inner ear was normal on both sides. These X-ray findings were favorable for being able to establish open ear canals and improve hearing. Vincent underwent surgery on one side that freed the malformed ossicles, reconstructed a new eardrum, and created a new ear canal. Audiometric testing now shows improved hearing in the operated ear.

Clipped!

John, age 55, complained of pain and hearing loss in his right ear. He told quite a story. While sitting at work one day, he got a persistent nagging itch in his right ear canal, so he straightened out a large paperclip and was using it to try to scratch the itch. Just then, his phone rang, startling him. With his sudden movement, his desk chair tilted backward! John felt a sudden sharp pain in his ear, followed by some dizziness. He later realized that he was not hearing well from that ear. A hearing test showed a mixed hearing loss, both conductive and sensorineural. Upon examination, the doctor found that John had an eardrum perforation and a disruption of the ossicles. In addition, it appeared that the stapes bone had actually been pushed into the inner ear. John underwent surgical repair of his middle ear bones and closure of the hole in his eardrum. This improved his hearing. However, some sensorineural hearing loss remains.

The Least You Need to Know

- Otosclerosis is one of the most common types of acquired hearing loss; often hereditary, it causes a conductive hearing loss.
- In the majority of cases, surgery to replace the stapes bone (stapedectomy) is successful in improving hearing in people with otosclerosis.
- Sticking anything long or sharp in the ear can result in accidental injury to the eardrum, middle ear bones, or even the inner ear.
- Injury to the ear due to pressure changes is called barotrauma.
- Problems during fetal development can cause congenital abnormalities of the middle ear that produce hearing loss.

Inner Ear Hearing Loss

3

Many problems can affect the inner ear, causing sensorineural hearing loss. We describe some of the more common problems in this part, which include two of the most common reasons for decreased hearing in adults—aging and noise exposure. We also explore a variety of causes of sudden hearing loss. Though not well understood, we shed light on what we know and what we can do about it. Finally, we devote two chapters to some specific diseases and tumors that can cause hearing loss, so you'll better understand these particular circumstances and the treatment options available.

Age-Related Hearing Loss

In This Chapter

- Hearing loss and age
- Possible causes of age-related hearing loss
- Prevention of hearing loss through diet and antioxidants
- Hearing improvement through the use of hearing aids and other devices
- Diabetes and hearing loss

According to the National Center for Health Statistics, hearing loss is the third most common chronic health condition facing seniors. High blood pressure and rheumatoid arthritis are the first two, and like these two conditions, age-related hearing loss can have a major impact on quality of life and psychological well-being. It can result in communication difficulties that in turn lead to poor psychosocial functioning, social isolation, loss of independence, and a higher incidence of anxiety, sluggishness, social disappointment, and possibly even a cognitive decline similar to dementia. We discuss these consequences of hearing loss in greater detail in Chapter 20.

One of us has a friend who tells the story of how when he was a boy, he heard his father and a workman who had come to the house yelling at each other. Frightened, he hid in his room. Only later did he realize that they weren't actually arguing—they were both just hard of hearing! It's not uncommon to hear an older person talking inappropriately loudly, most likely because he or she has a hearing loss.

In this chapter, we discuss the possible causes of age-related hearing loss, how it might affect you, and what might help prevent it. Is it in your genes? Can your diet affect your hearing as you get older? Is there any treatment for this type of hearing loss? Did you know that a now all-too-common chronic disease, diabetes, may be related to hearing loss? You don't have to be a senior citizen to learn a few things from this chapter.

It Happens to Most of Us

There appears to be a strong relationship between age and reported hearing loss. Of people between the ages of 45 and 64, 18 to 20 percent have a hearing loss; of people between the ages of 65 and 74, 25 to 40 percent have a hearing loss. Of those who are 75 to 84 years old, 50 percent have a hearing loss, and more than 75 percent of people 85 years and older have a hearing loss. *Presbycusis* is the medical term for this age-related hearing loss.

In 1999, the World Health Organization estimated that more than half a billion people worldwide over the age of 65 suffered from hearing loss. A global trend toward increasing life expectancies, populations, and median age in many countries (including the United States) is expected to at least double this number of people with age-related hearing loss in the near future, if not already.

DEFINITION

Presbycusis is the gradual deterioration of hearing as a result of natural degen-erative changes in the ear that occur mainly with aging. The word comes from the Greek *presbys,* which means "aged," and *akousis,* "hearing."

As you know from Chapter 1, the hearing process contains many steps. Sound is first picked up at the outer ear and then eventually sent along the hearing nerve to the central auditory center in the brain, where the information is processed. The two major aspects of hearing are awareness or detection (audibility) and understanding (processing). A person can be aware that something was said, but not always under-stand it. Presbycusis can impact both the detection and the processing of sound.

Age-related hearing loss can be mild, moderate, or severe. The loss is usually sym-metric or about the same in both ears. Because the loss is gradual, a person who has presbycusis might not realize his or her hearing is declining. Without good hearing, the ability to communicate with family, friends, co-workers, and strangers diminishes. This impairment in communication can result in misunderstandings, arguments, frustration, depression, and isolation. It's difficult to interact in social settings if the primary mode of communication is impaired. In senior living centers and nursing homes, activity directors often concentrate on group physical activities such as morning exercise programs that encourage social interaction but don't require good hearing to participate.

Presbycusis doesn't usually occur in isolation. Noise-induced hearing loss (see Chapter 8), a common cause of sensorineural hearing impairment, and ototoxicity (see Chapter 9) can be additional factors in creating hearing loss in the elderly. These conditions all produce sensorineural hearing loss that primarily affects high-pitched sounds. This means that when listening to sounds in the environment, it might be difficult to hear the nearby chirping of a bird, the ringing of a telephone, or the turn indicator in the car. Yet one might be able to hear the low-pitched sound of a truck or bus going by or the drums in a music performance. In conversation, a person with high-frequency hearing loss might have difficulty understanding a young child or a female speaker. Remember, vowels are primarily low-frequency sounds, while consonants are primarily in the mid-to-high frequencies of the speech range and are more likely to be adversely affected, especially in settings with background sound. We've discussed in several other chapters how difficult speech is to understand without hearing the consonants. This difficulty often goes unnoticed by the person with the hearing loss, but is quite apparent to family and friends.

HAVE YOU HEARD?

Older people diagnosed with age-related hearing impairment often report that they had never had an assessment of hearing function by their primary care physicians. This indicates that there may be an under-appreciation by primary care health-care providers of how great this problem is.

Age-related hearing loss is more common in men than in women. As mentioned in Chapter 2, it's often the wife or children who drag the husband or father to the hearing health professional's office seeking help. But whether the patient is male or female, it's quite common for the person to believe there is no real problem. The office is a quiet setting; the professional is speaking directly to him or her in a well-lit room; and the professional is projecting and probably using a well-enunciated speech pattern. In that setting, the response from the patient is "See, I told you I didn't have a hearing problem. Our difficulty in communicating must be your fault."

Well, anyone with a hearing loss might do well in the quiet office environment, but in the typical home and work environment that represents the real, noisier world, a hearing loss will most likely affect your ability to communicate with others. In the real world, the chips are stacked against you; a mild to moderate, sloping, high-frequency sensorineural hearing loss really does make it more difficult to understand the higher-pitched voice of your wife or perhaps your grandchildren. In the typical family setting, in the den watching television or in the kitchen while your wife (or you) moves around preparing for or cleaning up after the meal, that background noise makes it difficult to hear the higher-pitched consonants that are crucial to understanding. With a mild to moderate, high-frequency hearing loss, you'll have less difficulty hearing and understanding a low-pitched male speaker.

Whether you're a man or a woman with a hearing loss, what is the path that might save you the cost of marriage counseling? Acknowledge that you might have a hearing problem; see an ear doctor and have your hearing evaluated; and, if warranted, get treatment. (Keep reading to find out what the treatment options are.) In Chapters 19 and 20 we discuss the many things you can also do to improve your ability to communicate, even with a hearing loss.

Causes of Age-Related Hearing Loss

Sometimes hearing loss in the elderly is a conductive hearing disorder, meaning abnormalities of the external or middle ear cause the loss of sound sensitivity. Such abnormalities can include reduced function of the eardrum or reduced function of the ossicles that carry sound waves from the eardrum to the inner ear. Presbycusis most commonly arises from changes in the inner ear, but age-related hearing loss can also result from complex changes along the nerve pathways leading to the brain.

Inner ear changes that lead to sensorineural hearing loss from presbycusis involve varying degrees of hair cell (sensory) and cochlear nerve cell loss. Both types of loss are often found together. Studies of the temporal bone have shown that people with high-frequency loss patterns of presbycusis show degeneration of the stria vascularis, the part of the inner ear that contains many small blood vessels and is considered the engine of the ear; spiral ganglion cells, extensions of the cochlear/hearing nerve; and inner and outer hair cells, the sensory elements whose loss is associated with the severity of the hearing loss and that fine tune the sound signals. These changes occur primarily in the lower turn of the cochlea, affecting the high frequencies. The cochlear hair cells are formed in the fetus during the first trimester of pregnancy and, unlike a team sport in which injured players can be replaced, these cells can't be repaired or replaced once damaged (though researchers are working hard to see whether we can learn how to regenerate hair cells).

Changes with aging also occur in cells of the hearing pathway beyond the ear, leading to a decrease in the ability of the central auditory system to process sound—that is, to detect, locate, recognize, and understand the message. Aging creates a problem with the hearing decoder (the brain). Defects in the auditory centers of the brain can lead to greater difficulty in understanding speech for the elderly than what would be expected from the changes in detection levels alone shown on the audiogram. This is especially true in noisy environments requiring complex listening skills. Diseases that impair cognitive abilities (thinking, memory, attention, etc.) will also impair hearing.

Changes in the blood supply to the ear because of heart disease, high blood pressure, or vascular conditions caused by diabetes or other blood circulation problems can cause presbycusis. Because sound signals cross from the right to left and left to right sides as they travel from the ears to the brain's auditory center, the ability to hear is usually not affected after someone has a stroke (but the ability to understand can be). Diseases that involve the liver or kidney can create metabolic changes that speed up the progression of hearing loss in the elderly.

Exactly what causes these age-related changes in the hearing system is not really known, particularly in terms of genetic workings. The age when this process starts and how fast it progresses varies greatly among individuals. Similarly, the hearing function of the ear associated with these changes in the inner ear, such as worsened auditory thresholds and word recognition, also varies among individuals. In the past, presbycusis was often considered an inevitable consequence of aging. Current thinking recognizes that age-related hearing loss is affected by many factors, including both genetic and environmental influences such as noise, exposure to drugs or other substances that can damage hearing, and chronic medical conditions. Environmental influences on hearing impairment have been thoroughly studied, but we still don't know much about genetic factors that might play a role in hearing loss as we age. Studies using twins and families suggest there can be an inherited tendency to presbycusis in humans. Genetic studies with mice have found multiple genes playing a role in this disease. Currently many studies are in process trying to learn more about what genes might play a role in age-related hearing loss.

HAVE YOU HEARD?

A study by Brandeis University used twins to try to determine the role that genes play in age-related hearing loss. They looked at 179 identical and 150 fraternal male twin pairs, ranging in age from 52 to 60 years. About two thirds of the hearing loss in the subjects' better ears could be accounted for by genetic factors. The research findings suggested that middle-age and older people with a genetic tendency to hearing loss should be particularly careful about harmful noise and medications whose side effects could be detrimental to hearing. The lead author, who is an expert on the relationship between memory performance and hearing loss in older adults, also noted that even mild hearing loss can indirectly lead to declines in cognitive performance because intellectual energy normally used for high-level comprehension must be directed toward the effort for accurately hearing speech.

Treatment of Age-Related Hearing Loss

Because we have no specific known cause for presbycusis, we also have no specific treatment, so management is directed at preventive measures and methods to improve hearing.

Prevention

Certainly, protecting the ears from significant noise exposure can prevent hearing loss (see Chapter 8), and this is true at any age. But if you have a genetic susceptibility to age-related hearing loss, reducing potential exposure to noise may be particularly important as a preventive measure. Because the ear, like any other organ, depends upon blood supply and the oxygen it delivers to function, doing things to improve and maintain heart and lung function is also important. It's worthwhile to follow that now age-old advice to watch your weight; modify your diet to decrease the intake of sugar, salt, caffeine, fried and fatty foods; get moderate regular exercise; and don't smoke.

A significant amount of the three T's (Time, Talent, and Treasure) has been spent on trying to prevent the aging process. We've not yet managed to stop the process but perhaps have postponed the onset of the ultimate end. A nutritious diet and exercise help many people enjoy longer, healthier lives as a healthful, balanced diet provides the appropriate mix of protein, carbohydrates, and fat and contains the necessary vitamins, minerals, and fatty acids required for good health. We can use multivitamin and mineral supplements to enhance an inadequate diet. A poor diet certainly can lead to chronic serious diseases, some of which, by the time we're older, might affect hearing. Unfortunately, although a poor diet might ultimately contribute to poor hearing, a good diet won't necessarily improve hearing. In some ear diseases, such as Ménière's disease (Chapter 10), salt and caffeine can directly influence hearing. Decreasing salt and caffeine can control the symptoms of Ménière's, and in some people, hearing and tinnitus improve. In presbycusis, good nutrition can help prevent hearing loss, but don't count on it to restore hearing that is already gone. Some studies tout the benefits of supplements and herbal remedies in preserving hearing, but other studies have found no real benefits.

There are three major theories about what causes the changes our bodies face with aging. This isn't the place to explain them, but all three suggest that "free radicals" lead to cellular dysfunction and perhaps consequently, in the ear, to presbycusis. Free radicals are unstable molecules that can damage cells, proteins, and DNA by altering their chemical structure and have been linked to cancer, heart disease, and stroke. Antioxidants such as beta-carotene, lycopene, and Vitamins A, C, and E can "deactivate" these free radicals, so treatments that can reduce the production of free radicals could potentially help prevent the effects of aging, including presbycusis. Studies using rats have found that those treated with antioxidants (Vitamin E, C, melatonin) had improved auditory thresholds, while those treated with placebo had worse thresholds, similar in pattern to humans with presbycusis.

Unfortunately, the typical American diet contains less than the optimal amounts of Vitamin E, fruits, vegetables, nuts, and omega-3 fatty acids, such as fish oil—the food sources for antioxidants. It's been estimated that 95 percent of Americans have less than one helping of fruit or vegetables each day. A significant number of older adults fail to get amounts and types of food to meet essential energy and nutrition needs. Deficiencies of vitamins and minerals may affect as many as a third of all adults over the age of 65. Poor vitamin intake has been linked to chronic heart disease, cancer, and osteoporosis.

SOUND ADVICE

Smokers tend to have lower antioxidant levels in their blood and may be deficient in Vitamin C. If you smoke and have presbycusis, consider increasing your antioxidant defenses by including more of the appropriate foods in your diet. Better yet, stop smoking! Nicotine causes the blood vessels to constrict. Theoretically, this could lessen the blood supply to the inner ear, trigger the release of free radicals, and eventually damage hair cells, spiral ganglion cells, and the stria vascularis, causing hearing loss.

Hearing Improvement

If you have a hearing loss, there are things you can do to improve your hearing and your ability to communicate. If you let other people know you have a hearing loss, you can educate them about what they need to do for you to aide effective communication. By improving the conversational environment and learning to speechread, you can improve your hearing ability (see Chapters 19 and 20).

Devices to assist you in hearing and communicating are your primary option if you have presbycusis. These devices include hearing aids (Chapter 16) and other assistive listening devices (Chapter 17). Hearing aids are the most common assistive devices available to treat age-related hearing loss. They increase audibility, improving the ability to hear conversation. Modern technology has greatly changed hearing aids from those available only a decade ago. They can help you hear more by reducing background noise and amplifying speech sounds. And all of this comes in very small packages! But hearing aids can't improve the central processing of sound by your brain. Even a million-dollar hearing aid wouldn't help those who can hear but who are unable to process or understand what they hear.

There are now a wide variety of assistive listening devices available that help people use a telephone, watch television or movies, hear in the theater or auditorium, and listen in meetings and group discussions. Alerting and signaling devices can tell you someone is at the door, it's time to get up, or there might be a fire in the house.

Motivation and expectation are two important factors for a hearing aid user. People who seek hearing aid use on their own are more likely to be successful users compared to those who purchase a hearing aid just to please a spouse or family member. If you expect to hear "normally" while wearing a hearing aid, you'll be disappointed. It's unreasonable for someone with presbycusis to expect to have perfect hearing in settings where the speaker is truly mumbling or not projecting his or her voice; where there is significant distance between the speaker and the listener; if there's significant background sound; or when the hearing aid user is not tuned in or is tired, stressed, or concentrating on another activity. You must be willing to try some rehabilitation or training strategies involving you and your family to improve communication. Studies have shown that elderly adults who successfully use hearing aids experience an overall improvement in quality of life, family relationships, and feelings about themselves.

Activities with visual input can sometimes be helpful for the elderly person with hearing impairment. Speechreading (Chapter 19), closed captioning, and other alerting devices (Chapter 17) can improve the communication ability of the elderly. But remember that the elderly are also more likely to have visual problems such as cataracts, glaucoma, and macular degeneration. Simple alterations of the environment can improve the ability of seniors, as well as anyone with a hearing loss, to communicate (Chapters 19 and 20). For those of you with normal hearing, don't mistake hearing loss in your loved ones or friends for mental confusion or dementia.

HAVE YOU HEARD?

Here's an old joke. An elderly man had had serious hearing problems for a number of years. Finally, he saw an ear doctor, was tested by an audiologist, and was referred to a hearing aid dispenser to have hearing aids fit. With the hearing aids, his hearing was greatly improved. A month later he went back for a check-up, and the hearing aid dispenser said, "Your hearing is perfect. Your family must be really pleased that you can hear again." To this the man replied, "Oh, I haven't told my family yet. I just sit around and listen to the conversations. I've changed my will three times!"

Chronic Disease Related to Hearing

Because changes in the blood supply to the ear can cause presbycusis, any general health problems that affect circulation can potentially affect hearing. These include heart disease and high blood pressure, though these problems have not been specifically linked to hearing loss. One chronic disease, in particular, that is now thought to cause hearing loss is diabetes.

Diabetes is a chronic disease that affects both children and adults. The prevalence among older Americans is as high as 20 percent or more than 7 million people over the age of 65. The disease creates problems in both the circulatory and nervous systems. As a result of the changes in the small blood vessels of different organs, known diabetic complications include heart disease, kidney failure, blindness, and stroke. Many diabetic people also have hearing loss. A study funded by the National Institutes of Health found that people with diabetes are more than twice as likely as those without the disease to have hearing loss. It's not yet clear whether the hearing loss and diabetes are directly linked in a cause-effect relationship, but blood vessels and nerve cells, both of which can be affected by diabetes, are important to hearing. Inner ear function relies on a rich supply of tiny blood vessels. Nerve cell damage can cause the hearing signals from the cochlea to travel more slowly along the auditory nerve or result in slower processing of complex sounds such as speech in the brain.

LISTEN UP

If you have diabetes, ask your doctor to check your hearing or refer you for a hearing test and evaluation to obtain a baseline level. This should be a routine part of your diabetes care.

True Stories

There are millions of Americans who could tell you about their age-related hearing loss, and you undoubtedly know quite a few people yourself. Here we give you just a few stories that highlight some important points for you to keep in mind.

Judged a Success

Andrew, following his appointment by the governor, spent 15 years on the State Court of Appeals, then left the Court at age 68 to become an arbitration judge.

During his first case, he found himself having significant difficulty understanding the parties at the arbitration, particularly a young woman attorney. After the case, he made an appointment to have a hearing test, and his audiogram showed a mild high-frequency hearing loss. Concerned that he would have more trouble at the next arbitration, Andrew requested an evaluation for hearing aids. He was prescribed two behind-the-ear devices and used them around the house to become accustomed to them. When he wore them at his next arbitration, he was amazed at the ease with which he was able to hear all parties involved.

Eat, Drink, and Be Merry?

Paul retired from his accounting firm at age 60, and for the last 10 years, he's enjoyed his retirement by reading, golfing, and traveling with his wife. They ate and drank their way through several countries. His early years set the tone for the rest of his life. Paul was not an athlete; he sat at work. When golfing, he always used a cart, and he refrained from any exercise that required exertion. As a result, he was a big guy, although in his mind he wasn't overweight. In fact, he didn't understand why his physician, at each annual physical for the last 15 years, had told him it was important for him to change his diet, to decrease his alcohol consumption, and to begin to exercise. He figured modern medicine and his prescriptions would control his blood cholesterol and sugar levels (he was diabetic) and would allow him to continue to enjoy life. Unfortunately, in spite of using insulin, he began to have kidney and eye problems associated with his diabetes. He also began to notice more difficulty understanding his wife. A hearing test performed five years ago revealed that Paul had a mild to moderate high-frequency sensorineural hearing loss in both ears, and a recent test showed a further decline in his ability to hear. Though he was not enthusiastic about using hearing aids, he relented to his wife and daughter's wishes and obtained two aids. To his surprise, he found them extremely helpful.

She Doesn't Understand

Ruth spent most of her life working as a furniture manufacturer representative. She had no children of her own but did have a dozen nieces and nephews, so she was Auntie Ruth not only to her family members but also to all their friends. Though she had lived alone for several years, her house was a hub of family activity at least once a month. She marked the passage of time through her medical ailments. She had a hip replacement at age 65, hearing aids at 70, and cataract surgery at 75. All her family was looking forward to celebrating her eightieth birthday. Two of the nieces, who had been with her the most, noticed she wasn't understanding them as well as she used to. She still was mentally sharp; she played a mean game of bridge and occasionally took home winnings playing poker with the nephews. Her original hearing aids had been replaced at age 75, and she had obtained new aids only a year ago, but they didn't seem to provide as much benefit as the older aids had. Thinking new aids were needed, Auntie Ruth was taken to the audiologist for another hearing aid evaluation. The repeat test showed that her overall ability to hear had actually remained about the same, but her ability to process what she heard—her speech discrimination—had decreased. New hearing aid technology would provide some improvement, but they just wouldn't give as much benefit as she had once obtained, so communication strategies were discussed to help Ruth communicate better, especially at her large family gatherings.

The Least You Need to Know

- *Presbycusis* is the medical term for age-related hearing loss.
- Age-related hearing loss is usually sensorineural and can be mild, moderate, or severe.
- There can be an inherited tendency to presbycusis.
- Prevention is key, but the primary treatment is use of hearing aids.
- Possible prevention approaches include diet, exercise, and healthy habits, such as not smoking.
- Antioxidants found in Vitamin E, fruits, vegetables, nuts, and omega-3 fatty acids might help prevent damage to the inner ear.

Hearing Loss from Noise Exposure

In This Chapter

- What makes a sound "noise"
- Sounds that can cause noise-induced hearing loss
- Warning signs and symptoms
- Noise at home, at work, at play, in the environment, and in the military
- Ways to prevent noise-induced hearing loss

Noise-induced hearing loss (NIHL) is the second most frequent cause of hearing loss in the world, next to aging, but unlike hearing loss due to aging, at least at present, NIHL is a preventable disease. According to the National Institute for Occupational Safety and Health (NIOSH), nearly 10 percent of the total population in the United States is exposed to hazardous levels of noise in the workplace on a daily basis. Teenagers are also at great risk for NIHL if they listen to music at excessive volume levels for long periods of time, and everyone these days is plugged into cell phones and MP3 players or stereo headsets. Because of noise in our society, hearing loss is appearing much earlier in life than would have been expected just 30 years ago.

Damage to the inner ear from regular exposure to excessive sound levels over time or brief but intense sound, such as an explosion, can lead to permanent and debilitating hearing loss and tinnitus. The amount of damage depends primarily on the intensity of the noise and the length of the exposure. Temporary hearing loss can result from short-term exposures to noise, with normal hearing returning after a short period, but prolonged exposure to high noise levels over a period of time gradually causes permanent damage.

In this chapter, we describe how noise damages the ear, point out many of the sources of noise in our daily lives, tell you what sounds are unsafe, and describe warning signs that you may have or are developing NIHL. We provide tips on preventing further hearing loss, discuss hearing protection devices, and review federal requirements regarding noise in the workplace. We also provide some tips for parents about protecting their children's hearing.

We're Surrounded by Sound—Is It Noise?

The type of hearing loss we're talking about in this chapter is referred to as noise-induced hearing loss. But really, it should be called "sound-induced" hearing loss because the damage to the ear is based mainly on the loudness level of the sound and how long one is exposed to it, not other qualities of the sound. We all know that our children, or our parents, find the music we like distasteful and may refer to it as "noise." Yet we find it perfectly pleasant. So what makes something noise? And does that have anything to do with hearing loss?

HAVE YOU HEARD?

The most common theory about the origin of the word *noise* is that it goes back to the Latin *nausea*, which means "seasickness." Another theory connects it to the Latin *noxia*, meaning "a fault" or "offense." In either case, the implication is of something unpleasant.

Most of us probably think of noise in terms of how it affects us emotionally—is the sound pleasant or unpleasant? If unpleasant, we call it noise. But sounds that are soothing for some might be irritating to others. Scientists who study acoustics, or the characteristics of sound, define noise as complex sound waves with irregular vibrations and no definite pitch. From the point of view of its effect on hearing, noise is any sound that might cause damage to the ear because of its loudness level. Noise in our environment not only affects physical health but also has psychological and social implications. It affects our quality of life. It's a pollutant and a hazard to human health and hearing. In fact, some have described it as the most pervasive pollutant in America. Studies show that noise can have many negative effects on the human body besides affecting hearing.

Am I at Risk?

With prolonged exposure, sounds louder than 85 dB can cause permanent hearing loss. Factors that determine risk include the loudness, the duration of sound exposure, repeated or cumulative exposure, and personal susceptibility. The louder the sound, the shorter the duration of exposure that is needed to create hearing loss. The current definition of NIHL is based on chronic exposure to noise levels of between 85 and 140 decibels or an even brief exposure of greater than 140 decibels. The National Institute for Occupational Safety and Health (NIOSH) has developed guidelines for safe levels of sound exposure. These guidelines are stated in terms of the maximum time an individual can safely be exposed to different average levels of sound on a daily basis over a 40-year period. The table shows how long you could listen to a given decibel level before risking NIHL.

NIOSH-Recommended Decibel Exposure Guidelines

Sound Level	Safe Listening Time
85 dB	8 hours
88 dB	4 hours
91 dB	2 hours
94 dB	1 hour
97 dB	30 minutes
100 dB	15 minutes
103 dB	7½ minutes
106 dB	3¾ minutes

Exposure to 115 dB or greater may pose a serious health risk.

There's no exposure limit for sounds less than 85 dB in loudness; for sounds above 115 dB, you should have no unprotected exposure time. Note that for every 3 dB increase in sound level, the safe listening time is cut in half. Okay, so how do you know what level a given sound is? You could purchase a sound level meter and actually measure the sounds around you. But to make things easier, we've provided a chart of common sounds in Appendix C. Each sound is listed by decibel level based on the loudest it's likely to be. The chart also tells you how long you could listen before risking NIHL. Just to give you some sense of scale, a watch ticking or other just noticeable sound is about 20 dB. A whisper might be 30 dB, and normal conversation is around 60 dB. A power lawnmower is 90 dB; an ambulance siren is 120 dB; and a jet engine at take-off is 140 dB. Of course, the actual intensity level at your ear depends on the distance between you and the source of the noise, the make or model of a device, and many other factors.

> **LISTEN UP**
>
> If you have to shout or raise your voice above competing sound to be heard, you're likely in the danger zone above 85 dB. Such situations might arise at loud music performances (regardless of type of music), near power tools or loud vehicles, or even in some restaurants, especially those in which loud music is played.

There appear to be differences in personal susceptibility to NIHL. For example, among people working under the same noise conditions, some might suffer hearing loss while others have no problem. Studies in mice have found that a significant portion of the damage from NIHL can be attributed to inherited factors. Twin studies in humans suggest an inherited susceptibility of approximately 36 percent. That is, other factors are involved, but a person's genes might at least partially determine whether hearing damage occurs with exposure to hazardous noise. Researchers are currently working to discover which genes might be involved in NIHL.

Warning signs and symptoms of excessive noise exposure include the following:

- Sounds seem temporarily muffled or distorted (temporary threshold shift)
- Ringing or buzzing sensation
- Ear pain or discomfort after exposure
- Difficulty hearing in noisy environments
- Loss of high-frequency discrimination (speech sounds such as those represented by *s* or *f*)
- Sudden increase in sensitivity to sounds

If any of these symptoms last longer than one day, you should visit your doctor or an ENT specialist.

Sources of Noise

Let's take a brief look at some of the common problem sounds at home, in the environment, and at work. And let's include the special problems for military personnel.

Home and Lifestyle

Try making a list of the sounds that regularly occur in and around your home. There are many! Some of these sounds, though you don't think of them as "noise," can potentially damage hearing if you're exposed for too long or too often (see Appendix C). Common sounds usually just a little below 85 dB—the level at which damage is possible—include a ringing telephone, a hair dryer, a garbage disposal, an alarm clock, and a vacuum cleaner. A kitchen blender can make noise at 85 dB. However, you're not likely to listen to these sounds long enough to cause NIHL. Power tools are more likely to be in the damaging category. These include leaf blowers and power lawn-mowers at 90 dB. (If you're a gardener or landscape maintenance worker, you should be wearing ear protection).

HAVE YOU HEARD?

Did you know that a crying baby can produce sounds as loud as 110 dB, well into the extremely loud range and potentially damaging to hearing? Based on this maximum crying level, and assuming your ear is right next to the baby's mouth, the recommended exposure limit is two minutes a day! Fortunately, you're not likely to have such exposure over a 40-year period (though they do say that some people never grow up!).

Hobbies that can create noise-induced hearing loss or acoustic trauma include hunting or target shooting, do-it-yourself projects that involve nail guns, saws, or grinders, and recreational pursuits such as drag racing, motorcycling, and piloting private aircraft. Not only are many of these sounds in the potentially damaging range, but you also tend to have long-term continued exposure if these are activities you enjoy.

Perhaps the most widespread noise exposure related to lifestyle is exposure to music, whether through stereo speakers in the home, headsets or earbuds attached to a personal CD player or MP3 player, a car radio, or a live concert. If it's loud enough and the duration long enough, music of any type can lead to noise-induced sensorineural hearing loss. At full volume, MP3 players have been measured at up to 120 dB, and a rock concert can reach levels of 120 to 130 dB. Noise exposure adds up both with the time exposed as well as actual sound level, so if you work in a noisy environment and then go home and turn up the volume on your MP3 player or stereo, you're adding to the potential damage to your inner ear.

The Environment

Outside the home, we're also surrounded by sounds. Some of these are things we would all agree are "noise"—loud cars, motorcycles and diesel trucks accelerating (103 to 114 dB), or an ambulance siren (118 to 120 dB). You walk by a construction site where there are bulldozers, jackhammers, and generators, all above the extremely loud level of 100 dB. A bicycle horn or a balloon pop can be unbelievably loud (greater than 140 dB). Traffic and subway noises assault our ears daily.

Work

Noise is one of the most pervasive occupational health problems. It's a by-product of many industrial processes. Musicians or others in the music business whose jobs expose them regularly to loud sound are also at risk for occupational hearing loss. The Occupational Safety and Health Act of 1970 (amended 2004) was passed to lower the number of work-related injuries and deaths, including hearing loss. The Occupational Safety and Health Administration (OSHA) of the United States Department of Labor was created in 1971 to oversee and enforce the act. OSHA's hearing conservation program was designed to protect workers with significant occupational noise exposures from hearing impairment, even if they are subject to such noise exposures over their entire working lifetimes. We've taken the following information directly from OSHA's website to highlight some of the requirements employers must observe regarding hearing conservation.

Monitoring: Employers are required to monitor noise exposure levels in a way that accurately identifies employees exposed to noise at or above 85 dB averaged over 8 working hours (an 8-hour time-weighted average [TWA]). The exposure measurement must include all continuous, intermittent, and impulsive noise within an 80 to 130 dB range and must be taken during a typical work situation.

Audiograms: Employers must (with exceptions) provide baseline audiograms within 6 months of an employee's first exposure at or above an 8-hour TWA of 85 dB. They must provide annual audiograms within 1 year of the baseline. Employers must compare annual audiograms to baseline audiograms to determine whether the employee has lost hearing ability or experienced a standard threshold shift (STS). An STS is an average shift in hearing acuity in either ear of 10 dB or more at 2,000, 3,000, and 4,000 Hz. The employer must fit or refit any employee showing an STS with adequate hearing protectors, show the employee how to use them, and require the employee to wear them.

Hearing Protection: Employers must provide hearing protectors to all workers exposed to 8-hour TWA noise levels of 85 dB or above. This ensures that employees have access to protectors before they experience any hearing loss. Employees must wear hearing protectors under these circumstances: For any period exceeding 6 months from the time they are first exposed to 8-hour TWA noise levels of 85 dB or above, until their baseline audiograms; if they have incurred standard threshold shifts that demonstrate they are susceptible to noise; and if they are exposed to noise over the permissible exposure limit of 90 dB over an 8-hour TWA. Employers must provide employees with a selection of at least one variety of earplug and one variety of ear muff (see following text for more details). Most employers use the noise reduction rating (NRR) that represents the protector's ability to reduce noise under ideal laboratory conditions. If workplace noise levels increase, employers must give employees more effective protectors. The protector must reduce employee exposures to at least 90 dB and to 85 dB when an STS already has occurred in the worker's hearing. Employers must show employees how to use and care for their protectors and supervise them on the job to ensure that they continue to wear them correctly.

The Military

For people in the military, the possibility of being exposed to unprotected, high-intensity noise (acoustic trauma) markedly increases in a combat setting. Although the United States military issues state-of-the-art hearing protection, the reduction in sound level offered by these protective devices is about 25 dB, a level that's insufficient for the exposures experienced in a blast or firefight (greater than 183 dB). One study even found that 23 to 28 percent of recruits sustain a permanent threshold shift after basic weapons training. To help prevent hearing loss, the Army and Marine Corps have distributed thousands of pairs of special combat earplugs designed to block hazardous noise but still allow normal hearing. Other devices are currently being tested, such as a lightweight tactical communication headset with built-in high-level hearing protection.

HAVE YOU HEARD?

According to the Department of Veterans Affairs, hearing loss is the most common disability in the war on terror. Of the roughly 1.3 million troops serving in the Middle East (2009), approximately 70,000 are collecting disability for tinnitus and nearly 60,000 are being compensated for hearing loss. Reports from military audiologists confirm that 60 percent of military personnel exposed to blasts suffer a permanent hearing loss. For the first time ever, the Army has deployed audiologists to combat zones both in Iraq and Afghanistan. The intent is to educate and train troops on hearing protection and to monitor and treat soldiers' hearing problems.

A study of hearing loss among Navy personnel found it to be one of the most common disabilities among sailors. Enlisted sailors who spent at least half of a 30-year Navy career assigned to a surface warship had a 13 to 18 percent higher probability of hearing loss compared to those who spent their whole career in shore bases.

What Does Noise Do to My Ear?

When noise damage first occurs, it usually affects the part of the ear corresponding to the mid-frequency range (3,000 to 5,000 Hz). On an audiogram, this type of hearing loss configuration is commonly referred to as a "noise notch." If you have this notch and your hearing thresholds in this frequency range are greater than 25 dB, indicating below-normal hearing, you probably have a noise-induced hearing loss. Remember that these frequencies correspond to the region where consonant sounds are heard, so with this type of hearing loss you might have trouble understanding speech because it sounds "muffled."

Your hearing loss may or may not be accompanied by tinnitus—a ringing, buzzing, or fluttering in one or both ears (see Chapter 13). While normal hearing people can also have tinnitus, it's often a symptom of high-frequency hearing loss, such as that caused by noise exposure. Sometimes a short exposure to loud sound may cause only temporary hearing loss. This temporary hearing loss is referred to as a temporary threshold shift (TTS). You've probably experienced a TTS on any number of occasions. For example, after being at a loud concert, a loud movie, or a very noisy restaurant, you walk outside and feel like you just aren't hearing as well as usual. TTS usually disappears within 14 to 16 hours after overexposure to loud sound. But cumulative exposure to loud sounds eventually results in a "permanent threshold shift," that is, a permanent hearing loss.

LISTEN UP

If you think you're "getting used to" loud noises you routinely hear because they don't bother you as much, you've probably already suffered some hearing damage. Noise-induced hearing loss is usually gradual and painless. What you think of as "tuning out" the noise is more likely "wiping out" the hair cells of the inner ear!

Remember that most inner ear hearing loss is sensorineural, meaning damage to the sensory and/or nerve elements. Continuous low-level noise exposure damages the outer hair cells in the cochlea that particularly help us to hear speech in a noisy background as well as very soft sounds. This type of continuous noise results in biochemical changes in the sensory cells and neurons over time and produces the "typical" NIHL, with its associated high-frequency "notch." In contrast, brief but intense noise energy results in mechanical damage to the organ of corti, with threshold shifts occurring at frequencies above 2,000 Hz, and is referred to as "acoustic trauma." This type of noise exposure can be from chronic impulse noise (subsonic) or sudden blast exposure (supersonic). Studies in animals suggest that impulse noise is more damaging to the cochlea than continuous noise. Studies among United States Marines demonstrate greater degrees of permanent hearing loss for those exposed to armaments (weapons) than those exposed to continuous noise. You may know someone who has a hearing loss from gunfire near his ear—often a man who was or is in the military or who hunts or used to hunt, though women are increasingly joining this group.

Hearing Protection Devices

Hearing protection devices (HPDs) can significantly reduce the sound levels reaching the ear. These include foam earplugs, premolded earplugs, custom-molded earplugs, ear muffs, and in-the-ear monitors (IEMs).

Noise reduction ratings (NRRs) for foam earplugs range from 20 to 35 dB and provide greater reduction, or attenuation, at high frequencies than at low frequencies. Most foam HPDs are designed for one-time use, although there are reusable models. Fortunately, they're also inexpensive. You can buy an individual pair for 50 cents, a box of 10 pairs for about $3.50, or larger quantities such as 200 pairs for approximately $25.00. Many brands and styles are available. It's essential to insert the foam plugs both correctly and deep enough into the ear canal, or the noise reduction will be considerably less than that advertised.

SOUND ADVICE

Foam earplugs are easy to wear. Using clean hands, roll them into a crease-free cylinder. With your opposite hand, reach over your head and pull the top of your ear upward to help straighten your ear canal while inserting the rolled plug. After a moment, you should feel the plug unroll and expand, sealing your ear canal. Hold the plug in place with your fingertip for the time recommended on the label instructions. Always follow the manufacturer's instructions for earplug insertion; certain models or brands might require other methods for effective use.

Premolded earplugs are available in different sizes to accommodate small, medium, or large ear canals. Some people find they need a different size premolded plug for each ear! They're usually made from plastic, silicone, or rubber and are reusable and washable. Premolded plugs are also inexpensive (ranging from $2 to $10) and conveniently available online or at retail stores. Sporting goods stores sell special plugs for shooting and hunting.

Custom-molded earplugs are designed to provide equal sound attenuation for high and low frequencies and are reusable. Available with NRRs of 9, 15, or 25 dB, they are designed for people who rely on their ability to hear high and low frequencies without distortion, such as musicians and concert attendees as well as anyone who needs to hear accurately in high-noise environments (for example, music teachers, DJs, flight attendants, bartenders, waitresses, dentists, and dental workers). These HPDs are custom made by licensed hearing health-care providers and offer a comfortable fit and long-term wear. They range in cost from $170 to $225.

Ear muff–style HPDs are easy to take on and off, so they're ideal when frequent removal and replacement of hearing protection is necessary. They require a solid shell and acoustic seal around the ear to attenuate noise effectively, with typical NRRs of 20 to 30 dB. They can cost under $10 or more than $100 for high-end muffs with radio communication or UHF and VHF protection.

In-the-ear monitors combine the features of custom-molded HPDs and electronic earpieces and can be obtained from a licensed hearing health-care provider. IEMs attenuate ambient sound like a custom-molded HPD while allowing you to monitor signals routed to the IEM from a sound reproduction system. For listening with portable music devices, you can get noise-isolating ear phones for $50 to $100. For more serious music listening, prices range from $100 to $250. Customized in-the-ear monitors for musicians can range in price to more than $1,000.

Hearing Conservation Tips

Because noise-induced hearing loss is a preventable cause of hearing loss, you can protect your hearing, or, in other words, conserve your hearing by observing some general hearing conservation tips. We also offer some advice specifically for listening to music and pointers for parents to protect their children's hearing.

HAVE YOU HEARD?

Public awareness of the hazardous effects of noise is not as great as it should be, especially for non-occupational noise. To try to improve this situation, the fourth Wednesday in April has been declared International Noise Awareness Day (INAD) and has been celebrated for more than 15 years. As part of International Noise Awareness Day, a "Quiet Diet" is encouraged and is launched by observing 60 seconds of no noise from 2:15 to 2:16 P.M. The reduction, if not cessation, of everyday noises around us raises our awareness of the impact noise has on health and hearing. In addition, a number of organizations offer year-round hearing loss prevention education programs for teenagers, tweens, and young children, as well as for people in high-risk professions, such as the music industry.

General Tips

Here are some general things you can do:

- Avoid hazardous sound environments. If you must be in such an environment, wear hearing protection devices.

- Monitor sound pressure levels above 85 dB. Follow the general rule that if you have to raise your voice to be heard, you may be risking permanent hearing loss and should limit your exposure time. (See Appendix C for guidelines.)

- If you are "stuck" in a sound danger zone longer than the guidelines recommend, tone down the sound with earplugs or ear muffs. Whenever you can, carry your HPDs with you; you never know when you might find yourself in a loud noise environment.

- Take 15-minute "quiet breaks" every few hours if you're exposed to levels above 85 dB.

- Musicians and other live entertainment professionals should avoid practicing at "concert hall levels" whenever possible.

- Have a licensed audiologist check your hearing annually.

Hearing tests include pure-tone thresholds, middle ear function, otoacoustic emissions, and the "hearing in noise test" (HINT), which assesses speech perception in noise, similar to everyday listening situations (see Chapter 2). Otoacoustic emissions have been reported to be more sensitive to subtle damage in the inner ear than pure-tone thresholds. The HINT is better for indicating how well you hear in real-world situations. These tests together can give your hearing care provider important information for assessing your hearing health.

Listening to Music

Do you listen to music on a regular basis—through your car radio, portable CD player or MP3 player with headphones or earbuds, your powerful stereo speakers that are the centerpiece of your living room, or in a live concert setting? Or perhaps you make your own music. Music is one of our most frequent "noise" exposures, outside of the work setting, with more than just brief exposure durations.

For much of your music listening, one way to control the potential for NIHL is simply to turn down the volume knob! If you're using a headset, try getting earphones or earbuds with a good seal, making them similar to an earplug. Minimizing the background noise should allow you to listen to your music at a lower volume setting and still hear it well. One study has found that listening to a portable music player, with headphones, at 60 percent of the player's potential volume for one hour a day is relatively safe. Do you exercise at a health club or take an aerobics class? Talk to the instructor about turning down the music volume (or buy a pack of foam earplugs and offer them to all of your exercise buddies!).

If you enjoy live music concerts, be aware that sound levels can be extremely high, regardless of the type of music being played. Don't sit directly in front of a speaker while listening (or performing). The cheap seats might be better, but one study that examined sound intensity throughout a well-known concert hall found that sound pressure levels appeared equally hazardous in all parts of the concert hall. Regardless of how far you are from the stage, you should use earplugs at every type of musical concert. You can use custom-molded earplugs that provide flat attenuation if you're concerned that filtering some frequencies more than others might reduce your listening enjoyment. If you are one of those making the music, move away from onstage monitors or amplifiers, don't practice at concert levels, and turn down the amp on the electric guitar! And, of course, use an appropriate hearing protection device.

SOUND ADVICE

Always take earplugs to any music concert, whether its rock, jazz, folk, classical, alternative, rap, international, or any other kind of music. As more than one audiologist will tell you, earplugs are relatively inexpensive, while hearing aids can cost thousands of dollars.

Pointers for Parents

Hearing loss in children and teenagers is on the rise. According to a national study, an estimated 12 percent of children ages 6 to 19 already have NIHL. Loud noise can cause premature hearing loss, but we'll say it again—you can prevent it. It's important that children and teens develop good listening habits early and don't become conditioned to listening to sound at excessive levels. As a parent, take an active role in your child's hearing conservation and be aware of noise pollutants in his or her daily environment. Repeated and unprotected exposure to loud stereos, boom boxes, noisy toys, lawnmowers, farm equipment, or rock concerts can cause cumulative permanent damage to a young person's hearing. Make hearing conservation a family thing. When a child accompanies a parent to any activity or location with excessive noise, the entire family should wear ear protection.

Teenagers are reportedly at the greatest risk because this age group has a tendency to listen to music at excessive levels for long periods of time. One of the research audiologists at our institution says he tells his son, "If I can sing along with the song that you're listening to with your earbuds, and you're in the living room and I'm in the kitchen, it's way too darn loud." An MP3 player at full volume can be as loud as or louder than the average rock concert. Teenagers also like to talk on the cell phone for lengthy amounts of time. If they wear an earpiece for the cell phone, they need to be cautious (this goes for parents, too!). In a noisy mall, it's tempting to turn the volume up to what can be unsafe levels. Tell them to move to a quieter area while talking and keep the volume setting lower.

Don't think that noise is a problem you don't need to worry about until your child reaches the teenage years. Some toy sirens and squeaky rubber toys can emit sounds of 90 dB—as loud as a lawnmower and dangerous to a child's hearing. A noisy toy held directly to the ear, as children often do, can actually expose the ear to as much as 120 dB of sound—the equivalent of a jet plane or a rock concert. Noise at this level is painful and can result in permanent hearing loss.

Some of the toys recognized as a possible noise danger include cap guns, vehicles with horns and sirens, walkie-talkies, musical instruments, household toys such as vacuum cleaners, and toys with cranks. Parents who have normal hearing need to inspect toys for noise danger just as they would for small pieces that can be easily swallowed. Before buying a new toy, listen to it. If it sounds loud, don't buy it. Also examine toys already at home. You can always remove the batteries or discard toys that are too noisy and pose a potential danger to your child's hearing.

True Stories

Noise-induced hearing loss has no treatment other than using hearing aids when needed. So in this chapter, we're not going to give you any true stories. Rather, we want you to take the time to think about stories you may already know. Do you have a relative who was in the military who has told you that he doesn't hear well in one ear because of gunfire? Do you have a musician friend who has mentioned having tinnitus and seems to have some difficulty with high-frequency sounds? What about a neighbor who spends every afternoon working in his home workshop with power tools and doesn't seem to hear you when you say hello as he walks by? Do you come out of an action movie with your ears ringing and everything sounding muffled (remember TTS)? Did your grandmother used to work in a factory in the days before ear protection was required by OSHA, and, if so, how's her hearing?

The Least You Need to Know

- Noise is one the most frequent causes of hearing loss, but noise-induced hearing loss is preventable.
- "Noise" is any sound that might cause damage to the ear because of its loudness level.
- Sounds of 85 dB or louder are potentially damaging depending on the duration of exposure; if you have to raise your voice to be heard, you are likely in a sound environment of 85 dB or louder.
- Avoid hazardous sound environments or wear hearing protection devices.
- Be careful about sound level when listening to music, and always take earplugs to any concert.

Sudden and Drug-Induced Hearing Loss

In This Chapter

- Sudden hearing loss without a known cause
- Viral and bacterial causes of sudden hearing loss, including meningitis
- The many drugs that can cause sensorineural hearing loss, including antibiotics, chemotherapy agents, and pain killers
- Substances in the environment that can cause hearing loss
- Traumatic injury as a cause of sudden sensorineural hearing loss

According to the National Institute on Deafness and Other Communication Disorders (NIDCD), there are more than 100 possible causes of sudden deafness or sudden sensorineural hearing loss (SSHL). SSHL affects 5 to 20 of every 100,000 people. This is about 4,000 new cases a year in the United States, but many likely go unreported, so the actual number of people affected is probably higher. The cause of the sudden hearing loss is identified in only 10 to 15 percent of cases, and diagnosis is usually based on the individual's medical history. Possible causes include infectious diseases, trauma such as a head injury, abnormal tissue growth, immunologic diseases, toxic causes such as snakebites, ototoxic drugs (drugs that harm the ear), blood vessel problems, and neurologic causes such as multiple sclerosis.

In this chapter, we discuss some of the more common causes of sudden hearing loss (the most common being "unknown"!) and briefly describe symptoms and treatment. In particular, we tell you about some drugs and other substances that can potentially cause hearing loss, some of which may surprise you.

Sudden Unexplained Hearing Loss

As we said, the cause of most cases of sudden hearing loss is never known. Referred to as *idiopathic* sudden sensorineural hearing loss, it can affect anyone, but for unknown reasons it happens most often to people between the ages of 30 and 60. Even though the exact cause is unknown, idiopathic SSHL is considered a clinical diagnosis of its own, differing from other causes of sudden hearing loss. It has unique characteristics, but is ultimately diagnosed by ruling out other causes of hearing loss.

DEFINITION

Idiopathic means "of, relating to, or designating a disease having no known cause."

SSHL is defined as a loss of 30 dB or greater across at least three adjacent frequencies over a period of 72 hours or less. People report a sudden onset of hearing loss without being able to identify a cause such as an ear infection or loud noise exposure. Many people notice it when they wake up in the morning; others first notice it when they try to use the deafened ear, such as when they make a phone call. Some people notice a loud "pop" just before their hearing disappears. Fortunately, SSHL affects only one ear in 9 out of 10 people who experience it. The majority of people with SSHL develop tinnitus in the affected ear, and two thirds report symptoms of dizziness. Research suggests that the most likely causes of idiopathic SSHL are viruses, changes in the small blood vessels that supply the inner ear, or small tears in the membranes of the inner ear. But for any given patient, it typically remains unknown which of these causes, if any of them, is responsible for his or her sudden hearing loss.

LISTEN UP

Sudden sensorineural hearing loss can happen all at once or over a period of up to three days and should be considered a medical emergency. If you experience a sudden loss of hearing, you should visit a doctor immediately. Early presentation to a physician and early treatment improve the chances of hearing recovery.

If you go to the ear doctor to report a sudden hearing loss, your doctor will take a medical history and ask you questions about illnesses you've had, medications you might be taking, and even what you have eaten. You'll have a complete audiometric evaluation using the hearing tests described in Chapter 2. Because tumors of the hearing and balance nerve (see Chapter 11) can occasionally present with sudden hearing loss, the doctor will likely order an MRI to rule out this possibility, unless there is evidence of another clear cause. A tumor is unlikely to be the cause of your sudden hearing loss, but it's important to rule this out.

Two thirds of people with idiopathic SSHL recover spontaneously within two weeks of when the loss started. But we still don't know how to predict who will recover and who won't. For some, the hearing loss is permanent. Treatment for this condition is a 10- to 14-day course of oral steroids. People who can't tolerate steroids or who don't recover may receive steroid injections into the middle ear.

Viral and Bacterial Causes of Hearing Loss

Infections of the middle and inner ear can cause hearing loss. When infection, either viral or bacterial, reaches the inner ear, it causes labyrinthitis, or inflammation of the inner ear. Bacteria can be carried from the middle ear or the membranes that cover the brain. The viruses that cause mumps, measles, influenza, and colds can reach the inner ear following an upper respiratory infection.

Viruses

Viral labyrinthitis causes a sudden, unilateral (on one side) loss of balance function and hearing. You may experience severe, often incapacitating vertigo, frequently associated with nausea and vomiting. In fact, you may need to stay in bed until the symptoms gradually subside. The vertigo usually goes away after several days to weeks. But unsteadiness and vertigo when turning your head might last for several months. The hearing loss is usually mild to moderate and in the higher frequencies (greater than 2000 Hz). But any degree or type of hearing loss can occur. People who suffer this form of SSHL often report that it happened after having an upper respiratory tract infection.

Both mumps and measles can cause a virally induced hearing loss. Another form of viral labyrinthitis is herpes zoster oticus, also called Ramsay-Hunt syndrome. The cause is reactivation of varicella-zoster virus (the chicken pox virus) that can stay in the body and remain dormant for years after the primary infection. This is similar to what happens in shingles, when this virus becomes reactivated on nerves in other areas of the body and causes severe pain. The initial symptoms in the ear are deep, burning ear pain followed a few days later by a rash in the external auditory canal and concha. Vertigo, hearing loss, and facial weakness follow. Symptoms typically improve over a few weeks, but many people suffer permanent hearing loss and imbalance.

HAVE YOU HEARD?

Viral infections can also cause congenital hearing loss. Rubella and cytomegalo-virus (CMV) are the best-recognized viral causes of prenatal hearing loss. In other words, the viruses affect fetuses during pregnancy. We don't usually think of this as sudden hearing loss, because it presents itself as an existing condition in a newborn child.

Bacteria

Bacterial infections that have progressed to the inner ear are called suppurative labyrinthitis and can result in permanent hearing loss. The bacteria may have come from a middle ear infection (otitis media) or may be a consequence of meningitis (see the next section). The microorganism that causes syphilis, which has increased with the incidence of HIV, can also produce sudden hearing loss in the late stages of that disease. Bacterial toxins and inflammatory substances can also cross the round window membrane and cause inner ear inflammation without direct bacterial contamination. This condition, associated with acute or chronic middle ear disease (Chapters 4 and 5), is believed to be one of the most common complications of otitis media.

Profound SSHL, severe vertigo, ataxia (an inability to coordinate muscle activity), and nausea and vomiting are common symptoms of suppurative labyrinthitis. To treat suppurative labyrinthitis, antibiotics are given either by mouth or intravenously. If you have a middle ear infection with fluid (see Chapters 4 and 5), your ear doctor will also need to drain the fluid. With modern antibiotics, suppurative labyrinthitis is now relatively rare.

Meningitis

Both viruses and bacteria can cause meningitis, an inflammation of the membranes lining the brain. The most common causes of meningitis are viral infections that usually get better without treatment. Viral meningitis tends to develop in the late summer and early fall when viral infections are more common. It most often affects children and adults under age 30, with most infections occurring in children under the age of 5. Viral meningitis is most commonly due to enteroviruses, the viruses that also cause intestinal illness. Many other types of viruses can also cause meningitis.

Recently, West Nile virus, spread by mosquitoes, has become a known cause of viral meningitis in the United States. Viral meningitis is usually not serious, and symptoms typically disappear within two weeks with no lasting complications.

Bacterial meningitis remains a significant cause of SSHL, often profound. These infections are extremely serious and can result in death or brain damage, even if treated. Because bacterial meningitis can quickly become life-threatening, it is a true medical emergency and requires immediate treatment in a hospital. Early diagnosis and treatment are essential to prevent permanent neurological damage. In children, the risk of hearing loss secondary to meningitis is estimated to be 10 to 20 percent. Suppurative labyrinthitis caused by bacterial meningitis is usually seen in children younger than two years, which is the population most at risk for meningitis.

Bacterial meningitis usually affects both ears, while labyrinthitis from ear infections usually affects only one side. The bacteria known as meningococcus are the most common cause of bacterial meningitis in children and the second most common cause of bacterial meningitis in adults. Labyrinthitis ossificans (relating to bone growth) often follows suppurative labyrinthitis. This means that the cochlea becomes filled with bone, which makes placement of a cochlear implant (see Chapter 18) more difficult. So when bacterial meningitis is the cause of profound hearing loss, decisions regarding cochlear implantation must be made early.

Hearing Loss Due to Drugs and Other Substances

Ototoxic is the term commonly used to describe medications, drugs, cancer treatments, and other substances that can produce damage to the ear. The term means simply "toxic to the ear." Medications that are ototoxic have side effects that result in permanent or temporary sensorineural hearing loss, balance problems, or both. In fact, approximately 130 different drugs have known effects on the auditory system. The degree of toxicity varies, as does the onset of symptoms. Generally, larger doses, use of multiple ototoxic drugs, or underlying health problems that interfere with the metabolism of such drugs are more likely to cause side effects. In addition, some people also have more genetic susceptibility to ototoxic side effects.

Symptoms of ototoxicity include tinnitus, a sensation of ear pressure or fullness, SSHL, and dizziness or vertigo. Awareness of such side effects has led to improved treatment decision-making, including exploring other options that might be available and monitoring for side effects to minimize their impact. Considerable research is underway to increase understanding, prevention, and treatment of toxicity caused by such medications. Scientists are particularly interested in why the inner ear is more vulnerable to damage from these drugs than are other organ systems.

> **HAVE YOU HEARD?**
>
> Why would you be given a drug with the known side effect of hearing loss? As with many of life's decisions, it's a cost-benefit trade-off. For example, a particular antibiotic may be the best option to treat a potentially life-threatening infection, or you might need chemotherapy to treat life-threatening cancer. Unfortunately, the possible cost might be hearing loss.

If you are being treated with a medication known to have the potential to cause hearing loss, your hearing should be monitored. Baseline testing before administration of ototoxic agents should include full audiometric testing (see Chapter 2) including pure-tone air and bone conduction thresholds, speech reception thresholds, word recognition scores, and in some cases, high-frequency audiometry. Otoacoustic emissions and auditory brainstem response (ABR) testing are performed in people unable to complete full audiometric testing because of their age or underlying conditions. Testing is recommended up to six months after treatment.

You're encouraged to keep an active list of your medications. Many people take medications prescribed by a number of different physicians, so knowing one's medications helps to prevent unnecessary toxic exposure that can occur with use of multiple drugs.

Antibiotics

The aminoglycoside antibiotics, introduced in the 1940s, were the first drugs described as ototoxic. This class of antibiotics, given intravenously, is used to treat serious infections of the body, especially blood infections, often in newborn babies and children. The aminoglycoside antibiotics in common use today, in order of toxicity, include neomycin, streptomycin, kanamycin, gentamicin, amikacin, tobramycin, netilmicin, rinostamycin, and dihydrostreptomycin. Aminoglycoside antibiotics are widely used because they're easily administered (once daily dosing) and are relatively inexpensive. This makes these antibiotics very attractive for use in developing countries. Unfortunately, they don't come without serious side effects to the hearing and balance systems.

Aminoglycoside antibiotics damage outer hair cells at the base of the cochlea, resulting in high-frequency sensorineural hearing loss and tinnitus. They can also damage the balance portion of the inner ear, causing dizziness and imbalance, side effects that can occur immediately after taking the antibiotics or months later. These antibiotics are also toxic to the kidneys. But thankfully, the toxic effects of amino-glycosides are less likely to occur in children than in adults. If you receive treatment with this type of antibiotic, special precautions should be taken, such as monitoring blood levels of the antibiotic to avoid high doses, screening for impaired kidney function, and questioning about any family history of susceptibility because certain genetic factors make a person more susceptible to aminoglycoside toxicity. There is currently much research on how to prevent SSHL and dizziness from the use of aminoglycoside antibiotics.

Erythromycin is in a separate class of antibiotics and has been linked to reversible hearing loss occurring in the speech frequencies. Eardrops that contain these antibi-otics as one ingredient have a theoretical risk of toxicity because whatever reaches the middle ear can potentially reach the inner ear. It's believed that the drops can enter the inner ear through the round window membrane from the middle ear. Although most of the studies regarding ototoxicity of topical ear solutions have been done on animals, the FDA has still issued guidelines for the use of topical antibiotic ear prepa-rations. These guidelines include the recommendation that no eardrops be used that have the potential for ototoxicity because they might reach the inner ear, but that if such drops are used, the patient must be made aware of the ototoxic potential. If the eardrum is intact, there's no risk because the drops won't reach the middle ear. Still, it's recommended that the drops be stopped as soon as the infection has been cleared. Before your doctor prescribes antibiotic eardrops, you must be evaluated to ensure there aren't any holes in your eardrum, changes due to ear surgery you may have had, or anatomic defects that could increase the possibility of inner ear exposure.

Diuretics

Some diuretics, also called water pills, can be ototoxic. These are the diuretics called the loop diuretics. Their name comes from the part of the kidney on which they work. Furosemide (Lasix), ethacrynic acid (Edecrin), bumetanide (Bumex), torsemide (Dermadex) and mannitol (given only by intravenous injection) are examples of loop diuretics. These drugs are used to treat medical conditions including hypertension, congestive heart failure, and kidney failure, but they're also known to cause SSHL, tinnitus, and vertigo. They cause sensorineural hearing loss by acting on the part of the inner ear that's responsible for maintaining the proper balance of different electrical charges in the fluids of the inner ear. They can also cause some damage to the hair cells.

The hearing loss caused by diuretic toxicity tends to be permanent, whereas the tinnitus and vertigo are more likely to be reversible. These diuretics must be used in doses that are proper for your kidney function level so that your kidneys can metabolize the drug and prevent its accumulation in the body. Unless medically necessary, you should not use diuretics at the same time as other drugs that might increase their toxicity; for example, with the aminoglycoside antibiotics discussed in the previous section.

Cancer Treatments

Platinum-based chemotherapy agents, including cisplatin and carboplatin, are used to treat a wide range of cancers. Potential side effects of this class of chemotherapy drug include sensorineural hearing loss and tinnitus. The hearing loss caused by these drugs usually starts in the very high frequencies. As toxic levels of the drugs accumulate, the hearing loss can move to the frequencies we use for speech and other sounds. The drugs exert their toxic effects on the part of the inner ear that's responsible for maintaining the proper balance of different electrical charges in the fluids of the inner ear (the same part of the ear affected by loop diuretics) as well as on the outer hair cells of the inner ear. People undergoing chemotherapy must be monitored with hearing tests prior to, during, and after treatment. Some studies have found that people at either end of the age spectrum—children and the elderly—are particularly susceptible to SSHL from platinum-based chemotherapy agents.

LISTEN UP

Scientists have discovered that there's a relationship between noise exposure and the toxic effects of platinum-based chemotherapy. That is, noise can increase the amount of hearing loss the chemotherapy might cause. It's recommended that children undergoing treatment with these drugs avoid excessive noise exposure. Keep things quiet!

In addition to chemotherapy drugs, radiation therapy used to treat cancers of the head and neck can also have ototoxic effects on the inner ear. Radiation is administered to try to avoid exposing the inner ear, but this can still occur and can result in sensorineural hearing loss. The higher the radiation dose, the greater the degree of hearing loss that occurs. The hearing loss is usually limited to the side of the head being irradiated. Occasionally, radiation can affect the middle ear, causing an inflammatory response that can lead to scarring and interfere with the efficient conduction of sound from the external ear through the middle ear to the inner ear. If a significant conductive hearing loss occurs, treatment options include hearing aids or middle ear surgery.

Organ Transplant Drugs

Patients undergoing organ transplantation must take drugs after the transplant to suppress the immune system so that their bodies do not reject the transplanted organ. There is increasing evidence that some of the drugs used as immunosuppressants can affect hearing. A few examples of the drugs implicated in producing hearing loss are cyclosporine A, OKT3 (a monoclonal antibody), and tacrolimus. In most of the cases reported, the hearing loss was sudden but was usually reversible if the dose of the medication was adjusted or the patient was switched to a different immunosuppressive drug.

Pain Medications

Chronic and overuse and/or abuse of medications, called analgesics, for pain relief can cause sudden hearing loss. One of the most common of these is the seemingly benign aspirin. Aspirin can cause reversible SSHL and tinnitus if taken in high doses (20 to 30 tablets per day). The compound in aspirin that causes these effects is salicylic acid. This wonder drug is a naturally occurring compound and comes from the willow tree. Inner ears that are damaged from salicylic acid show a variety of different types of damage when viewed under the microscope, including some of the same types of damage as caused by the ototoxic drugs we've already discussed. But stopping the use or lowering the dose of aspirin usually leads to a reversal of the hearing loss.

One commonly used type of prescription pain reliever is a combination of two medications, hydrocodone and acetaminophen, distributed under brand names such as Vicodin, Hydrocet, Lorcet, Norco, and their generic counterparts. Overuse of these drugs (20 pills or more a day for several months or more) can lead to rapidly progressive and irreversible hearing loss. In many cases, this hearing loss is profound, which means that the only possible treatment is surgical placement of a cochlear implant (Chapter 18).

HAVE YOU HEARD?

In September 2008, Dr. John House of House Clinic and House Ear Institute wrote an essay titled, "House vs. House: Vicodin Addiction and Hearing Loss" (available online). He was referring to the popular TV show *House* in which the main character, Dr. Gregory House, is addicted to Vicodin. The real Dr. House said, "I have a very real concern about a message and theme that runs through each episode. It is not his poor bedside manner. It is not his mistreatment of residents. It is his addiction to Vicodin that is the problem. Here at the House Clinic, my colleagues and I have seen a significant number of patients who have become addicted to Vicodin and have gone completely deaf …. It is bad enough that the show depicts a doctor treating patients while addicted to a serious narcotic, but Vicodin is ototoxic, which means, if abused, it can cause irreversible and total hearing loss."

Other Substances

Among newer drugs that have been found to cause hearing loss are those used to treat erectile dysfunction. Drugs such as Viagra, Cialis, and Levitra are known to cause sudden blindness. They've recently been shown to be associated with SSHL as well.

Certain toxins, both naturally occurring and human-made, can cause sudden hearing loss. Methylmercury, lead, carbon monoxide, industrial solvents such as styrene, and other toxins have been linked to hearing loss. One source of mercury in the environment is in fish, and fish raised in fish farms are not exempt from this risk. In general, larger fish have a higher mercury load. Two of the fish highest in mercury content are swordfish and shark. Most of the time, the hearing loss caused by high mercury levels in the body are subclinical, meaning they're not detected by traditional auditory testing. A good rule of thumb is not to eat fish more than two or three times a week to avoid mercury poisoning or poisoning from some of the other toxic compounds that can build up in fish.

One final compound that is known to cause tinnitus, vertigo, and hearing loss is quinine. Quinine is a naturally occurring substance found in the bark of the cinchona tree. Quinine's primary use is as a drug to treat malaria, but other uses include treating restless leg syndrome. Quinine affects both the outer hair cells of the cochlea and the auditory cortex of the brain to produce its toxic effects. Luckily, the hearing loss, tinnitus, and vertigo associated with quinine toxicity are reversible, usually within one week of stopping the drug.

Traumatic Injuries

Traumatic forces on the inner or middle ear can cause sudden hearing loss. When we discussed damage to the middle ear from temporal bone trauma and barotraumas (or injury caused by pressure changes) in Chapter 6, we told you that these sources of injury can sometimes produce sensorineural hearing loss as well. Blunt trauma of the type that occurs during motor vehicle accidents or penetrating trauma from gunshot wounds can result in fractures of the temporal bones, and fracture lines can go straight through the inner ear, resulting in a profound SSHL. Barotrauma can also cause sudden changes in hearing. In addition to hearing loss, pressure changes can also affect the balance organs, which is especially dangerous if a scuba diver becomes disoriented underwater.

The inner ear requires a good blood supply, so a stroke can result in hearing loss. Because the inner ear blood vessels also feed the organs of balance, someone having a stroke might also experience sudden onset of dizziness or vertigo. The treatment for stroke doesn't change regardless of hearing loss symptoms, as it's focused on preventing immediate progression of the stroke and on preventing recurrence in the long term.

HAVE YOU HEARD?

Lightning kills more people annually than do tornadoes, hurricanes, or winter storms. Of storm-related hazards, only flash floods cause more annual deaths than lightning. Approximately 50 percent of lightning victims suffer ruptured eardrums, causing a conductive hearing loss, and temporary hearing loss and tinnitus affect most survivors of lightning strikes. But lightning can cause permanent sensorineural hearing loss, affecting either the inner ear, the auditory cortex in the brain, or both.

True Stories

As you now know, many things can cause a sudden sensorineural hearing loss. Most of these are things over which you have no control, but let us give you just a few examples of SSHL from our patient files.

It's More Than the Flu

Jaime recently finished the eighth grade and was looking forward to going to high school in September. Just before her family's scheduled summer vacation, she caught a bad cold that persisted and worsened with a fever above 103°F and muscle aches all over her body. Her pediatrician became concerned when she complained of a severe headache along with a stiff neck, so the pediatrician admitted Jaime to the hospital for workup for possible meningitis. When the lab results from a spinal tap revealed changes consistent with bacterial meningitis, the doctor ordered appropriate antibiotic medication. During Jaime's first night in the hospital, she woke up just before sunrise with severe dizziness, ringing in both ears, and an inability to hear. An MRI done that morning didn't reveal any tumors or serious middle ear disease, but a screening hearing test performed at the bedside showed significant hearing loss in both ears. Because her headache and flu-like symptoms were improving and her dizziness had lessened, she was discharged from the hospital the following day with home health treatments. A hearing test done at the ENT's office revealed a moderate-severe sensorineural hearing loss in both ears. Hearing aids were prescribed and she was given loaner aids to try. Eight weeks following the meningitis, a repeat MRI showed her inner ears to be clear of any scar tissue. A repeat hearing test showed that the moderate-severe loss had persisted. The hearing aids did provide significant benefit, and three months after onset of her hearing loss, Jaime was fitted with two digital hearing aids of her own.

Lost the Competition, and That's Not All

Jane, 28 years old and an experienced rider, was thrown from her horse during a competition, and a CT scan of her skull revealed a fracture of the temporal bone. She had been wearing her helmet and had no other obvious problems but noticed she couldn't hear in her right ear. She had blood in her middle ear that, like a bruise, resolved after a few weeks. However, her hearing was still reduced, and a hearing test confirmed a severe sensorineural hearing loss. Because she has normal hearing in her left ear, Jane has chosen not to use a hearing aid at this time. But she has made her family and friends aware of her loss and asks them to speak to her "good" side.

You Abuse, You Lose

Suzanne, a retired nurse, worked on a rehabilitation ward for years before injuring her back while lifting a patient, and has had chronic back pain since that injury. Although she's had multiple back surgeries, her debilitating pain has persisted. She recently came to the otology clinic complaining of loud tinnitus in both ears and a complete loss of hearing that occurred suddenly. When an audiogram showed a profound hearing loss in both ears, she was placed on high-dose steroids in an attempt to improve her hearing and even underwent the injection of steroid directly into her middle ear. Despite these measures, her profound hearing loss persisted. Upon further questioning, she acknowledged that she'd been taking up to 40 Vicodin pills per day to control her chronic back pain. Her MRI scan was normal, and doctors concluded that she had sudden sensorineural hearing loss from Vicodin toxicity. Unable to benefit from hearing aids, she underwent cochlear implantation and is currently getting very good results from her implant.

Fishing for Answers

John, a very fit and health-conscious man in his 30s, had noticed a gradual decline in his hearing over the past six months. His audiogram showed a flat sensorineural hearing loss across all frequencies as well as a decrease in his word understanding. He was treated with steroids and took potent vitamins but had no improvement in his hearing. During one of his return visits to the clinic, the discussion turned to John's health-conscious lifestyle and the diet that he follows as part of that lifestyle. When it turned out that John's primary source of protein was fish—he was a pescatarian—and his favorite fish was swordfish, he was sent to the laboratory to have special blood tests performed, one of which was for detection of the level of mercury in his blood. The results showed that the mercury level in John's blood was sky-high, so his doctor concluded that the toxic effects of mercury poisoning were causing his hearing loss. John stopped eating all fish immediately, and over the course of the next several months his hearing returned to almost normal levels.

The Least You Need to Know

- Most sudden sensorineural hearing loss is idiopathic—the cause remains unknown.
- Viruses and bacteria can cause labyrinthitis, inflammation of the inner ear leading to sensorineural hearing loss.
- Aminoglycoside antibiotics and chemotherapy agents may be necessary to treat life-threatening conditions but can cause SSHL, so hearing should be monitored closely while on these drugs.
- Overuse of certain pain medications can result in profound SSHL.
- Environmental toxins, such as mercury, can cause hearing loss at high levels.

Inner Ear Fluid Imbalances

In This Chapter

- Ménière's disease and cochlear hydrops
- Causes of inner ear fluid imbalances
- Drugs and diet to control Ménière's disease symptoms
- Surgical procedures for the vertigo caused by Ménière's disease

Most sensorineural hearing loss either stays the same for long periods of time or gets worse very slowly. However, the two types of hearing loss due to inner ear fluid imbalance—*Ménière's disease* and *cochlear hydrops*—are different from other types of sensorineural hearing loss. In these two disorders, the hearing loss tends to change or fluctuate. On a given day, the hearing may change considerably from better to worse and even back to better. In both Ménière's disease and cochlear hydrops, symptoms of fullness in the ear and tinnitus also usually accompany the changing hearing. These two disorders are thought to be caused by excess fluid in the inner ear.

The National Institute on Deafness and other Communication Disorders (NIDCD) estimates that there are currently about 615,000 people with diagnosed Ménière's disease in the United States, and 45,500 newly diagnosed cases occur each year. In this chapter, we describe the clinical symptoms of Ménière's disease and cochlear hydrops, what is known about their causes, and the variety of treatments for these disorders.

DEFINITION

Ménière's disease is a disease of the inner ear thought to be caused by fluid imbalances in both the organ of hearing and the organ of balance. It results in episodes of vertigo as well as hearing loss and tinnitus or ear fullness.

Hydrops is an excessive accumulation of fluid in any of the tissues or cavities of the body. **Cochlear hydrops** is the presence of excess fluid, called endolymph, in the cochlea, or organ of hearing of the inner ear. It produces symptoms of fluctuating hearing loss and tinnitus or ear fullness.

Symptoms and Diagnosis

There is no objective test, such as a blood test or x-ray, that we can use to determine whether someone has Ménière's disease or cochlear hydrops. To diagnose these disorders, doctors use several procedures, including a medical history interview and physical examination, hearing and balance tests, and possibly an MRI (to rule out other causes).

If a patient relates a history of fluctuating hearing loss, has had at least two episodes of severe, violent vertigo lasting at least 20 minutes each time, and has tinnitus or a feeling of pressure in the ear, a diagnosis can be made of Ménière's disease. Frequently, dizziness or imbalance also occurs.

LISTEN UP

Many types of dizziness are misdiagnosed as Ménière's disease. Unless an individual has had at least two spells of true vertigo severe enough to stop all activities for at least 20 minutes, hearing loss that may fluctuate, and either tinnitus or ear pressure or both, he or she probably does not have Ménière's disease. The symptom of ear fullness alone may indicate a problem with the outer ear (ear wax, for example) or middle ear (fluid behind the eardrum), as well as the inner ear.

Occasionally, fluctuating hearing loss, head noise, and ear pressure occur without vertigo or dizziness. This variation is called cochlear hydrops. Some doctors and researchers think cochlear hydrops might be a beginning phase of Ménière's disease. About a third of people first diagnosed with cochlear hydrops are later diagnosed with Ménière's disease, yet many other patients never get the vertigo that defines Ménière's disease. In the remainder of this chapter, we refer mainly to Ménière's disease. But all discussions regarding medical treatment and treatment specifically for the hearing loss seen in Mènière's disease also apply to cochlear hydrops.

HAVE YOU HEARD?

The dizziness we now associate with Ménière's disease was actually described in the 1830s by observing pigeons! A researcher intentionally produced injury to different parts of the balance mechanisms of the inner ears of pigeons and then observed that they showed signs of imbalance. Thirty years later, in 1861, a French physician named Prosper Ménière first associated dizziness in humans with the inner ear. Later, the condition of fluctuating sensorineural hearing loss, episodes of vertigo, and head noise was named for him—Ménière's disease.

The changing or fluctuating hearing loss associated with Ménière's disease and cochlear hydrops can make them difficult to diagnose at first. A patient might tell the doctor that he or she has a hearing loss, but upon testing, all hearing levels are normal. On another day, the same type of hearing test might find an objective, obvious hearing loss. It's often necessary for the doctor to obtain a number of hearing tests on different days to make the diagnosis of Ménière's disease or cochlear hydrops.

In both disorders, the hearing goes up and down. But over time, the hearing loss may get worse so that the "good" hearing isn't quite as good as the previous time and the "bad" hearing is worse than the previous time. Eventually, the hearing fluctuation may stop, and the individual may be left with a permanent, nonchanging hearing loss. One goal of treatment is to "stabilize" the hearing so it stops getting progressively worse. Fortunately, rarely do Ménière's disease or cochlear hydrops cause someone to go deaf or lose all useful hearing.

The symptoms of Ménière's disease often seem to start suddenly and can occur daily or as infrequently as less than once a year. Vertigo, often the most unbearable symptom of Ménière's disease, usually involves a whirling dizziness that may force one to lie down. These vertigo attacks, which may come with little or no warning, can lead to severe nausea, vomiting, and sweating. Many people with Ménière's disease may also experience some dizziness when they change position, such as suddenly turning the head toward the side with the ear that has Ménière's, but this type of dizziness usually lasts only seconds and is not as severe as the spinning dizziness of vertigo.

Some people with Ménière's disease have attacks that start with tinnitus, a loss of hearing, or a full feeling or pressure in the affected ear before the vertigo occurs. It's important to remember that all these symptoms are unpredictable. Usually, an attack lasts several hours, and people experience these discomforts in differing degrees and at different time intervals. Some people may feel slight vertigo a few times a year. Others may be occasionally disturbed by loud, uncontrollable tinnitus while sleeping. Some disease sufferers may also notice a hearing loss and feel unsteady all day long for some period of time. Other occasional symptoms of Ménière's disease include headaches, stomach discomfort, and diarrhea. A person's hearing tends to recover between attacks but over time becomes worse.

A few people experience what are informally known as drop attacks—a sudden, severe attack of dizziness or vertigo that causes the sufferer to fall if not already sitting down. The experience may be like a feeling of being pushed or pulled. Some patients may find it impossible to get up for some time, until the attack passes or medication starts to work.

The following findings about Ménière's disease come from various studies:

- It's a little more common in women than in men.

- On average, symptoms first occur between the ages of 30 and 50 but can start much younger or much older.

- Most of the time, symptoms occur only in one ear. Over time, some people (about 20 to 40 percent) get symptoms in their second ear.

- Dizziness, ear fullness, and tinnitus have each been reported as the very first symptom by an equal number of people with the disease. One of these symptoms is likely to start before the first attack of vertigo.

- The first vertigo attack often occurs only a few days after the very first symptom. But a few people didn't get a second symptom until many years later.

LISTEN UP

Pay careful attention whenever you have a Ménière's disease vertigo attack to see whether you can identify any warning signs that an attack was coming. You may be able to find some triggers, such as diet, stress, and so on, that you can avoid.

Causes of Ménière's Disease

Ménière's disease is diagnosed as a clinical disorder; that is, the diagnosis is based entirely on the patient's symptoms. It is called "idiopathic" (of unknown origin), meaning that at the present time, we don't truly know what causes it. However, we do know a great deal about this condition.

Fluids in the inner ear chambers are constantly being produced and absorbed by structures that are part of the hearing and balance system. Any disturbance in this delicate relationship results in the overproduction or underabsorption of the fluids, which leads to increased fluid pressure—that's the hydrops that we briefly explained earlier.

So how does the increased fluid pressure cause the symptoms of Ménière's disease? Two different types of fluids in the inner ear have different chemical compositions and are separated by a membrane. An increase in one of the fluids can cause the membrane to balloon out. Eventually, the membrane may rupture, or the distended membrane itself may leak, allowing the two different fluids to mix. Many scientists believe this mixing can produce the symptoms of the disease.

But what causes the malfunction in the production or absorption of fluid? Current thinking is that something may cause inflammation of the structures that produce and absorb the inner ear fluids, perhaps in a patient with a genetic tendency for this problem. A variety of things might cause this inflammation, triggering the onset of the disease. These triggers could include a long-lasting viral infection of the inner ear, allergies, an autoimmune reaction, or metabolic abnormalities such as hypoglycemia (low blood sugar) or thyroid disease. It is also possible an affected patient may be born with a structural abnormality in the inner ear that is more likely to result in Mèniére's symptoms.

Medical Treatments

Treatment of Ménière's disease is usually medical but, in severe cases, may be surgical. Surgical treatment is not used for the hearing loss associated with either Ménière's disease or cochlear hydrops, and the medical treatment of cochlear hydrops is the same as that we describe for Ménière's disease. Medical treatment is aimed at improving the inner ear blood circulation and controlling the fluid pressure changes of the inner ear chambers. Surgical treatment, described in the following section, is used only for the vertigo of Ménière's disease.

Medical treatment of Ménière's disease varies with the individual patient, depending upon what the suspected cause is, how serious the symptoms are, and how often the symptoms occur. Treatment generally consists of medications to stimulate the inner ear circulation, decrease the inner ear fluid pressure, or prevent inner ear allergic or inflammatory reactions.

Steroids, Diuretics, and Other Drugs

The most common treatment for Ménière's disease is the use of diuretics or water pills, medications most often prescribed for the treatment of high blood pressure. They work by stimulating the kidney to get rid of more sodium in the urine than under normal circumstances. Patients with Ménière's disease are believed to have an abnormal balance of sodium and potassium in the inner ear fluids. Removing more sodium from the body than is normal can help draw out some of this excess sodium from the inner ear, which may reduce the fluid pressure and improve or stabilize hearing, reduce tinnitus, and decrease or stop attacks of vertigo. For the same reason, patients are advised to follow a low-salt diet (the salt in food is sodium chloride).

Medications that relax the blood vessels in the body, called vasodilators, are also commonly used to stimulate the inner ear blood circulation. Histamine, a chemical commonly released in allergic reactions, is sometimes given either in tablet, drop, or injectable form to treat the disease. It's thought that the histamine relaxes the blood vessels in the inner ear and also has an effect on the transmission of balance signals in the brain and inner ear. Substances that constrict the blood vessels have an opposite effect and should be avoided or limited in the diet. Unfortunately, these substances include caffeine and nicotine—commonly consumed by many people.

Steroids (strong anti-inflammatory drugs) are being used more and more for a "rescue" treatment of Ménière's disease if other medical treatment fails. This treatment can be in either pill form or by injections through the eardrum, called intratympanic. A patient with the disease will probably obtain at least temporary relief of symptoms with the use of steroids, but sometimes this benefit is long-lasting. Steroids taken by mouth are often prescribed for a period of one to four weeks. The dose starts high and then is gradually decreased. Steroid pills do have potentially serious side effects, including osteoporosis (thinning of the bone), increased blood sugar, insomnia, weight gain, increased risk of glaucoma and cataracts, and even emotional changes. The pills probably will take a little longer to work than injecting steroids through the eardrum, but they may give a longer benefit.

Usually done in an otolaryngologist's office, intratympanic steroid injections can be given as a single injection or multiple times over a few days to a few weeks. Injections may give more rapid improvement than pills because the amount of steroid absorbed into the inner ear is higher. First, the patient lies down, and the eardrum is made numb so the injection is not too uncomfortable. After the injection, the patient continues lying down with the injected ear facing up for 20 to 30 minutes, which helps increase the absorption of the steroid into the inner ear. Possible complications of intratympanic injections include a hole in the eardrum (which might have to be repaired surgically), infection, and a small risk of steroid-produced symptoms throughout the body such as those seen with use of steroid pills.

In addition to these drug treatments, there are several investigational treatments for which evidence of effectiveness is still lacking. This includes antiviral medications if a viral trigger for Ménière's disease is suspected and also some nutritional substances.

Low-Salt, Low-Caffeine Diet

It's commonly recommended that people with Ménière's disease avoid excess salt in the diet, and we encourage patients to monitor their salt intake by reading labels on food packaging. Ideally, patients should try to keep their sodium intake between 1,500 and 2,000 milligrams a day. In addition to a low-salt diet, they should avoid caffeine. This includes coffee, tea, and chocolate (oh, no!).

In Appendix D we provide some tables that can help you determine what foods to avoid on a low-salt diet and how much sodium or caffeine is contained in many common foods and drinks.

Allergy Treatment

There appears to be a link between Ménière's disease and allergic reactions to inhaled substances (pollen, pet dander, grasses, etc.) or food in some patients. Among our patients, 41 percent of those with Ménière's disease have had a positive test for inhalant allergies; another 17 percent say they have allergies but have not been formally tested. In contrast, only 14 percent of the overall United States population has been diagnosed with allergy by a physician.

Treatment with some form of anti-allergy medications for the vertigo of Ménière's disease is very common. These medications include antihistamines such as prescription-strength meclizine, Benadryl, and Dramamine. Other antihistamines such as Phenergan and Compazine are often recommended to treat the nausea associated with Ménière's disease. Most oral medications used to treat Ménière's disease don't seem to have any effect on the hearing loss but are useful for treatment of vertigo. Interestingly, the newer, nondrowsy antihistamines, used in the treatment of the nasal symptoms of allergy, don't appear to help the symptoms of Ménière's disease at all.

There is now considerable experience using either allergy injection therapy for inhaled allergies and/or dietary treatment of suspected food allergies in patients with

Ménière's disease. This form of allergy treatment has been shown to help reduce the severity and the number of attacks of vertigo in patients who also have allergy. The allergy treatment may also help stabilize hearing—note that here we mean to keep hearing from getting worse, not actually to improve it. Some scientists don't think enough good studies have been done yet to really prove that allergy treatment can help Ménière's symptoms. But if you have allergies that are bothering you anyway, you might find that specialized treatment for those allergies can also help your Ménière's disease. Detailed information on the treatment of allergies in patients with hearing loss is presented in Chapter 12.

The Role of Stress

For decades, many patients have commonly mentioned that their symptoms of hearing loss and vertigo get worse during times of emotional stress. Remember, stress is not just an emotional state but also results in the release of many chemicals in the body that elevate blood pressure as well as produce other physiological effects. Some of the physical reactions to these chemicals, although we don't know which ones, may contribute to making disease symptoms worse during stressful times. While no studies have proven this relationship, it certainly wouldn't hurt (and might help) a person with Ménière's to participate in activities that relieve stress, such as regular exercise (the specific exercise should be based on how much dizziness or imbalance one has) or meditation.

HAVE YOU HEARD?

In the early 1970s, many doctors (especially in England) believed that Ménière's disease was a psychosomatic disorder, meaning it was caused by psychological factors. One of the reasons for this belief was that patients with Ménière's disease often came into the office rather hysterical about their problem. To study this, patients were given tests that appeared to show they had some psychological abnormalities, but these studies had many flaws. So our institution asked two clinical psychologists to really study this issue carefully. When they did, they found that, yes, people with dizziness scored differently than people without dizziness on a variety of tests about anxiety, stress, and other psychological characteristics. But those with Ménière's disease were no different from people who had dizziness from other well-known ear diseases. They concluded that Ménière's disease was not psychosomatic, but rather somatopsychic—that the possibility of having an attack of dizziness or vertigo at an inopportune time (for example, while driving or standing at the top of some stairs) could lead one to feel a bit hysterical!

Surgical Treatments

Surgical procedures are not useful for improving or stabilizing the hearing loss associated with either Ménière's disease or cochlear hydrops. But surgery can help greatly when medical treatment fails to relieve the severe attacks of dizziness. With a number of different effective surgical procedures available, the choice depends on the individual patient and the amount of hearing loss already present, age, and other factors.

Reducing Inner Ear Fluid Pressure

The endolymphatic sac shunt operation, which is usually performed under general anesthesia on an outpatient basis, drains excess fluid (endolymph) from the inner ear. The surgeon makes an incision behind the ear and performs a mastoid operation (mastoidectomy, see Chapter 4). A microscopic tube is inserted into the structure that produces and absorbs endolymph for the inner ear (the endolymphatic sac) to drain out any excess fluid. This tube is left in place permanently.

HAVE YOU HEARD?

Alan Shepard was the first American (and the second person) in space when he flew a manned space flight in May of 1961. But he was grounded from 1963 to 1969 because of Ménière's disease! After Dr. William House performed a new surgical procedure he had developed—an endolymphatic sac shunt—Shepard was able to return to active astronaut status. In 1971, as part of the Apollo 14 mission, he became the fifth man to walk on the Moon (where he famously "played golf"). Dr. House and his wife were invited to watch the lift-off, and Shepard spoke to them from space.

A shunt operation usually is chosen if a patient's hearing is still good in the involved ear. Some permanent additional hearing loss occurs in about 5 percent of patients as a result of this surgery, but total loss of hearing from the operation occurs very rarely—only in about 1 percent of patients.

Cutting the Balance Nerve

The vestibular or balance nerve (part of the eighth cranial nerve, which also includes the hearing nerve) is responsible for sending the signals to the brain from the balance mechanisms of the inner ear. Normally, these impulses to the brain come in equal amounts from both the right and left inner ear. When one inner ear is not function-ing correctly, the brain receives nerve impulses that are no longer equal, causing it to perceive this information as distorted or off balance. The brain then sends messages to the eyes, causing them to move back and forth abnormally (called *nystagmus*) and making the surroundings appear to spin.

DEFINITION

Nystagmus is an involuntary rhythmical or jittery oscillation of the eyeballs. The direction and type of eye movements help doctors to diagnose the source of dizziness.

The brain can eventually become used to and ignore abnormal or unequal impulses from the inner ears. Called compensation, this is more likely to happen when the signal from one side is nearly all or totally gone rather than when the nerve fires sometimes and not at other times. Because of this, an operation to cut the balance nerve on the malfunctioning side nearly always prevents any further attacks of severe vertigo. However, some dizziness or unsteadiness may continue for a number of weeks or months until the brain adapts. Although balance after this operation is not normal, it does prevent vertigo.

Several different surgical procedures can be used to section, or cut, the vestibular nerve, all performed under general anesthesia. Two procedures are used when hearing is good in the involved ear. In the retrolabyrinthine procedure, an incision is made behind the ear, a mastoidectomy (see Chapter 4) is performed, and the balance nerve is cut before it enters the inner ear. This procedure requires some hospitalization. Up to 2 percent of people may develop a severe hearing impairment in the operated ear because of the surgery. A middle fossa nerve section requires an incision above the ear, where the balance nerve is cut before it enters the inner ear. The stay in the hospital is usually five to seven days, and up to 5 percent of patients may develop a severe hearing impairment in the operated ear.

For people who already have a severe hearing loss, surgeons might use a translaby-rinthine labyrinthectomy and section of the vestibular nerve. Through an incision behind the ear, a mastoidectomy is performed, the inner ear balance chambers (the semicircular canals) are removed, and the balance nerve is cut. This procedure, which requires the patient to stay in the hospital for a few days, results in total loss of hear-ing in the operated ear. It also frequently results in a temporary increase in dizziness. The translabyrinthine labyrinthectomy procedure is usually performed only if other surgery has not been successful.

Patients who have ongoing balance problems, and especially those who have required surgery, should consider balance training or therapy (called vestibular rehabilitation) with a qualified therapist. These are often physical therapists or others who have had specialized training in balance rehabilitation. This training can speed up the process of compensation, getting the brain to ignore the unequal input that causes dizziness. Vestibular rehabilitation may be helpful even in those who do not have surgery.

Risks and Complications of Surgery

There are a number of possible complications from the surgeries for Ménière's disease, which your doctor will discuss with you in detail for the specific procedure you are going to have performed. Following is an overview of possible complications:

- Hearing loss. Further hearing impairment in the operated ear may occur following any of the procedures and is the expected result following some.

- Tinnitus. Tinnitus usually remains the same as before surgery. If the hearing is worse following surgery, tinnitus may be more noticeable.

- Taste disturbance and mouth dryness. These problems are not uncommon for a few weeks following surgery, and in some patients, this disturbance lasts longer.

- Weakness of the face. Because the facial nerve travels through the ear bone (see Chapter 1), temporary weakness of one side of the face is a possible complication of many types of ear surgery but occurs infrequently. Permanent paralysis of the face is extremely rare. If it does happen, eye complications could develop, requiring treatment by an eye specialist.

- Spinal fluid leak. All the operations described above result in a temporary leak of cerebrospinal fluid (fluid surrounding the brain). This leak is always closed before the end of surgery. Uncommonly, the leak reopens, and further surgery may be necessary to stop it.

- Infection. Infection is a rare occurrence following dizziness surgery. But if it happens, it could lead to meningitis, an infection in the fluid surrounding the brain, which might require staying in the hospital longer for treatment.

- Hematoma. A collection of blood under the skin at the site of the incision develops in a small percentage of patients, which can prolong hospitalization and healing. If this complication occurs, it may require another operation to remove the clot.

Other Treatments

There are several other treatments that are currently used for Ménière's disease aimed at reducing the vestibular symptoms. These include a chemical means of destroying the balance nerve and a device intended to reduce the inner ear fluid pressure. And let's not forget that hearing loss from Ménière's or cochlear hydrops might be helped by using a hearing aid. We discuss these treatment options in the following sections.

Injections Through the Eardrum

A relatively newer treatment being used increasingly for the vertigo associated with Ménière's disease is to inject a powerful antibiotic, gentamycin, through the eardrum. Gentamycin is usually used as a life-saving drug for severe infections, and as you learned in Chapter 9, it's ototoxic. Usually, the effects of gentamycin are seen first on the balance nerve, and only later after longer use does it cause sensorineural hearing loss. Some doctors realized that this meant perhaps it could be used to intentionally destroy or damage much of the balance function of the inner ear and yet not harm hearing. So instead of surgery to cut the vestibular nerve, small injections of gentamycin are made through the eardrum where it can be absorbed directly into the inner ear. Unfortunately, there has been some significant hearing damage from the gentamycin in up to 30 percent of patients, and hearing loss can range from mild to deafness.

A major advantage of gentamycin treatment is that it can be given as an outpatient procedure in a physician's office. It may be given in multiple, small injections to try to decrease the potential for damage to the hearing nerve. It's usually recommended for those patients who have uncontrolled vertigo not helped by medical treatment and who already have some significant loss of hearing in the involved ear. We usually do not recommend this treatment for people with good hearing in the ear that has the disease because there is a greater risk of increased hearing loss than with surgery. But in people with other medical conditions that make them poor candidates for surgery, gentamycin may be the best alternative for controlling vertigo, even with the increased risk of some loss of hearing.

Devices

A low-pressure pulse generator, called the Meniett device, is another fairly new treatment for the dizziness symptoms. This small, table-top device delivers a wave of low-pressure pulses to the inner ear through a tympanostomy tube, which is placed in the eardrum (see Chapter 6) using local anesthesia in the otolaryngologist's office.

Then a small, rubber air tube from the Meniett is placed into the ear canal, and pulses of low pressure are generated. These pulses are thought to produce pumping movement in the inner ear fluids in a way that reduces the extra fluid pressure that might cause the symptoms of Ménière's disease. The patient can use the device at home for three to five minutes three times per day. Patients receive varying degrees of relief from the device, ranging from complete relief to no improvement at all. The Meniett device has not been shown to improve hearing levels but rather is a treatment for vertigo or dizziness.

Many patients with Ménière's disease benefit from the use of a properly fitted hearing aid. All patients with Ménière's disease or cochlear hydrops have sensorineural hearing loss; this is part of the definition of these disorders. In some cases, the hearing loss may fluctuate and then revert to completely normal hearing, but in other cases, the hearing loss may fluctuate and eventually result in permanent sensorineural hearing loss. Fortunately, it's the uncommon patient who progresses to total deafness.

Hearing aid evaluations in these patients are challenging for the audiologist because the hearing loss can seem different on different days. Such patients often tell the otolarygologist, "I tried hearing aids, and they didn't work for me." The most beneficial hearing aid for these people is likely one that has different programs or levels of amplification that the wearer can choose depending on how much the hearing is fluctuating on a given day. Once the audiologist or hearing aid dispenser has determined how much a person's hearing fluctuates, he can use that information to program the hearing aid. We discuss hearing aids in detail in Chapter 16.

True Stories

Here are some patient stories to help you better understand the diagnosis and treatment of Ménière's disease and cochlear hydrops. Notice that although these cases represent a range of ages, there are no children or senior citizens, as both diseases typically start in adulthood and before age 50.

It's the Chinese Food!

Joanna, a 47-year-old woman, had been diagnosed with Ménière's disease on her right side only a year ago. Despite being treated with a diuretic and advised to follow a low-salt diet, she had problems with her hearing fluctuating. After careful questioning, it seemed the worst problems occurred on weekends. More questioning revealed that every Friday night, she and her husband went out for Chinese food. She always asked for low-sodium soy sauce because of her diagnosis, but low-sodium soy sauce still contains a whopping 700 mg of sodium per tablespoon! Realizing this, Joanna was encouraged to change her food preference to another variety. After she began using available information (like the tables in Appendix D) to determine her sodium intake and has restricted it to no more than 1,500 mg per day, her hearing has remained stable.

No Infection, but Injection

Roger was a 55-year-old man with a long history of Ménière's disease in the left ear when he was referred to us. He was using diuretics and following a low-sodium diet, and he had ruled out allergies finding none, but he continued to have three spells of disabling vertigo each month. Upon examination, he had only 20 percent remaining hearing in his left ear. He also had a mild high-frequency loss in the right ear that did not fluctuate. Because of the severe loss already present in his left ear, we treated him with gentamycin antibiotic injected through the eardrum. He has had no vertigo for three years now, and has no further loss of hearing in the left ear. He wears a small hearing aid in the right ear to help his high-frequency loss.

It's Not Always Ménière's Disease

Brianna, a 39-year-old patient, had fluctuating hearing in her right ear. She did complain of ear fullness and tinnitus on the right side, but she'd never had any vertigo. Often, she noticed her ear symptoms when she was experiencing asthma and nasal congestion from her allergies. Her internist had told her she had Ménière's disease and that she "should live with it." She was also told she would eventually lose all her balance and go deaf on that side. Our testing showed that she had a mild to moderate sensorineural hearing loss in the right ear and normal hearing on the left. Allergy testing showed moderate to high sensitivity to grass, tree, and weed pollens, dust mites, house cats, and wheat. We correctly diagnosed her with cochlear hydrops in the right ear, allergic rhinitis, and asthma and started her on diuretics, a low-sodium and wheat elimination diet, and allergy shots. Five years later, she has never developed vertigo, has had improved hearing in her right ear, and has minimal symptoms from her asthma. She has a hearing aid she keeps for times when her hearing is worse, and she uses occasional antihistamines before going to a home with a cat.

A Hearing Aid Got the Job Done

Jenny was a 24-year-old woman referred for problems with hearing. Having been diagnosed with Ménière's disease two years before we saw her, she wanted to know if there was a surgery that could help her hearing. She had had difficulty during her last year of college, having always to sit in the front row because of her hearing loss. Now she was in her first job (in marketing) and was afraid she wouldn't be promoted. She hadn't had any vertigo for three years, and she had begun taking a diuretic. But she'd been told "there was no treatment for hearing loss with Ménière's disease." Hearing tests showed she had fluctuating hearing loss in both ears, ranging from a mild hearing loss on a "good" day to a moderate loss throughout all the frequencies on her "bad" days. It's true: no surgery could help her hearing, but we fitted her for programmable hearing aids (she decides which program to use on a given day), and she has now been promoted in her job!

The Least You Need to Know

- Ménière's disease and cochlear hydrops are thought to be caused by fluid imbalances in the inner ear.
- Ménière's disease symptoms include vertigo, hearing loss, and tinnitus and/or ear fullness.
- Diuretics and a low-salt, low-caffeine diet are the first line of treatment for both Ménière's disease and cochlear hydrops.
- If medical treatment does not work, surgery or intratympanic injections of gentamycin can be used to eliminate severe attacks of vertigo.
- A hearing aid, especially a programmable device, can help hearing loss from Ménière's or cochlear hydrops.

Tumors of the Temporal Bone

In This Chapter

- Acoustic tumors and their removal or treatment
- The importance of tumor size
- Different surgical approaches to remove these tumors
- The role of radiation therapy
- Risks and complications of treatment
- Other tumors that can affect hearing and their treatment

The temporal bones sit on each side of the skull and enclose the hearing and balance organs. Next to the temporal bone is an area called the cerebellopontine angle (CPA). This area, between the brain and the skull, contains the hearing and balance nerves as well as the nerve that controls facial movement and sensation. A person with a diagnosis of a tumor in the CPA most likely has what we commonly call an acoustic tumor.

These tumors are nonmalignant fibrous growths originating from the balance or vestibular nerve and do not spread or metastasize to other parts of the body. Because acoustic tumors are located deep inside the skull and are adjacent to vital brain centers in the brainstem, they affect surrounding structures in the brain that control vital functions. The brain is not invaded by an acoustic tumor, but the tumor pushes on the brain as it enlarges. As it grows, the tumor typically first affects hearing because it protrudes from the internal auditory canal into an area behind the temporal bone. The internal auditory canal (IAC) is the bony channel connecting the CPA to the structures of the temporal bone. The seventh (facial) and eighth (hearing and balance) cranial nerves travel through the IAC as they move from the inner ear to the brain. The internal auditory canal is the site of development of acoustic tumors.

When large acoustic tumors cause severe pressure on the brainstem and cerebellum of the brain, they threaten vital functions that sustain life.

Before we continue, let's insert one note about terminology. Acoustic tumors are more correctly or technically called vestibular schwannomas because these tumors arise from specialized cells known as Schwann cells and almost exclusively involve the vestibular division of the hearing and balance nerve (the eighth cranial nerve). However, historically, people have called these tumors acoustic tumors or, occasionally, acoustic neuromas. In this book, we call them acoustic tumors because they primarily affect hearing.

Acoustic tumors constitute 6 to 10 percent of all brain tumors and are found in roughly 1 of every 100,000 people per year in the United States. This translates to about 2,500 to 3,000 newly diagnosed acoustic tumors per year. Symptoms may develop at any age but usually occur between the ages of 30 and 60. Unilateral (on one side) acoustic tumors are not hereditary. Several other kinds of tumors also occur in the area of the temporal bone and can affect hearing and balance or facial function. In this chapter, we discuss acoustic tumors in some detail and touch briefly on other kinds of tumors as we tell you about the surgical approaches for removing tumors from this area of the head, the relationship of size of tumor to surgical approach and possible outcome of surgery, the risks and complications of surgery, and other approaches such as radiation therapy.

Acoustic Tumors

The treatment goal for any benign brain tumor is to eliminate the tumor while preserving neurological function. Because of their location near delicate brain structures, acoustic tumors are a complex treatment problem. Specialized professionals provide the best care for someone with an acoustic tumor, as this is one of the few types of brain tumors that must be attended to by physicians who specialize in and frequently treat this condition.

Because acoustic tumors are located deep inside the skull and are adjacent to vital brain centers, their first signs or symptoms usually are related to ear function and include tinnitus and often disturbances in hearing on one side as well as unsteadiness or loss of balance. As these tumors grow larger, they involve other surrounding nerves having to do with more vital functions. Headaches may develop as a result of increased pressure on the brain. If allowed to continue over a long period of time, this pressure on the brain can eventually result in death.

LISTEN UP

Severe symptoms such as headaches, staggering, and mental confusion can indicate an increase of intracranial pressure. Immediate attention is required because this pressure can be a life-threatening complication.

In most cases, acoustic tumors grow slowly over a period of years, but sometimes the rate of growth is more rapid. Symptoms can be mild or severe, and multiple symptoms might develop rather rapidly. Although many people have hearing loss on one side, head noise, and balance difficulties, rarely are these symptoms due to an acoustic tumor. But everyone with these symptoms should have a very careful evaluation. Today, the most common method of diagnosing an acoustic tumor is by a detailed MRI of the head. In some cases, the tumor becomes relatively large before a definite diagnosis is established, but the problem must be faced as it exists at the time of diagnosis. Whatever risks are necessary to remove one of these tumors, they're less than the risks of leaving the tumor untreated.

Preserving life is the most important objective of treatment. A secondary objective is to preserve as many vital structures as possible, and many patients resume a completely normal life following treatment. Some people experience minor physical handicap; a few may suffer a physical handicap that persists. In the following paragraphs, we discuss three treatment options: watchful waiting or observation, surgery, and radiation therapy. The choice of treatment is based on tumor size, hearing in the ear at time of diagnosis, patient age and health, and, of course, patient preference.

Size of Tumor

Risks and complications of acoustic tumor treatment vary with the size of the tumor: the larger the tumor, the more likelihood of complications and of serious complications as well. Tumor size is reported using the metric scale, usually as centimeters (cm) or millimeters (mm) of the longest portion of the tumor (we measure in three different planes) or sometimes as volume (cm^3). If you can picture size better in inches, there are 2.54 cm per inch.

We classify tumors as small, medium, or large. Here are the details:

- Small tumor—Confined within the internal auditory canal that extends from the inner ear to the brain. Small tumors are either totally within the IAC (and if so, they are called intracanalicular) or up to 1.5 cm.

- Medium tumor—Has extended from the IAC into the brain cavity but has not yet produced pressure on the brain itself. Size is greater than 1.5 cm and less than 3 cm.

- Large tumor—Has extended out of the IAC into the brain cavity and is large enough to push on the brain. Tumors this size can sometimes produce pressure on the brain called hydrocephalus. Size is typically greater than 3 cm.

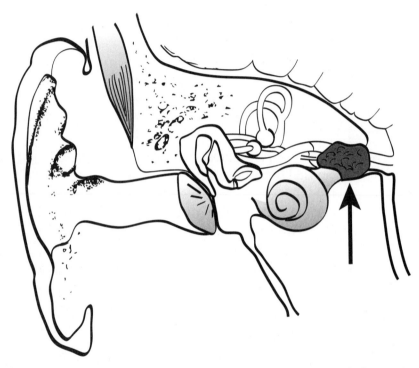

Drawing of a small acoustic tumor within the internal auditory canal, showing its proximity to the cochlea and inner ear structures.

Watchful Waiting

In most cases, it's definitely best to treat a growing tumor actively by surgical removal or by stopping its growth with radiation treatment. But for some people, monitoring the tumor at regular intervals to be sure it isn't growing can be an appropriate alternative. This approach, referred to as watchful waiting or observation, is usually used only in older patients who might be poor surgical candidates or those with other medical problems that make having surgery undesirable. Watchful waiting is not "doing nothing." The patient must have follow-up MRIs of the head, using contrast material, as often as every six months for the first year after diagnosis. If the tumor hasn't grown, repeated MRIs are done at the doctor's discretion, perhaps as often as yearly. Any change in symptoms also calls for an MRI to check for tumor growth. Because these tumors can grow rather suddenly, great care must be taken to treat the tumor before it's so large that complications are more likely. Remember, the smaller the tumor at time of active treatment, the better the outcome of treatment is likely to be. On the other hand, some tumors do not grow or grow only very slowly.

Surgical Approaches

To accomplish the preservation of life with a minimum of physical disturbance, a team of surgeons and assistants carries out the surgery—as well as the pre- and postoperative care—for patients with acoustic tumors. This team includes an internist, an anesthesiologist, a specially trained surgical nurse, a neurosurgeon, and a neurotologist (ear specialist who performs surgery related to inner ear and nerve problems).

The removal of an acoustic tumor, whether large or small, is a major surgical procedure, with possibilities of serious complications, including death. The risk involved in the removal of these tumors must never be minimized. The choice of surgical approach depends upon the size of the tumor and amount of remaining hearing. It's possible to save hearing in only a minority of cases; if hearing preservation is successful, the preserved hearing will not be better than the preoperative level and may be worse. The larger the tumor is, the lower the chances for hearing preservation. In some cases with poor preoperative hearing or a larger tumor, it's better to sacrifice the hearing in order to remove the tumor. All the following procedures are performed with the patient under general anesthesia. The surgeons look through an operating microscope and use special equipment to monitor the facial and possibly hearing nerves to prevent injury.

Translabyrinthine approach: This involves an incision behind the ear. The mastoid bone, which is a part of the temporal bone, and the inner ear structures are removed to expose the tumor, which is usually completely removed. Rarely, in a partial removal, a small fragment of tumor may be left. The opening in the mastoid area where bone was drilled out is filled with fat taken from the abdomen. This is inside the skull and can't be seen from the outside. The translabyrinthine approach sacrifices the hearing mechanisms of the inner ear, so the ear is made permanently deaf. We remove most large tumors by this approach, as well as smaller tumors in ears with little hearing remaining.

Middle fossa approach: An incision is made above the ear, and the brain in this area is lifted to expose the tumor. The tumor is completely removed in most cases. Every effort is made to preserve the hearing and still remove the tumor. Even in very small tumors (less than 1 cm), the tumor involves the hearing nerve or the artery leading to the inner ear in 40 percent of cases, so total loss of hearing occurs in the operated ear. As the tumor enlarges, the likelihood that it will involve the hearing nerve or cochlear artery increases. By the time the tumor is 2 cm, hearing loss nearly always occurs. We use this approach for small or smaller medium tumors in patients with useful hearing in the operated ear.

Retrosigmoid approach: An incision is made behind the ear, and the brain is depressed to expose the tumor, which we completely remove in most cases. This approach, like the middle fossa approach, includes an effort to preserve the hearing and still remove the tumor. In about 50 percent of cases, total loss of hearing in the operated ear results. Following this approach, some patients may experience persistent headaches. This approach we use for select small or medium tumors when the patient still has some useful hearing in the ear to be operated. The position and shape of the tumor, as well as the preference of the surgical team, are the criteria surgeons use when deciding between this approach and the middle fossa approach.

Partial removal of the tumor, regardless of its size, is necessary in rare cases if the patient's responses during surgery indicate disturbance of the vital brain centers that control respiration, blood pressure, or heart function. In this case, it's sometimes necessary to stop the operation before we can remove the entire tumor. Usually partial removal restores these vital brain center functions. However, they sometimes don't recover completely. If a tumor is only partially removed, the surgeon will tell you. It's possible that the remaining portion of the tumor may gradually enlarge and once again produce symptoms. If this happens, a later operation might be necessary. Usually the first operation reduces the size of the tumor enough that it has a chance to separate from the vital brain centers, and it can therefore be successfully removed at a later date (four to six months). In other cases, watchful waiting again comes into play.

Radiation Therapy

In recent years, some neurosurgeons have used stereotactic radiation therapy to treat acoustic tumors. This type of radiation therapy is different from radiation used for cancer; it's highly focused on the tumor, with only low levels of radiation affecting most of the brain. This type of treatment has proved effective for certain patients. Tumors up to 3 cm (small or medium) have been treated with radiation. While patients of all ages can be treated, stereotactic radiation therapy may be best for older patients because the long-term effectiveness (20 years or more) has yet to be determined. As with surgery, there are risks to hearing and to the facial nerve.

Several devices and methods are currently being used for carrying out stereotactic radiation therapy. Single-dose treatment is performed on a single day; fractionated therapy is carried out over the course of multiple days. There are theoretical advantages and disadvantages to each of these methods. For patients who choose or require stereotactic radiation therapy, we prefer Gamma Knife radiosurgery, which uses a single-dose procedure. This is considered the gold standard of radiation treatment for acoustic tumors because it's been used for the longest period of time and for by far the greatest number of patients. That is, there's more experience with this type of radiation treatment, so we know more about what to expect. *Gamma* refers to the type of radiation. Gamma rays "slice" through the tissues and bone of the skull to the site of the tumor without an actual incision. The term radiosurgery has stuck, even though the tumor is not actually being surgically removed. Because acoustic tumors are benign growths, many physicians do not routinely advise radiation treatment as it is not risk-free and does not result in disappearance of the tumor. After this treatment, some patients have experienced continued tumor growth that required surgical removal. In such cases, it can be more difficult to avoid surgical complications due to the effects of the radiation and the scar tissue it creates.

Risks and Complications of Surgery

It's not possible to list every complication that might occur before, during, or following a surgical procedure, but we can give you some idea of the risks and complications peculiar to acoustic tumor treatments. Mostly we discuss the risks of surgery, as this is the most common treatment for these tumors, but we briefly discuss the risks and complications of radiation therapy as well.

Hearing loss: In patients with small tumors, it's sometimes possible to save the hearing while still removing the tumor. When tumors are larger, however, the hearing is usually lost in the involved ear as a result of the surgical procedure. The hearing loss may be related to loss of blood supply to the inner ear, either through spasm or interruption of the supplying artery, or as a result of injury to the hearing nerve. Following the surgery in these situations, the patient hears only with the remaining good ear. Many people function quite adequately with only one hearing ear. We've discussed unilateral hearing loss (loss in one ear) in several other chapters of this book and later briefly discuss the hearing impairment following tumor removal.

Tinnitus: Tinnitus remains the same as before surgery in most cases. If the patient had tinnitus before surgery, it will most likely remain after surgery. In 10 percent of patients, the tinnitus may be more noticeable.

HAVE YOU HEARD?

In one study from our clinic, the majority of people who had tinnitus before surgery for acoustic tumor removal told us that it rarely went away after surgery but did sometimes improve (that is, decrease) in severity. About half the people who did not have tinnitus before surgery said they had some after surgery, but it was usually considered mild.

Taste disturbance and mouth dryness: Taste disturbance and mouth dryness is common for a few weeks following surgery, but in 5 percent of people, this disturbance lasts longer. Specialized nerve fibers travel with the facial nerve and carry our taste sensation from the front two thirds of the tongue back to the brain. Any irritation of this nerve during surgery leads to problems in taste or causes the mouth to feel overly dry.

Dizziness and balance disturbance: In acoustic tumor surgery, it's necessary to remove part or all of the balance nerve and, in most cases, to remove the inner ear balance mechanism. Because the tumor usually damages the balance system, tumor removal frequently results in improvement in any preoperative unsteadiness. But dizziness is common following surgery and may be severe for a few days. Imbalance or unsteadiness when the patient moves his or her head can occur until the normal balance mechanism in the opposite ear—along with the three other components of the balance system, the eyes, muscle-joint sense (proprioceptive system), and the brain—compensates for the loss in the operated ear, usually in one to four months. A few people say that they continue to notice unsteadiness for several years, especially when they're tired.

Occasionally, the blood supply to the cerebellum—the portion of the brain responsible for coordination—is decreased by the tumor or the removal of the tumor. Difficulty in coordination in arm and leg movements, a condition called ataxia, may result, but this complication is extremely rare.

Facial paralysis: Acoustic tumors are in intimate contact with the facial nerve, which closes the eye as well as controls the muscles of facial expression. Careful tumor removal, with the help of an operating microscope and facial nerve monitoring, usually results in keeping the nerve intact, but nerve stretching may result in swelling of the nerve, which may lead to temporary facial nerve dysfunction. Swelling of the facial nerve can occur because the tumor in the IAC has been pushing and distorting the nerve. Weakness, when it occurs, is usually temporary and can range from slight to total paralysis of one side of the face. It may last for 6 to 12 months. A few people experience permanent weakness. If it becomes certain that facial nerve function will not recover (approximately 1 to 2 percent of cases), a second operation called an *anastomosis* may be performed to connect the facial nerve to a nerve in the neck.

DEFINITION

Anastomosis is a process whereby cut ends of a nerve are sutured together. For the facial nerve, this can include reconnecting the two injured ends or splicing a graft in between the two injured ends when the nerve has actually been cut at surgery. More often, it is reconnecting one end of a different nerve to the end of the facial nerve.

In 1 to 2 percent of cases, the facial nerve passes through the center of the acoustic tumor. On occasion, the tumor may even originate from the facial nerve, a condition called facial nerve neuroma (more on this later in the chapter). In either instance, it's necessary to remove all or a portion of the nerve to accomplish tumor removal. When this is necessary, it may be possible immediately to reconnect the facial nerve or to remove a skin sensation nerve from the upper part of the neck (the greater auricular nerve) or from the leg (the sural nerve) to replace the missing portion of the facial nerve. When it's not possible to reconnect or replace the facial nerve, a second operation may be performed at a later time to reanimate the face. One option is called a facial-hypoglossal anastomosis, connecting the nerve of the tongue to the facial nerve, which restores some tone to the face and the beginning of a smile. Another option is called the facial reanimation operation. One of the chewing muscles (the temporalis muscle) is attached to the muscles of the face to help move them.

Nerve fibers responsible for eye tearing also travel with the facial nerve. If facial paralysis develops following surgery, the eye can become dry and unprotected because the eyelid is stuck open, and care by an eye specialist may be required. It can be necessary to use artificial tears, to tape the eye shut, or to use a moisture chamber or eye patch. When prolonged facial nerve paralysis is expected, an eye specialist may insert a spring eyelid closing device, a gold weight, or place a contact lens. This keeps the eye moistened as well as providing comfort and improved appearance.

Brain complications and death: Because acoustic tumors are located adjacent to vital brain centers that control breathing, blood pressure, and heart functions, as the tumor enlarges, it may become attached to these brain centers and become intertwined with the blood vessels supplying these areas of the brain. If the blood supply to vital brain centers is disturbed, serious complications may result: loss of muscle control, paralysis, even death. In the modern era of medicine and with the aid and availability of MRI scanners, these tumors are usually detected before they become so large that they impinge on vital structures. In our experience, death occurs very rarely as the result of acoustic tumor removal.

Spinal fluid leak: Acoustic tumor surgery results in a temporary leak of cerebral spinal fluid—the fluid that surrounds the brain. Prior to the completion of surgery, this leak is closed with fat removed from the abdomen. Occasionally—in 5 percent of patients—this leak reopens and further surgery is necessary to close it.

Infections occur in less than 1 percent of patients following acoustic tumor surgery. Infection is usually in the form of meningitis, an infection of the fluid and tissue surrounding the brain. If this complication occurs, the hospital stay will be longer. Treatment with high doses of antibiotics is used to treat the meningitis, and complications from antibiotic treatment are rare.

Other complications: Rarely, acoustic tumors may contact the nerves that supply the eye muscles, facial sensation, the mouth, and throat. These areas may be injured, causing double vision; numbness of the throat, face, and tongue; weakness of the shoulder; weakness of the voice; and difficulty swallowing. These problems may be permanent but are extremely rare in the modern era. Headache following acoustic tumor removal is common immediately after surgery. In some cases, headache may be prolonged. Low back pain can occur due to blood within the fluid space around the spinal nerve roots, but this is usually temporary and responds to heat and physical therapy. Bleeding and brain swelling can develop after acoustic tumor surgery; if this occurs, a subsequent operation may be necessary to reopen the wound to stop the bleeding and allow the brain to expand. This complication can result in paralysis or death; again, it's extremely rare these days.

Risks and Complications of Radiation Therapy

Radiation therapy also has risks as hearing loss, facial paralysis, and serious complications have also occurred after therapy. Because tissue exposed to the radiation dies gradually, hearing loss and other complications may not appear immediately but rather over a longer period of time. In addition, there is a risk that the radiation treatment may lead to development of a cancerous lesion many years later. The frequency of occurrence of this problem is not yet known because radiation treatment for acoustic tumors has been in use for a relatively short time. Although the chances of this are remote, if it does occur, such tumors can be fatal.

Hearing Impairment Following Treatment

Following middle fossa and retrosigmoid acoustic tumor surgery, the operated ear sometimes becomes deaf, but it always becomes deaf following translabyrinthine surgery. If the patient's hearing has deteriorated prior to surgery, as is common, the person is already aware of problems such as locating the direction of sound, hearing a person on the deaf side, and—usually the major problem—understanding speech in difficult listening situations. Someone with such a hearing impairment must learn to watch a speaker carefully, using the eyes to help the brain understand words that may sound very much the same but appear different on the lips, for example: *pope, coke, soap, dope, cope.* (Read Chapter 19 regarding speechreading and other hints for communicating effectively with a hearing loss.)

Considerable help also may be obtained with a contralateral routing of signal (CROS) aid. The CROS aid is an instrument that receives sound on the deaf side, amplifies it, then routes it to the good-hearing ear. Along the same principle as a CROS aid, a bone-anchored hearing appliance (Baha) improves hearing sensitivity. A Baha uses a titanium screw implanted into the bone behind the ear. After this screw becomes integrated, a vibrating hearing aid is attached to the screw. The vibrating hearing aid stimulates the cochlea on the good side, allowing sound detection from the deaf side. The Baha implant can be placed at the same time as tumor removal or at a later time. We discuss both of these devices in Chapter 16.

Neurofibromatosis Type II

In rare cases, a person might have bilateral acoustic tumors—tumors on both sides. This is the hallmark of a disease called neurofibromatosis Type II (NF2). The incidence of NF2 is one in 33,000 to 40,000 live births. Early diagnosis using gadolinium-enhanced MRI and techniques of hearing preservation surgery have improved our ability to prevent total hearing loss while completely removing the tumors. Because this is a genetic disease, with a dominant inheritance pattern, family screening and DNA analysis have increased early diagnosis.

HAVE YOU HEARD?

Half of the individuals with neurofibromatosis Type II have inherited the disorder from an affected parent; half seem to have a mutation for the first time in their family. Each child of an affected parent has a 50 percent chance of inheriting the disorder.

Unlike those with a unilateral vestibular schwannoma, people with NF2 usually get symptoms in their teens or early adulthood. They frequently also develop multiple brain and spinal cord tumors. NF2 tumors may affect the nerves important for swallowing, speech, eye and facial movement, and facial sensation. Determining the best management of the acoustic and other tumors is more complicated than deciding how to treat a unilateral acoustic tumor. Treatment options to be considered include the following:

- Hearing preservation surgery with total tumor removal.

- Observation without surgical intervention.

- Surgical decompression of the tumor without completely removing it.

- Retrosigmoid surgery, with partial tumor removal.

- Translabyrinthine total tumor removal (with no preservation of hearing).

- Auditory brainstem or cochlear implantation. For people with larger tumors or no useful hearing, the auditory brainstem implant allows restoration of some auditory function when the tumor is removed.

- A cochlear implant (in selected cases) can be used with good results (see Chapter 18).

Meningiomas

Another type of tumor found in the area of the temporal bone or CPA is called a meningioma. Unlike acoustic tumors, meningiomas arise not from a nerve but rather from a different type of cell. These cells come from the special covering of the brain and actually arise within the structures that are responsible for recirculating cerebral spinal fluid back to the blood vessels. Meningiomas are distinguishable from acoustic tumors in many cases by their characteristics on MRI results. But, on occasion, a tissue diagnosis, or *biopsy*, is required to distinguish between an acoustic tumor and a meningioma.

DEFINITION

A **biopsy** is a procedure for obtaining a tissue sample to be examined by a specially trained physician known as a pathologist. The pathologist determines the origin of the tissue to aid in making a diagnosis. Obtaining the sample may require surgery or may be done using a long needle, depending on the location of the tumor. Obtaining a tissue sample from a tumor inside the skull, such as a meningioma, requires surgery.

It's not uncommon for someone with a meningioma to have some of the same symptoms (hearing loss, balance difficulties, and headaches) as a person with an acoustic tumor. One difference is that meningiomas do start from other regions of the brain while acoustic tumors are limited to the CPA region.

Facial Nerve Neuromas

A nonmalignant fibrous growth may develop in the facial nerve itself, producing a gradually increasing facial nerve paralysis. Facial nerve neuromas occur infrequently and the exact incidence is not known. While acoustic tumors are much more common than facial nerve neuromas, it's not entirely possible to distinguish between the two different tumor types on MRI results. As a result, we counsel patients who plan on undergoing surgery for acoustic tumors about the possibility of the tumor actually representing a facial nerve neuroma.

Removal of a facial nerve neuroma requires severing the facial nerve. As we mentioned earlier, it's often possible to perform an anastomosis between the two cut ends of the facial nerve at the time of surgery using a skin sensation nerve from the neck. Total paralysis will be present until the nerve regrows through the graft, which usually takes 6 to 15 months. There will be some permanent facial weakness. When the tumor destroys the portion of the facial nerve nearest the brain, a hypoglossal-facial nerve anastomosis procedure is necessary (we discussed this earlier in this chapter). Removing a facial nerve neuroma, like an acoustic tumor, may require removal of the inner ear structures. If this is necessary, it results in a total loss of hearing in the operated ear and temporary severe dizziness. Continuing unsteadiness is uncommon.

Other Tumors

Other types of tumors also occur within the cerebellopontine angle. Names you may hear from your doctor include: epidermoids, schwannomas from other cranial nerves, vascular (blood vessel) tumors, arachnoid cysts, hemangiomas, dermoid tumors, chordomas, and metastatic lesions. These are uncommon and their treatment varies, depending on the patient and the usual range of variables considered when any tumor or illness is diagnosed and treated.

True Stories

Unfortunately, tumors do develop in the temporal bone and adjoining areas. Although these are relatively rare compared to the many other causes of hearing loss, we provide you a few patient stories to illustrate their diagnosis and treatment.

A Slow Decline

Anne, a 45-year-old teacher and mother of two, had, for the past year, been noticing a gradual decline in her hearing on the left side. She didn't think much of it at first but eventually decided to have it checked out. When she was ultimately sent to see an ear specialist, she had a hearing test performed, which showed that more than 50 percent of her hearing was gone on the left side. When an MRI scan showed a 2.5 cm tumor of the cerebellopontine angle, an acoustic tumor, Anne elected to undergo surgical removal via a translabyrinthine approach because her hearing was already poor. Immediately following surgery, Anne's facial nerve was working properly, though she did have dizziness and nausea. She stayed in the hospital for a total of four days and had only mild dizziness when discharged. An MRI scan performed six months after surgery showed no remaining tumor. Anne's facial nerve has continued to work properly, and she is now considering a Baha hearing aid to help improve her hearing.

Leaks Happen

Raymond, a 27-year-old airline pilot, noticed some slight ringing in his right ear and a drop in his hearing. When a hearing test at work found an asymmetric (unequal in the two ears) hearing loss, Raymond was promptly sent to an otologist. An MRI scan revealed a large, 4.2 cm acoustic tumor on the right side. Raymond had little useful hearing on the right and so elected to undergo a translabyrinthine approach for removal of the acoustic tumor. Postoperatively, he had some unsteadiness and continued ringing on the right side, but he did well and went home on the fifth postoperative day. One week later, Raymond reported the presence of clear fluid coming from his nose. A test revealed the fluid to be cerebral spinal fluid, so Raymond had a second procedure in which his ear canal was closed completely and packing was placed in the middle ear to help prevent further leakage of the CSF. He recovered well from this procedure and has not had any further problems.

Save the Hearing

A 57-year-old woman, Marianne, presented with a several-month history of tinnitus in her left ear. Her doctor sent her to an ENT specialist who ordered an MRI scan of her brain. When a 1 cm mass was detected in the left internal auditory canal, she was then referred to an otologist who ordered an audiogram. Her hearing was at a near normal level in the left ear. After consultation, Marianne decided to have total surgical removal of the tumor via a middle fossa approach to try to save her hearing. Her tumor was completely removed, and her facial nerve function was perfect after surgery. Hearing was preserved within 10 percent of her preoperative level on audiogram. She spent five days in the hospital (including the day of surgery) and was back to work after a 1-month recovery period at home. She had no residual problems after surgery, and her tinnitus was not bothersome.

Don't Wait; Radiate

David, an 84-year-old, had several medical problems, including diabetes, hypertension, coronary artery disease, and chronic obstructive pulmonary disease. His hearing had dropped over the years, and a recent hearing test revealed a significant difference in the hearing on his right side as compared to the left. An MRI scan showed a 1.5 cm acoustic tumor on the right side. Given his age and other health problems, radiation treatment was recommended because David didn't want simply to observe the tumor with repeat MRI scans every year. Following his treatment, David had no worsening in his hearing. He did complain of some slight unsteadiness but has been able to maintain a modest degree of activity. Repeat MRI scans show that during the two years since treatment, the tumor has maintained its size and has not grown. Continued surveillance will be required to determine whether any changes in tumor size or shape occur.

The Least You Need to Know

- Acoustic tumors, also called vestibular schwannomas, are benign and do not spread to other parts of the body.
- Acoustic tumors are most commonly treated by surgical removal, though in some cases radiation therapy or watchful waiting may be options.
- The smaller the tumor at the time of surgery, the less the chance of complications.

- Hearing impairment on the side of the tumor is frequently present before surgery but may become worse after surgery, or the operated ear may be deaf after surgery.
- Other tumors, such as meningiomas and facial nerve tumors, can also affect hearing and balance as well as facial nerve function.

Other Issues of Hearing Loss

4

We're all familiar with the sneezing and respiratory distress that allergies can cause. But hearing loss? It's possible! We talk about how allergy can affect all the different parts of the ear. We also explore tinnitus or head noise. Tinnitus, often a symptom of other causes of hearing loss, can be extremely troublesome on its own, so we look at the many treatment options available.

Because hearing loss in children creates problems in addition to the problems adults experience, here in Part 4 we take two chapters to look at the situations and decisions that parents may face as they deal with—or determine whether there is—hearing loss in a child.

Hearing Loss Due to Allergies

12

In This Chapter

- The symptoms of allergy
- The effects allergies can have on the ear
- Hearing loss caused by the body overreacting to itself
- Determining one's allergies
- Treatment of allergy

Allergy is the term we use to describe an overreaction of the body to a substance that is normally harmless, and this substance to which the body overreacts is called an allergen. An allergen causes the immune system to produce antibodies (proteins) for protection from what it thinks is a harmful substance. A person can be exposed to an allergen in several ways, including breathing it in (inhalant allergy), eating it (food allergy), or touching it (contact dermatitis) to cause symptoms. Often, people inherit a tendency to develop allergies. If one parent or sibling is allergic, it's estimated that the chance of a child having allergy is 40 percent. If both parents or a parent and sibling are allergic, the chance of allergy in a person is about 70 percent!

Contrary to popular belief, many children don't "outgrow" their allergies. The symptoms may simply change, such as from nasal congestion to asthma. An adult just diagnosed with allergic disease often has a history of childhood allergies that may or may not have been treated. He or she might have had allergies as a child, but the symptoms weren't even recognized as being allergic. A person may have been told he or she had ear infections, chronic tonsillitis, or some other symptom but didn't realize these were suggestive of allergies.

In this chapter, we tell you briefly what the symptoms are, how the body produces an allergic reaction, and how allergy can affect all three major parts of the ear—external, middle, and inner. We also describe the different types of allergy as well as how to diagnose the specific substances to which you're allergic. And we discuss ways to treat allergies in general, as well as treatments aimed at an individual's specific allergic symptoms and allergens.

Symptoms of Allergy

Approximately 14 to 20 percent of Americans suffer from "hypersensitivity" diseases, another term for allergy, with the head and neck being the most commonly affected areas. Although the nose is the organ most commonly involved in allergic reactions, an allergy can affect multiple organs in the body, including the ear. Nasal congestion, runny nose, polyps (benign growths) in the nose, itchy and puffy eyes, frequent sore throats, asthma, skin rashes, and behavioral problems such as hyperactivity in children may be symptoms of allergy. Symptoms can occur in almost all systems of the body, including the outer, middle, and inner ears.

After a person's first contact with an allergen causes the immune system to react, later contact with that same substance causes an additional boosting of the immune response. This response is sometimes too much and can cause tissue damage. These exaggerated reactions, or sensitization, which are based on the body's normal means to combat infections, are called hypersensitivity reactions. They may occur a short time after a first exposure to the allergen, or it may take years of exposure to occur, which can make it difficult to self-diagnose one's specific allergens.

Types of Allergies

We mentioned in the introduction that a person may have contact with an allergen by breathing it in, eating it, or touching it. In the following sections, we discuss the three types of allergies—inhalant, food, and contact dermatitis—and tell you about some of the most common allergens of each type.

Inhalant Allergy

Reactions to allergens breathed in through the nose cause symptoms of inhalant allergy. An allergic reaction may develop after repeated or lengthy exposure to allergens such as pollens, dust, molds, animal dander, or other substances breathed in. Symptoms of inhalant allergy can last year-round or may be just seasonal.

HAVE YOU HEARD?

Hay fever (technically, allergic rhinitis) is a form of inhalant allergy due to weed pollen released in the late summer and fall. "Hay fever" is an old term. Because hay was cut in the fall—the same time weeds were pollinating or reproducing—people thought the sneezing and other symptoms were due to the hay! These autumn symptoms often improve in colder climates after the first frost.

There really is no hypoallergenic dog (no, not even Bo Obama). The allergenic part of animals is the dander—minute particles from hair or skin) that all dogs and cats shed. Some just shed less than others. The reaction of an allergic person to an individual dog or cat may vary greatly, but all dogs and cats do shed.

When the nose or lungs come in repeated contact with allergens, the immune system makes a high level of a blood protein (or antibody) called immunoglobulin E (IgE). The IgE attaches to special allergic cells, called mast cells, found throughout the body. When the allergen enters the respiratory tract, a change occurs in the mast cell's outer membrane, causing the cell to release inflammatory substances, called mediators, that produce allergic symptoms. One of the best-known mediators is called histamine; it causes itching, mucous secretion (for example, runny nose), sneezing, and nasal congestion. This is why an antihistamine is frequently prescribed for allergy symptoms. Other mediators that produce symptoms are also released with an allergic reaction.

Food Allergies

You might be surprised to know that common foods you eat frequently are the ones most likely to cause symptoms of food allergy. Allergens taken into the digestive tract can cause allergic symptoms such as nasal congestion, hives, or ear infections. Each year, millions of Americans have allergic reactions to food. Although most food allergies cause relatively mild symptoms, some food allergies can cause *anaphylaxis*, a severe reaction that is rapid in onset and may cause death if not treated immediately.

DEFINITION

Anaphylaxis (also called anaphylactic shock) is a sudden allergic reaction that is severe and involves the whole body. Tissues in different parts of the body release histamine and other substances, causing difficulty in breathing and other symptoms. Food allergy is believed to be the leading cause of anaphylaxis outside the hospital setting, causing an estimated 50,000 emergency room visits each year in the United States.

For reasons that aren't clear, the incidence of food allergies is increasing in the United States, especially in children. Although you could be allergic to any food, such as fruits, vegetables, and meats, eight foods account for 90 percent of all food allergic reactions. The United States Food and Drug Administration (FDA) officially lists these as: peanuts, tree nuts, eggs, milk, shellfish, fish, wheat, and soy. Additionally, the FDA lists sulfites (chemicals often found in food flavorings and color). In other countries, because of differences in the genetic makeup of the citizens and different levels of exposure, the official allergen list differs. For example, Canada recognizes all eight of the allergens recognized by the United States but also recognizes sesame seeds as a common allergen.

Did you know that most children with allergies develop food allergies before they develop inhaled allergies? Common signs of food allergies in young children can include (but are not limited to) the following:

- Frequent ear infections.

- Frequent "colds," although it's common for young children to have more colds than adults or older children.

- Eczema, a rash that often develops on the face, inside areas of the arm, and behind the knees.

- Being a "fussy" eater.

Nonfood substances, such as penicillin or sulfa, or chemicals such as food preservatives, can cause inflammation resulting in similar symptoms. It's also possible to experience adverse effects from foods that seem like allergic reactions but are not technically allergy. For example, if you get a rash when eating a large amount of shellfish, strawberries, or tuna but no symptoms with a smaller amount, this is probably not a true allergy. Digestive problems from milk are more likely due to a lactose intolerance than to an actual food allergy.

HAVE YOU HEARD?

Pistachios, mangoes, and poison ivy are all related to each other in terms of allergy. Some people can eat mangoes with no difficulty. But if they touch their mouths to the skin of the mango, they develop a rash similar to poison ivy on the mouth that usually requires steroid cream or pills to clear up.

Contact Dermatitis

Contact dermatitis is a rash or swelling caused by direct contact of an allergen with the skin. Poison ivy, nickel earrings, wool shirts, or certain ear drops may stimulate a cell called the T-lymphocyte to release allergic mediators that affect the skin. The resulting rash may last for weeks or months after exposure. Sometimes these rashes are misdiagnosed as a skin infection and treated with antibiotics. One tip for telling the difference between infection and contact dermatitis is that although contact dermatitis is uncomfortable, the skin rash is generally not painful as it is in an infection.

Contact sensitivity to metals used in earrings, especially nickel and chromium, occurs frequently. Treatment is to use earring posts of surgical stainless steel, or in more extreme cases, 14-karat or higher weight gold or titanium. Too bad, you might just have to have solid gold earrings!

Allergy and the Ears

As we noted, allergy can affect any of the three basic parts of the ear—the external ear, middle ear, or inner ear. In the following sections, we describe the wide variety of ways that allergy can affect each part of the ear.

External Ear

Ongoing itching or frequent infections of the ear canal may be due to allergy. Chronic otitis externa (see Chapter 3), characterized by a red, scaling, itchy rash, may involve either the auricle (outer visible part of the ear) or the external ear canal. Often an infection is suspected, and so ear drops are prescribed. The auricle or canal may become sensitized to the antibiotic in the ear drops, making the problem even worse. Ear drops containing neomycin are especially known for doing this. The skin will get red and swollen, but, unlike an infection, there is little pain. Usually, stopping use of the drops solves the problem. However, it may be necessary to apply steroid drops or lotion for a short period to soothe and reduce the swelling. It may also be necessary to have a doctor clean the ear canal.

Some people develop contact sensitivity to the plastic used in hearing aid earmolds, the custom-fitted piece that fits in the ear canal. The resulting rash and swelling occurs only in the areas of skin in direct contact with the earmold. Unfortunately, this can prevent successful use of the hearing aid. The problem can usually be solved by having the hearing aid dispenser or manufacturer boil the offending earmold for

30 seconds to make it less irritating. Another option is to substitute a less reactive plastic for the earmold. Many alternative materials are available from most earmold laboratories, such as UV Lucite and silicone. In severe cases, the earmold may be plated with a thin film of gold over the area in contact with the skin.

SOUND ADVICE

One of our patients wanted to save time when told about boiling the earmold to make him less sensitive to the material, so he decided to do it himself instead of taking it back to the dispenser. After throwing the whole hearing aid into the boiling pot of water, he had to buy a completely new aid—made of a less reactive material, of course! Don't try to do this yourself.

In children, the outer ear may occasionally turn bright red after eating foods to which they're allergic. But unlike when there's an infection, there's no pain. Elimination of the food or foods after the allergy is diagnosed will eliminate this problem.

A dermatophytid reaction is an unusual problem that can affect the outer ear. People with this problem actually have a fungal infection somewhere else, often under the toenails, to which they eventually develop an allergic sensitivity. The allergic reaction can cause a scaling, very itchy rash in the outer ear canal and/or the auricle, possibly interfering with hearing aid use. The fungus is at the foot, but the allergic reaction is in the ear—that's why we call this foot and ear disease! The treatment starts with diagnosing the particular fungus to which the patient is allergic, followed by both allergy treatment to desensitize to this fungus and treatment by a dermatologist for the primary fungal infection.

Middle Ear

Repeated ear infections and long-standing fluid behind the eardrum (otitis media with effusion (OME)) are often due to allergy. Both of these are more common in children than in adults. There's a relationship among upper respiratory tract infections (such as colds and flu), allergy, and poor Eustachian tube function, which is the primary cause of OME. As noted in Chapter 6, OME is the most common cause of hearing loss in children today. Scientists think that allergy plays a role in more than half of children with fluid in the ear severe enough to require surgery for placement of ventilation tubes. The highest incidence of OME coincides with the time of year when dust and mold counts are highest, and these are common allergens.

LISTEN UP

If a child doesn't have a cleft palate or other known factor that increases the risk of OME but has required more than one set of PE tubes, allergy should be considered. One child was referred for diagnostic testing for allergy only after having had 14 sets of tubes! She didn't require any more surgery after beginning allergy shots.

At birth, children are normal nose breathers, so parents should have a child who usually breathes through the mouth evaluated. Chronic nasal congestion is often seen in children with OME because allergy plays a role in both. In many children with enlarged adenoids—the lymph tissue found on the back wall of the throat—allergy is also believed to play a role.

The role of food allergy in causing OME is rarely discussed. But the younger the child who develops OME and also has a family or other history of allergy, the more suspicious you should be of foods rather than inhaled allergens as a possible immune trigger. After determining what food(s) the child is allergic to, eliminating them from the diet often dramatically reduces symptoms.

Most children with OME due to allergy also have other symptoms such as hay fever or asthma. The antihistamines and oral decongestants commonly used to treat nasal allergies don't have any known effect on the ear or the Eustachian tube. It's also not known whether nasal steroid sprays and other sprays used for nasal allergies and asthma help OME. This question is a subject of research at the present time. But many studies show the benefit of allergy shots in certain patients with inhalant allergy and middle ear disease. Steroid pills can help relieve symptoms of OME in many people, but the side effects of steroids make their use in children inadvisable most of the time. Use of oral steroids by children can affect growth, thin the skin, and make the child more susceptible to infections.

Another common symptom of ear allergy, especially in adults, is an ongoing feeling of ear fullness or pressure, which is due to Eustachian tube dysfunction, especially if one has a history of past or current nasal allergy. Allergy can sometimes cause the effects of Eustachian tube problems (see Chapter 6).

Inner Ear

Most sensorineural hearing loss is due to aging or noise exposure. However, in some cases, dizziness, ear fullness and pressure, tinnitus, and sensorineural hearing loss can be due to underlying inhalant or food allergies. Ménière's disease in one or both ears (see Chapter 10) may sometimes be aggravated or triggered by allergies. A person could have a possible allergic link to inner ear symptoms if any of these situations applies:

- A known history of allergy and either Ménière's disease or cochlear hydrops.

- Hearing loss and/or dizziness that seem to be related to the time of year (seasons) or eating certain foods (other than salt) or are accompanied by other symptoms of allergy such as nasal congestion.

- Autoimmune inner ear disease (see the following paragraphs) that improves with steroid treatment.

As in OME, most medicines we use for treatment of nasal allergies do not help inner ear symptoms, with the exception of oral steroids. Steroid nasal sprays are not absorbed into the body enough to reach the inner ear. Antihistamines do not "dry up" inner ear fluid, although the older antihistamines that cause drowsiness can help reduce symptoms of dizziness and vertigo in Ménière's disease. But allergy treatment has been shown to improve vertigo, result in less hearing loss (stabilize hearing), and improve quality of life in people with some inner ear diseases.

Autoimmune Inner Ear Disease

Autoimmune inner ear disease (AIED), while not technically allergic, is believed to be caused by the body's immune system attacking the inner ear and damaging the hearing and sometimes the balance nerve. AIED occurs when the body produces an immunological or inflammatory reaction to itself, instead of reacting to an external substance. In most cases, we don't know why this occurs. Some people with AIED may also have symptoms in other parts of the body caused by an overly active immune system, including arthritis, skin rashes, or damage to internal organs. The symptoms of inner ear involvement by an autoimmune disease are similar to those of other inner ear disorders. This can include fluctuating hearing, often with dizziness or vertigo and/or ear fullness. Symptoms usually occur in both ears in a short period of time.

Diagnosis of Specific Allergies

The specific allergens that cause allergic reactions can be diagnosed by skin testing, blood tests, or a challenge test. Blood tests are also used to aid the diagnosis of autoimmune inner ear disease.

Skin Testing for Inhalant Allergies

To identify inhalant allergies, small amounts of allergens representing things you might breathe in are injected in rows on the forearm, the upper arm, or sometimes the back causing little bumps called wheals to form on the skin at the injection sites. After 10 to 20 minutes, these wheals are measured. Certain larger wheals indicate an allergy to the substance injected at that area. The wheal size helps the doctor determine how sensitive you are and at what strength your allergy shots for treatment should start if you're going to have treatment.

In Vitro Test

An in vitro test, meaning "in a test tube," is a blood test sometimes used to diagnose food and inhalant allergies (also sometimes called a RAST test, which stands for radioallergosorbent). It measures antibodies (such as IgE) to specific allergens and may be used to determine one's sensitivity to inhalants and some forms of food allergy.

Challenge Test for Food Allergies

Skin testing can help to diagnose food allergies. Many patients crave foods to which they are allergic, and a doctor may take a food history from them to identify some of these. But a challenge test may be necessary to determine exactly what foods cause the allergy symptoms. Foods to be tested may either be eaten or injected in a purified form (as with skin testing for inhalant allergies). When the food has been absorbed, the allergic patient may develop common symptoms of allergy such as nasal stuffiness, a change in hearing, or ringing in the ears, or a skin test wheal has grown significantly after 10 to 20 minutes. The test is done under the watchful eye of the allergy clinic staff so any severe reactions can be quickly treated.

Blood Testing for Autoimmune Disease

The diagnosis of AIED is made first by the patient-reported history and the finding of a rapidly progressive (developing over several weeks to a few months) worsening or very unstable hearing level, which is usually in both ears. The suspected diagnosis is supported by obtaining special blood tests to show evidence of antibody increases to inner ear or other tissue often seen in patients with this disorder. Blood testing may also indicate evidence of autoimmune problems in other areas of the body, such as the skin or a kidney.

SOUND ADVICE

If you have chronic, poorly controlled asthma, your doctor might consider obtaining a CT scan or x-ray of the sinuses. Ongoing sinus disease, called chronic sinusitis, may not necessarily produce facial pain at first. If the upper airway (nose and Eustachian tube) is not healthy, the lower airway and the lungs may have very significant symptoms. Chronic sinusitis can have an allergic cause.

Medications and Non-Specific Allergy Treatment

Mild allergic symptoms don't require specific testing for diagnosis when the symptoms can be well controlled with some combination of antihistamines, prescription nasal sprays, decongestants, and, of course, avoiding known allergens. Side effects of oral antihistamines may include dry mouth, difficulty urinating, and drowsiness. Newer antihistamines, which often don't produce drowsiness, can be effective for the symptoms of dripping nose and itching but don't help relieve nasal congestion unless they are combined with an oral decongestant.

Antihistamines may also be sprayed into the nose as a non-addicting nose spray. Used this way, they can reduce nasal congestion as well as the itching, sneezing, and runny nose symptoms commonly seen in allergy. Most of the prescription nasal sprays for allergy are mild topical steroids and can be very effective for most nasal allergy symptoms, including congestion, dripping, and itching, but be aware that they really do take several hours to have an effect on symptoms. Side effects from steroid and antihistamine nasal sprays include occasional nosebleeds, headaches, or nasal crusting.

Decongestants shrink swollen tissue such as the mucous membrane of the nose and are often combined with antihistamines. Side effects include insomnia, increased blood pressure, rapid heartbeat, and potential prostate obstruction in men. Because of these side effects, they shouldn't be taken for a lengthy period of time.

Excellent measures to avoid contact with allergens (called environmental control) include the use of a central or room-size air purifier with a high-efficiency particulate filter (HEPA) to remove the microscopic allergens such as pollen or mold spores. Other air purifiers with ozone production can actually be harmful to the health of the respiratory tract. Impermeable mattress and pillow covers to lessen exposure to dust mites are inexpensive and quite useful. Information on other products such as those designed to make animal dander less allergenic and kill molds that grow in living spaces can be obtained from your otolaryngologist, allergist, or through environmental supply manufacturers.

To avoid allergens, of course, one must know what they are. We had one patient who was sure she was very allergic to her synthetic knitting yarn. It turns out her knitting club was held at the home of a friend with six cats! Moving the location of the knitting club "cured" her problem with her yarn.

SOUND ADVICE

Pollen counts are highest between 5 and 10 in the morning. To avoid exposure, keep windows closed, particularly during these hours. The counts are also higher on windy days, so use air conditioning or ceiling or floor fans as an alternative to open windows for ventilation during these times.

Kick the dog or cat out of the bedroom!

The strongest indicator that mold contamination is in a room is the musty smell. To live, mold needs some organic debris, a source of moisture, and low light. Many molds are black in color, but a black color doesn't necessarily make one mold more toxic than another. Some things to do to reduce chances of exposure to mold and mold spores include: using exhaust fans in bathrooms to reduce humidity; using mold-killing solutions in bathrooms and shower stalls; replacing bathroom carpets with tile or linoleum; never putting away wet shoes or clothing; using exhaust fans in the kitchen to remove cooking steam and food vapors; repairing water leaks; using a dehumidifier to keep the relative humidity low (40 to 50 percent is recommended) and deter mold growth. If you have mold allergies, be alert to their possible presence.

Specific Allergy Treatment

More severe or chronic allergic symptoms and those not controlled by medication—especially those involving the inner ear—may require tests to identify the specific allergen. The type of treatment depends on the underlying cause and may involve desensitization (in the form of allergy shots), avoidance of exposure to an inhalant allergen, dietary elimination of food allergens, or medications.

Inhalant Allergy

If your doctor suggests desensitization therapy for inhalant allergies, once or twice a week you'll be given injections that contain purified extracts of the allergens to which you're sensitive, based on your test results. The injections stimulate the immune system to produce specific antibodies and protective agents that help block the production of allergic symptoms. Shots are often recommended for moderate to severe, perennial symptoms that don't respond to environmental control or medication. This is especially important for inner ear symptoms of allergies because there is no time of year when you can do without your hearing.

It's important to be treated by a physician who is highly experienced in the testing and treatment of allergic diseases. The risk of side effects from shots include skin irritation or bumps, increased symptoms (until the dose is properly adjusted and monitored), anaphylactic shock, and in very rare cases, death. Although the liquid in allergy shots is often termed serum, it's actually a mixture of extracts of common airborne allergens. There's no risk of transmission of HIV or other blood-transmitted diseases.

Sublingual immunotherapy (SLIT) refers to allergen desensitization given in a drop form underneath the tongue. The drops contain extracts of inhalant allergens or, occasionally, food allergens and are held in the mouth for several seconds to a few minutes and then swallowed or spit out. While this treatment, rather than injections, is being used in Europe in almost half of the immunotherapy patients, it's not approved for routine use in the United States. Clinical studies are currently being performed in the United States to evaluate the effectiveness of this form of treatment. So far, it doesn't appear that the results from SLIT are as long-lasting as those obtained by inhalant allergy shots.

Food Allergy

For food allergies, the primary treatment is to avoid the foods that cause allergic reactions. Called an elimination diet, this allows the body to decrease its sensitivity to these foods. In a small percentage of people, the food allergies remain fixed and symptoms will always be produced after eating the food, even after long periods of elimination from the diet. Fortunately, this type of food allergy is relatively rare. For most people, taking about three to six months off from eating the allergic food will do the trick. After the symptoms are improved, a challenge test will be given again. If no symptoms are produced, the food can be put back into the diet, eating the food no more than one day out of every four. In addition to dietary elimination, a patient will be asked to vary the other foods in his or her diet to prevent new food allergies from developing.

Contact Dermatitis

Your doctor will try to determine what substances may be causing your symptoms and have you avoid contact with them. The doctor may also prescribe an anti-inflammatory medicine (a steroid) in pill, cream, or drop form to help decrease the inflammation.

Autoimmune Inner Ear Disease

The most effective treatment for AIED is use of steroids. While short courses of a few days to weeks may be helpful, it's common to require high doses of steroids given for several weeks or even months to obtain improvement of very unstable AIED. Side effects of steroids may include insomnia, skin rash, early onset of osteoporosis, and glaucoma. Along with, or in place of, steroids, it may be necessary to use other medications that suppress or change an overly active immune response. These medications are often used in other forms of autoimmune disease such as rheumatoid arthritis but are used off-label for AIED (that is, the doctor prescribes it even though it has not been approved by the FDA for that purpose). Affected patients may have improved hearing and balance after treatment.

A patient might need to be tested for allergies if his or her history suggests the presence of, past history of, or strong family history of allergy in order to lessen overall inflammation in the body. This is especially a consideration in those patients with AIED who can't get off of steroids without a significant increase in hearing loss or dizziness and/or vertigo.

Surgery

Surgical placement of a ventilation tube in the eardrum can treat ear symptoms due to allergy, such as OME. Surgery to control dizziness is necessary at times, even though the underlying problem started as a result of an allergy. Chronic infection in the middle ear space may also develop in some patients as a result of underlying allergy. In some cases, this infection can only be eliminated by a surgical procedure. Following surgery, the underlying allergic problem itself should be treated to prevent the symptoms from recurring. In unusually severe cases of AIED in which the hearing loss becomes profound in spite of medical treatment, cochlear implant surgery can be performed to restore a useful level of hearing.

True Stories

Once again, we searched our patient files for some stories to help illustrate the different ways that allergy can affect the ear and hearing. Here are just a few.

Treat the Allergy, Stop the Fluid

Twelve-year-old Isabelle was referred for the placement of PE (ventilation) tubes for recurrent fluid in her middle ear space. When meeting her, the physician noticed that Isabelle didn't breathe through her nose at all, but rather through an open mouth, which her parents said was normal for her. Her past history revealed she'd had 14 sets of tubes from various doctors and had also had her tonsils and adenoids removed. Her first set of tubes was done at age nine months. Despite this, she had fluid behind both eardrums. Allergy testing found she was moderately allergic to many inhaled allergens, so she started on allergy shots. Because the fluid had been behind her eardrums for more than three months, she also had surgery to drain it, and PE tubes were again put in place. Now, five years later, fluid has never recurred. The tubes that were placed have fallen out, and she remains fluid free, with normal hearing.

Pop Go the Ears

John, a 22-year-old man, wanted to be a commercial pilot. He always had problems with ear clearing during plane flights, but he could finally get them to clear with effort. When he came in for an evaluation of this problem, he had no evidence of fluid behind the eardrums or swelling of his nasal tissue. His hearing was normal, but he did have abnormalities on his tympanogram, a test that measures Eustachian tube function. Both of his parents had a history of allergy, although they had never taken shots. He had been treated with various antihistamines and nose sprays, with no help. We performed skin tests for specific allergies and found he was allergic to a number of things, including milk. He started on immunotherapy (allergy shots) and was asked to eliminate milk products from his diet. Now, two years later, he has his pilot's license and is set to receive his instrument rating. He has to "pop" his ears by swallowing during descent but now is always able to get them to clear.

Contact

Rachel was a 32-year-old hearing-impaired woman. Her loss was discovered at age 6, and she had worn hearing aids ever since. She came in because of pain and draining from her ear when she wore her hearing aid. On exam, she had a rash or redness only in her ear canal and the bowl of her outer ear and only where her hearing aid earmold touched. She had a less allergenic earmold made and is now able to wear her aids comfortably. She had worn the same type of material in her hearing aid molds for years, but eventually became allergic to them.

Pollen and the Inner Ear

Richard, a 40-year-old man, has cochlear hydrops involving his right ear. He wears a hearing aid and takes a diuretic on a regular basis, but he had problems each year with unstable hearing, requiring steroid injections or oral steroids. On reviewing his records, it appeared that his reduced hearing always occurred in the spring and fall. He was tested for allergies and found to have reactions to the pollens released in the fall (weeds) and the early spring (trees). Treated with allergy shots, he now has had stable hearing, with minimal fluctuation, for more than three years.

The Least You Need to Know

- Allergy can affect the external, middle, or inner ear, causing hearing loss and other ear symptoms.
- An individual can be allergic to something he or she breathes (inhalant allergy), eats (food allergy), or touches (contact dermatitis); a person can also be allergic to him- or herself (autoimmune).
- Mild allergy symptoms can be controlled well with antihistamines, nasal sprays, and by avoiding the allergens.
- Moderate to severe allergies should be specifically diagnosed by testing and treated with desensitization allergy shots (immunotherapy) or food elimination diet.

Tinnitus or Head Noise

13

In This Chapter

- The many characteristics of tinnitus
- The causes and types of tinnitus
- Treatments for tinnitus
- Helpful hints for dealing with your tinnitus

Many people hear sounds when there's no apparent external cause for the sound. In fact, this happens to almost everyone on rare occasions. But if you hear such sounds frequently or if they last more than a few minutes, you may have tinnitus (pronounced either TIN-it-us or tin-NIGHT-us). Tinnitus, often called head noise, is common (see Chapter 2). According to the National Institute on Deafness and Other Communication Disorders, in 2001, roughly 25 million Americans experienced it. More recently, the American Tinnitus Association (ATA) puts the number at 50 million people.

Most studies find that 10 to 15 percent of adults have tinnitus, but it's more common with increasing age (probably because of increased hearing loss and other illnesses with age). Tinnitus is most often associated with hearing loss; about 80 percent of people with a hearing loss, regardless of cause, also have tinnitus. And it tends to be more common in some types of people—men, Caucasians, and those with age-related hearing loss. Also, people exposed to loud noises for long periods of time and those with post-traumatic stress disorder (PTSD) are known to be prone to it.

Although loud tinnitus might sometimes interfere with hearing, it doesn't in itself cause hearing loss (even though it's common for people with tinnitus to feel that it affects their hearing). It's important to understand that tinnitus is a symptom and not a disease. But because so many people with hearing loss have tinnitus and need to understand it, we include it in this book. In this chapter, we take a look at the characteristics of tinnitus, its possible causes, and the wide variety of treatments that we've found useful. We also point out some things you can do to help yourself deal with your tinnitus.

Characteristics of Tinnitus

Tinnitus, although often described as "ringing in the ears," can also present as a buzzing, hissing, seashell sound, roaring, humming, or pulsation. It might be constant or intermittent, loud at times and barely noticeable at others, but usually it's most noticeable when the environment is quiet. It may or may not be associated with hearing impairment, but most people with hearing loss (80 percent) have tinnitus as one symptom. Only about 5 to 10 percent of people with tinnitus have normal hearing on an audiogram. If you have both hearing loss and tinnitus, don't worry. The severity of your head noise is not related to the future course of your hearing impairment. Many people with tinnitus mistakenly fear that they're going to lose their hearing.

HAVE YOU HEARD?

Many notable people have reported having tinnitus. Some of those who have been cited publicly include musicians Beethoven, Eric Clapton, Barbara Streisand, Neil Young, Paul Simon, Pete Townshend, and Roger Miller; painters Vincent van Gogh, Michelangelo, and Francisco de Goya; radio and television personalities and actors Garrison Keillor, Steve Martin, Leonard Nimoy, Tony Randall, and William Shatner; and public and historical figures Ronald Reagan, Alan Shephard, Joan of Arc, and Martin Luther. And many, many more!

Questionnaires designed to assess tinnitus usually ask what kind of sound you hear and how severe it is, how loud it is, how much it interferes with daily life, how often it occurs, how long an episode lasts if it's not constant, where the sound is localized (for example, in your ear or in your head), and whether it interferes with your sleep. There are also tests, referred to as "tinnitus matching," that try to determine the pitch of the sounds you are hearing and how loud the sound is compared to your hearing thresholds. Because many of the causes of hearing loss affect both ears, many people with tinnitus hear it in both ears. But it can affect just one ear. Some people actually describe it as centered in their head or are unable to localize it to one side or the other.

Most people who experience tinnitus are not bothered greatly by it. Usually, they're not aware of it and only notice it when they listen for it or when they're in very quiet situations. We all learn to ignore many of the sounds around us. For example, we usually don't hear the refrigerator noise or the fan on our computer until we listen for it. After time, the brain is able to adjust for these environmental sounds and ignore them.

But some people with tinnitus (about 20 percent) are severely disturbed by it, because it's so severe it interferes with their daily activities. With severe tinnitus, a person may find it difficult to concentrate, work, or even sleep. In fact, nearly half of people who complain of severe tinnitus report sleep disturbances. Sleep deprivation can be one of the primary effects of tinnitus and can cause an individual to have trouble focusing and to become angry and frustrated. There may be associated anxiety or depression which tends to aggravate the tinnitus, and then the reaction to the tinnitus increases the anxiety or depression. In other words, a vicious cycle can develop of increased tinnitus, increased anxiety or depression, and a worsening of the tinnitus.

Forms of Tinnitus

In many cases, the cause of tinnitus is considered idiopathic—doctors can isolate no cause. That is true for both forms: subjective and objective. The most common form, in 98 percent of cases, is subjective, which means that you hear the sound but others cannot. Tinnitus that an observer can hear is called objective. In other words, some causes of tinnitus actually produce a sound that a doctor can hear with a listening device.

Subjective Tinnitus

Most people with subjective tinnitus have a sensorineural hearing loss; a few have a conductive hearing loss (for example, from fluid in the middle ear, ear wax, or a hole in the eardrum). As you now know, there are many causes of sensorineural hearing loss, but those most likely associated with tinnitus include noise-induced hearing loss, age-related hearing loss, inner ear infections, trauma such as head injury, tumors of the hearing nerve, Ménière's disease, and some ototoxic medications.

When hearing loss is caused by ear trauma, you'll usually notice the tinnitus in both ears because both ears are usually exposed to the same noises, drugs, and other influences. Loud noise exposure is a very common cause of hearing loss with accompanying tinnitus. In the rare case of an acoustic tumor, tinnitus is usually noticed just in the one ear with the tumor. It can also occur with some neck injuries or in people with temporal mandibular joint (TMJ) pain. In this case, hearing is usually normal, and the tinnitus improves when the underlying condition responds to treatment.

Stress is present in everyone's life periodically, and stress factors that might cause or aggravate existing tinnitus include chemical stress, acoustic stress, physical stress, and emotional stress. Examples of chemical stress include ingesting aspirin in high doses, caffeine, or some drugs used for chemotherapy. Many examples of very loud sounds in our everyday lives can increase tinnitus. Fatigue, a form of physical stress, often contributes to the perception of it as your tinnitus may seem louder at the end of the day or after you've had some physical exertion. At times, tinnitus may in itself lead to depression as in the vicious cycle of anxiety, depression, and increased tinnitus. And many changes in life, especially with aging, cause emotional stress. Illness, retirement, loss of function, loss of a spouse or friend, and reduced social activity can lead to mood swings, depression, and anxiety. This emotional stress can affect tinnitus and exacerbate your negative reactions to it.

LISTEN UP

Aspirin in high doses (20 to 30 tablets per day) can cause temporary hearing loss and tinnitus. Reducing the dose usually leads to a return of hearing and resolution of the tinnitus. More than 300 prescription and over-the-counter medications list tinnitus as a side effect, including powerful aminoglycoside antibiotics and quinine.

Where Is the Sound Coming From?

What produces subjective tinnitus is not fully understood. It's a perceived sound in the brain just like all sound. Special kinds of brain scans called functional MRI and positron emission tomography (PET) show areas of increased activity of the auditory cortex of the brain in people with severe tinnitus. But where in the auditory system does the sound stimulus start? There are a number of different theories about this, which involve the hair cells, the auditory nerve, and the central auditory nervous system, including the auditory cortex.

One theory suggests that tinnitus is generated in the brain or central pathways leading to the brain. When the tinnitus is associated with hearing loss, the cochlea is no longer sending the normal signals to the brain. It's as if the brain becomes "confused" by this and develops its own noise to make up for the lack of normal sound. Researchers have found that tinnitus most often continues even after the hearing nerve is destroyed when removing acoustic tumors. So the sound must be coming from somewhere more central than the cochlea.

Another study found that when college students with no tinnitus were placed in a soundproof, echo-free chamber, 93 percent reported hearing a buzzing, pulsing, or whistling sound. When left with absolutely no sound input, our brains may create some. On the other hand, profoundly deaf people don't often have tinnitus! In sensorineural hearing loss that is not profound, there's usually damage to the hair cells in certain areas. Some scientists suggest that neurons that send signals toward the brain may trigger abnormal auditory sensations at frequencies near the area of damaged hair cells because of biochemical changes to the hair cells. That is, in this case, the tinnitus is generated at the cochlea.

Objective Tinnitus

Your ear doctor may actually be able to hear your tinnitus by listening with a small tube that goes into your ear on one end and the examiner's ear on the other. Or the doctor might use a stethoscope to listen by placing it over the bone behind your ear or over the upper neck. The causes of objective tinnitus are either vascular or muscular.

The carotid artery, which supplies blood to your brain, runs very close to the inner ear. The jugular vein that drains blood from the brain is also located close to the middle and inner ear. So it's surprising that we don't always hear blood coursing through these vessels! Pulsatile tinnitus is usually related to blood flow. Causes of this kind of tinnitus include pregnancy, anemia (lack of blood cells), overactive thyroid, or tumors involving blood vessels near the ear. Pulsatile tinnitus can also be caused by a condition known as benign intracranial hypertension, which is an increase in the pressure of the fluid surrounding the brain. When a plaque forms in the artery or when the jugular bulb is enlarged, you might hear a pulsating sound in the ear. This is objective tinnitus. Another rare cause of objective tinnitus is a vascular tumor in or near the ear. These tumors cause a pulsating, rhythmic sound in the involved ear that is synchronous with your heartbeat. In most cases, removing the vascular tumor relieves the tinnitus.

LISTEN UP

If you have vascular tinnitus due to plaques in the carotid artery, you should see a vascular surgeon for further evaluation and possible treatment. This is one of the few situations in which tinnitus may be a symptom of a potentially serious problem.

Another form of objective tinnitus is muscular. Remember those two small muscles in the middle ear, one attached to the first middle ear bone and the other to the third bone (see Chapter 1)? These muscles contract when the ear is exposed to loud noise, and immediately after the loud sound stops, the muscles relax. Occasionally, you might develop a sporadic rhythmic contraction of one of these muscles, which causes episodes of clicking and fluttering in the ear. If it's bothersome, your doctor can prescribe muscle relaxant medications. In rare cases that don't resolve, the tendon to these muscles can be cut surgically. This surgery is performed under local anesthesia through the ear canal.

A third muscle (levator palatine), located in the roof of the mouth, lifts the soft palate and briefly opens the Eustachian tube. When you swallow or yawn, the Eustachian tube opens briefly to equalize the pressure in the middle ear (see Chapter 4), and it's not unusual to hear a soft pop when the tube opens. Rarely, a condition occurs in which this muscle goes into a series of rhythmic contractions (called clonus), causing a staccato popping in the ear. Someone sitting close to you might even hear the popping sound. When this happens, it's possible to see the clonic contractions of the palate that are synchronous with the popping. Again, muscle relaxant medications may help, but for a rare case that doesn't resolve itself, Botox can be injected into the muscle to weaken it and prevent the contractions.

Jaw joint misalignment problems or muscles of the ear or throat "twitching" can cause clicking types of objective tinnitus. At times a blockage of the ear by wax or an inflammation in the middle ear can also cause a pulsation or throbbing in that ear. Removing the wax or treating the inflammation with appropriate medications usually cures this.

SOUND ADVICE

One survey of people with tinnitus found that the average length of time they waited to seek medical attention was five years! By then, 60 percent thought they had a serious medical problem and more than half thought they would go deaf. Both of these are misconceptions in nearly all cases. If you have tinnitus, see an ear doctor and find out its possible cause. At the least, this could save you a lot of worry and stress. At best, it might be treatable.

Treatment

Remember, tinnitus is a symptom, not a disease. There's not one specific treatment to relieve it. If you have tinnitus, see an otologist for a complete evaluation to determine the cause of the tinnitus. This exam will help identify any underlying physical problems that might be treatable either medically or surgically. The evaluation will include a history of the tinnitus (answering questions such as those we mentioned earlier about your tinnitus), general health, and any history of hearing loss. You'll have a complete hearing evaluation including pure-tone air and bone conduction tests and a speech discrimination test (see Chapter 2), and your doctor might order other tests based on your history and the findings of your hearing test. Some clinics may also do some tests to determine the pitch and loudness of your tinnitus and other specialized tinnitus tests.

Depending on the results of your tests and examination, treatment for your tinnitus may be recommended. Immediate treatment can be performed, for example, to remove impacted earwax or drain fluid from the middle ear. If something like this is the cause of your tinnitus, you might leave the doctor's office essentially cured! But in most other cases, the treatments that we describe below don't actually cure tinnitus. The goal of these treatments is to reduce your perception of the tinnitus so that it bothers you less and has less of an impact on your life.

Hearing Aids

Tinnitus is perceived as being louder in quiet situations. By increasing the level of background sound, it's possible to achieve a decrease in the strength or apparent loudness of the tinnitus. Only rarely is it possible to suppress tinnitus perception completely this way, but some decrease of the tinnitus is possible by enriching the auditory background. If you have a hearing loss, amplification of the auditory background by the use of hearing aids can be helpful. The hearing aids can help both your hearing loss (and improve communication ability) and the tinnitus by increasing the input to the ears.

Sounds of nature as well as music have been shown to be effective in reducing stress, lessening sleep problems, improving a sense of well-being, and bringing on positive changes in cognitive function (memory, attention, and so on). Sound that you associate with positive memories, especially music, is particularly helpful. Hearing aids can enhance these positive effects by increasing the pleasurable perception of these sounds. Even if you have a mild hearing loss or function fairly well with your hearing loss, you might find a hearing aid beneficial for your tinnitus. It can reduce some of the stress associated with hearing loss and amplify background sounds to make your tinnitus less noticeable.

SOUND ADVICE

Using your hearing aids to amplify background sounds won't help at night because most people don't try to wear their hearing aids to bed. Instead, some people find it helpful to have some sound in their bedroom at night to increase the auditory input and help reduce the level of their tinnitus. This could be a fan, air filter, radio, or noise-making machine.

Tinnitus Maskers

For unexplained reasons, most people find listening to an external sound, even noise, less offensive than listening to their tinnitus. The general principle of using external sounds to cover up or mask tinnitus has been used to develop a device that you can wear to provide masking sounds, even if you don't have a hearing loss and wear a hearing aid. These are worn at ear level and produce a broadband sound that might reduce or even eliminate your perception of tinnitus (called partial masking and complete masking). Tinnitus maskers look like a hearing aid and emit a sound into the ear; you can adjust the frequency and loudness of the sound to match your tinnitus. If you have a hearing loss, you can use a tinnitus instrument, which is a combination of a hearing aid and a masker. The hearing aid helps amplify sounds of the speech frequencies, and the masker blocks the usually higher frequencies of the tinnitus.

Medications

Medications can be helpful to some people with disturbing tinnitus, but unfortunately, no single medication works for all cases. Some people seem to respond to vitamin therapy or the use of certain herbs such as ginkgo biloba. But there's little scientific evidence that these treatments actually affect the tinnitus any more than a placebo. The same is true of the many remedies advertised to treat and "cure" tinnitus. Among the types of medications proposed to relieve it are antianxiety drugs, antipsychotics, sedatives, antidepressants, antihistamines, and anticonvulsants—a lot of *anti*'s! However, most scientifically sound clinical studies of these various drugs have shown little conclusive evidence of benefit for tinnitus.

Two medications that might be helpful in selected cases of severe, bothersome tinnitus are amitriptyline and nortriptyline, generic names for a class of antidepressants. But in addition to treating depression, they've been shown to be effective in some patients with chronic pain and with tinnitus. They are centrally acting, meaning they affect the part of the brain that intensifies the perception of pain, and in this case, tinnitus. The doses used for tinnitus are less than doses used for treating depression.

Many people with severe, disturbing tinnitus awaken frequently during the night and have difficulty going back to sleep. Because one side effect of these drugs is sedation, they're usually prescribed to be taken at night, so this might help reduce your tinnitus and allow you to sleep through the night. Sometimes, anxiety has a strong affect on tinnitus. In this case, a low dose of a mild antianxiety medicine such as alpraxolam (Xanax) helps to reduce the anxiety and the perception of the sound. Some people find this helpful in the evening to help sleep, others use it during the day when anxiety is a greater problem.

Relaxation Techniques

As stress and tension aggravate tinnitus, when the muscles of the scalp or the jaw muscles are tight, your tinnitus is likely to seem louder. There are a number of relaxation techniques that can help reduce your stress (or the effects of stress on your body). For example, biofeedback is a treatment to reduce anxiety by teaching you to relax certain muscles and increase blood flow. An electrode attached to a muscle on your forehead and a temperature sensor on your fingertip provide feedback to show when you're succeeding in relaxing. When you've learned to consistently reduce muscle tension and increase blood flow to the skin, you might find your tinnitus is reduced. Other forms of relaxation that might be helpful include activities such as yoga, regular exercise, meditation, and, perhaps, psychotherapy. But like most of the other treatment modalities for tinnitus, scientific studies of the effect of relaxation have yielded mixed results.

Tinnitus Retraining Therapy

If you're one of those people who is unable to ignore tinnitus, some techniques have been developed to train the brain to ignore it.

HAVE YOU HEARD?

In the early 1980s, researchers noted that the majority of people with tinnitus develop a tolerance to it and learn to accept it as part of their environment within a year. They also noted that people associated more problems with the tinnitus when they had experienced it for only a short period of time. That is, an adaptation seems to take place that causes tinnitus to be less of a problem over time.

Tinnitus retraining therapy (TRT) is a program based on the idea that the brain is flexible and can adapt to different situations. The term for this phenomenon is habituation. The TRT program consists of two components: counseling and education to help you learn effective coping techniques and sound therapy. The premise behind TRT is that with proper counseling, education, and understanding, the brain is able to habituate or get used to a sound pattern to both reduce anxiety and allow you to focus your attention away from the tinnitus. TRT assumes that the negative emotional reaction to tinnitus is largely a conditioned response that intervention can change.

During the sound therapy component, you wear a tinnitus masker device that presents a soft sound in the ear so you can barely hear both the tinnitus and the sound generated by the masker. This, combined with the adaptation techniques taught during the counseling sessions, allows your brain to de-emphasize the importance of the tinnitus. The goal is habituation—the gradual reduction or elimination of the annoyance and the conscious perception of tinnitus. An audiologist or professional who has received specialized training in this area teaches the counseling sessions. If you're interested in this treatment, your otologist can make a specific recommendation and referral for it.

A number of other specific tinnitus treatments involving counseling and sound therapy include music therapies, the Neuromonics device and program, phase shift tinnitus reduction, desensitization, pink noise therapy, dynamic tinnitus mitigation system, and auditory integration training. For all these treatments, the use of properly fitted hearing aids should be beneficial if you have a hearing loss in addition to your tinnitus. These therapies are all intended to take advantage of the brain's plasticity to adapt to the unwanted sound.

Cognitive-Behavioral Therapy

Counseling is usually a component of all tinnitus treatments, but some methods use specific psychological techniques. One that has been used effectively in pain management and also applied to tinnitus is called cognitive-behavioral therapy. The goal is to identify negative behaviors, beliefs, and reactions that you might have to your tinnitus and help you substitute more appropriate and positive reactions. Psychologists usually perform this type of therapy, but some audiologists have received training in this approach because they work with patients to provide auditory rehabilitation.

Other Treatments

In recent years, a variety of other treatments for severe tinnitus have been tried, which include transcranial (through the skull) electromagnetic stimulation, transmastoid (through the bone behind the ear) ultrasound masking treatment, transtympanic (through the eardrum) low-dose laser treatment, and many more. Again, there is as yet little scientifically valid evidence that these treatments are effective.

HAVE YOU HEARD?

The United States Department of Veterans Affairs considers tinnitus a disabling condition. United States military veterans can submit claims for tinnitus if they believe noise exposure during their military service caused it. An approved claim usually results in monthly disability compensation payments.

Help Yourself

You can find lots of advice and tips online about how to help yourself deal with tinnitus. The American Tinnitus Association (www.ata.org), one of the largest organizations that deals specifically with tinnitus, gives these tips, among others:

- **Diagnose and understand your tinnitus.** Don't panic. Tinnitus is usually not a sign of a serious, ongoing medical condition. Check things out. The sounds you hear may actually be normal sounds created by the body. Review your current medications (prescription, over-the-counter, vitamins, and other supplements) with your doctor to find possible causes of your tinnitus. Be a detective. Keep track of what triggers your tinnitus.

- **Find good treatment and take care of yourself.** Find ways to eliminate or reduce some stress in different parts of your life. Pay attention to what you eat. One by one, eliminate possible sources of tinnitus aggravation, e.g., salt, artificial sweeteners, sugar, prescription or over-the-counter medications, tobacco, and caffeine. However, don't stop taking medications without consulting your doctor first. Don't give up on a treatment if it doesn't work right away. Some can take quite a while to have a positive effect. Protect yourself from further auditory damage by avoiding loud places and by using earplugs when you can't avoid loud noise.

- **Recognize that your attitude matters.** Don't create negative forecasts for your tinnitus. Counting on a better future can help you create one. Take heart. In many cases, people with tinnitus habituate to it—they get used to it and notice it less than at first. Be involved in your recovery. Consider yourself part of your treatment team; your thoughts and feelings count. Don't waste time blaming yourself. The causes of tinnitus are varied and difficult to determine.

- **Line up support.** Locate people who understand your struggles, and learn that you're not alone. Have people in your life who, though they can't see or hear your tinnitus, understand that you have it. Find a support group that will truly understand your struggles with tinnitus and help you sort out useful from useless information. Educate your family, friends, and co-workers about tinnitus; tell them about the conditions and settings that are difficult for you. Ask them for their support.

True Stories

These cases from our patient files illustrate how real people describe their tinnitus, some of the causes of tinnitus, and what treatments we used.

A Double Role for Hearing Aids

John, who was 50 years old, began to notice a high-pitched buzzing in his ears. When he consulted an otolaryngologist, he reported that he'd spent most of his life hunting and working with power tools. A hearing test showed that John had a moderate high-frequency hearing loss due to his past noise exposure. He actually wasn't aware of the hearing loss, but his family complained that at times he didn't seem to hear them. John's only real complaint was the tinnitus that bothered him during the day. We counseled John about using ear protection in the future and prescribed hearing aids to amplify the higher frequencies. In addition to helping his hearing, John found he wasn't aware of the tinnitus while wearing the hearing aids.

No, You Don't Have a Tumor

Susanna, a 35-year-old aerobics instructor, sought help for an intermittent but severe left-sided head noise, which seemed to increase late in the afternoon toward the end of her workday. Her classes were filled with college students and booming music. Susanna's hearing test did show a mild loss at 4,000 Hz, greater on the left side than the right. Although this pattern could be due to noise exposure, a rare cause for one-sided tinnitus and an asymmetric hearing loss is an acoustic tumor. To rule this possibility out, the ear doctor ordered an MRI scan, which fortunately was normal. The doctor reviewed with Susanna methods of coping with the tinnitus, including biofeedback training and use of a Neuromonics device. The doctor also suggested that she lower the music volume and use ear protection while instructing. On follow-up, Susanna's tinnitus was still present but didn't bother her as much. She felt relieved that the MRI proved there was no serious problem in her head.

The Chicken or the Egg?

Bob, 63, had a mild, very high-frequency hearing loss that didn't affect his under-standing of speech. The cause of hearing loss was probably normal age-related deterioration. But he was very disturbed by tinnitus as it affected his ability to sleep at night and his concentration during the day. He had been to many physicians, tried various herbal remedies, and also tried acupuncture, to no avail. He could go to sleep without difficulty, but would wake at 2 or 3 A.M. and not be able to return to sleep. Bob was aware that he was depressed and very anxious and believed the tinnitus caused these feelings. On careful questioning, the otologist found that Bob had recently lost his job and was very concerned about his finances, so he prescribed a mild antianxiety, antidepressant medication and referred Bob for counseling. After several weeks, Bob was able to adapt to the tinnitus and learned to ignore it most of the time. However, the tinnitus still becomes loud when he's under stress.

Subject and Objective

Jane, a 52-year-old English teacher, noticed a pulsatile sound in her right ear that seemed to have gotten louder over the last several months. She also had a sense of fullness in her ear but no significant hearing problem. Her internist saw a bluish mass in her middle ear on the right side and referred her to the otologist who recognized the vascular mass as a glomus tympanicum, a benign growth that has a rich blood supply. Often, a pulsating objective tinnitus is the first sign of these tumors. A CT scan showed the tumor was only in the middle ear. Surgery was performed under general anesthesia as an outpatient, and the vascular tumor was successfully removed. Postoperatively, Jane's tinnitus and fullness on the right were gone.

The Least You Need to Know

- Tinnitus is a symptom, not a disease.
- About 80 percent of patients with hearing loss have tinnitus; only 5 to 10 percent of people with tinnitus have normal hearing on an audiogram.
- Hearing aids can help not only your hearing but also your tinnitus.
- Most people learn to ignore their tinnitus, but for those with severe, disturbing tinnitus, although there's not a certain cure, there are a wide variety of treatments to try.
- When stress is a factor in your tinnitus, reducing it with a variety of relaxation techniques may be helpful.
- Various sound therapies have been developed to take advantage of the plasticity of the brain and its ability to adapt to the tinnitus.

Hearing Problems in Children

14

In This Chapter

- The many causes of hearing loss in children
- Screening for hearing loss in the newborn baby
- Recognizing symptoms of childhood hearing loss
- Testing infants and young children for hearing loss
- The effects of differing degrees of hearing loss on children

Children, like adults, can have hearing loss caused by problems in any part of the ear, but hearing loss in children can have different consequences. Some adults can function adequately in their daily lives with mild or even moderate hearing loss, but even a small amount of hearing loss in children requires attention and intervention.

Children use their hearing to learn language, to learn to speak so they are easily understood, to pay attention and learn in school, and to make friends. Kids with normal hearing learn most of their words and proper grammar by overhearing what their families and people around them are saying, not by being taught each word or sentence directly. But a child who has any amount of hearing loss is less able to hear others talking. As a parent, a first reaction to this statement might be, "Whew, now I don't need to worry so much about what I say in front of the kid!"

If a child can't hear the speech of others, he or she is at risk for getting behind in development of speech and language. The greater the hearing loss, the greater is this risk. Medical treatment or properly fit hearing aids at the earliest possible time are crucial for the hearing-impaired child in developing speech and language and succeeding in school. This means that a parent must be alert to the signs of hearing loss, and appropriate testing must be performed.

In this chapter, we discuss the types of hearing loss that occur in children, some of the warning signs to look for if you suspect a hearing loss in your child, the differences in testing hearing in children versus adults, and the ways hearing losses of different degrees may affect a child.

Types of Hearing Impairment

In previous chapters, we described how different problems with the external, middle and inner ear can cause hearing loss. The sections below discuss these same issues but with special attention to children.

External and Middle Ear Impairment

As established in Chapter 1, abnormalities in the outer or middle ear can cause conductive hearing loss. Many of the same things that cause conductive loss in adults can also occur in children and usually produce a mild to moderate hearing loss.

Problems in the external ear canal can include earwax or foreign objects (yes, children will stick pencil erasers, beads, or other small items in their ears!). They may also get "swimmer's ear," an infection in the ear canal. These conditions are usually easily solved with a visit to the doctor (see Chapter 3). Damage to the eardrum from a perforation due to injury (such as pushing a cotton swab against it) or from a middle ear infection may heal on its own or be repaired by a surgeon. In rare cases, a child's ear canal never fully develops before birth, a condition called atresia. Atresia can sometimes be corrected surgically, although often children with atresia use a type of hearing aid called a bone conduction hearing aid (see Chapter 16).

Problems in the middle ear can include otitis media (middle ear fluid) or abnormalities with the bones that conduct the sound to the inner ear. Middle ear fluid is very common in young children and can cause mild to moderate hearing loss that comes and goes (see Chapter 6). This can usually be treated medically or with insertion of ventilation tubes into the eardrums. If the middle ear bones, or ossicles, become disconnected or if they become fused and don't vibrate normally, a surgeon may be able to repair the damage and restore hearing (see Chapter 5).

Inner Ear Impairment

Problems in the inner ear can be present at birth or acquired as a result of illness or injury to the very delicate inner ear structures. It can affect both ears equally, be less severe in one ear than the other, or be in only one ear and not the other. Sensorineural hearing loss cannot be corrected with medicine or surgery, although several surgically implantable devices can help some children who cannot benefit from conventional hearing aids (see Chapter 18).

Some examples of causes of sensorineural hearing loss in children include the following:

- Certain illnesses the mother might have had during pregnancy, such as rubella (a type of measles), toxoplasmosis (a disease caused by a parasite), and cytomegalovirus (or CMV, a mild infection in the mother that can cause severe complications for her baby)

- Lack of oxygen at birth

- Certain illnesses the child might develop, such as meningitis

- Accidents resulting in skull fracture or injury to the head

- Certain medications (usually used only with very serious illness) that can be harmful to hearing or ototoxic

- Exposure to very loud noise, such as a firecracker at close range, or repeated exposure to loud noise over time, such as shooting guns, amplified music, or loud equipment

- Hereditary factors and congenital abnormalities of the inner ear.

HAVE YOU HEARD?

How can it be that so many children with hearing loss are born into families where there is no history of hearing loss? In some cases the loss is genetic, but the gene causing the hearing loss is recessive. A recessive gene is one in which two copies of the gene (one from each parent) are required before the trait it carries can show up. If both parents do carry a defective gene, each of their children has a one in four (25 percent) chance of receiving defective copies of the gene from both parents, resulting in hearing loss, in this case. If the baby receives only one copy of the gene (from one parent), he or she will not have hearing loss, but is a carrier and could potentially pass the gene on to his or her own children. (But those children will not have the condition unless the other parent also transmits the defective gene). Two parents who have this kind of hearing loss will have children with hearing loss—because neither of the parents has a normal copy of the gene.

The inner ear has many, many different structures that can be congenitally mal-formed. There can be bony abnormalities of the cochlea and also abnormalities of the structures housed inside the bony cochlea. Many inner ear abnormalities are named after the scientists who first described them. Probably the most common form of inner ear abnormality in children with congenital profound deafness is called Schiebe dysplasia (*dysplasia* meaning abnormal development or growth of tissues, organs, or cells). Though extremely rare, there can be a complete absence of inner ear structures (Michel deformity); the cochlea can appear as a single cavity (cochlear aplasia); only a small, simple cochlea might develop (cochlear hypoplasia); or there can be a small cochlea with incomplete or none of the usual internal divisions of the cochlea (Mondini deformity). Besides abnormalities of the cochlea, the internal auditory canal (IAC) can be enlarged or narrowed. A narrow IAC can also be associated with a failure of the hearing nerve to develop.

LISTEN UP

Someone with a Mondini deformity or other congenital inner ear malformation is at increased risk for developing meningitis or perilymphatic fistula and may also be predisposed to develop a cerebrospinal fluid (CSF) leak. Children with one of these congenital malformations should avoid contact sports because of the increased risk of CSF leak following even a minor head injury. Middle ear infections must be treated aggressively because of the increased risk for menin-gitis. Parents should also consider genetic counseling after a careful analysis of their family history.

Newborn Hearing Screening

Knowing early that a child has a hearing loss and providing early treatment is criti-cal to successful development of language. Fortunately, no child is too young for a hearing test. Most states now require universal newborn hearing screening (UNHS), which allows professionals to identify hearing loss and begin the process of fitting appropriate hearing aids within weeks of a baby's birth. UNHS means the comple-tion of one or more objective, physiologic tests to determine hearing status in each ear for all newborn babies, regardless of risk factors, before they leave the hospital or birthing center.

In the past, only babies born with conditions that put them at high risk for hearing loss were screened. This meant that about 50 percent of newborns with hearing loss were being sent home without the hearing loss being detected—nearly 6,000 babies each year. On average, hearing loss in children was first identified at age 2½ to 3. Some children had hearing losses that were not identified until they were five or six years old. Now, the majority of states require newborn hearing screening, and some additional states have voluntary programs. Many hearing-impaired infants are now identified at a few weeks of age. The Joint Committee on Infant Hearing and the United States Public Health Service's Healthy People 2010 health objectives recommend that all newborns be screened for hearing loss by one month of age, have diagnostic follow-up by three months, and receive appropriate intervention services by six months of age!

HAVE YOU HEARD?

In 1993, less than 5 percent of all infants were screened for hearing loss before leaving the hospital. Today, more than 90 percent of newborns are screened before hospital discharge. Approximately 1 to 3 percent of those screened require referral for further diagnostic evaluation.

Early hearing screening (followed by complete testing if the baby does not pass) is especially important if there are any known risk factors for hearing loss. One such factor is family history: did a close relative have a hearing loss other than that associated with older age—especially a childhood sensorineural loss? Other risk factors include low birth weight or birth problems requiring a stay in the neonatal intensive care unit (NICU), treatment while in the NICU with assisted ventilation or medications known to cause hearing loss, or presence of high bilirubin in the blood (jaundice). Risk of hearing loss might also be greater in children with abnormal facial features (including deformed outer ear or cleft palate).

Screening doesn't pick up very mild loss, and it doesn't show the degree of loss or whether a loss is present at all sound frequencies or only at some frequencies. If the baby has a response, that doesn't rule out very mild loss or loss only at certain frequencies. If there is no response, the loss could be moderate or profound or any degree in between.

Some children are born with normal hearing, but hearing loss begins later or gets worse with time. Parents need to continue to be alert to possible hearing loss even if a baby passes the screening test (see next section for warning signs). Hearing loss can develop as a result of a head injury or as a result of chemotherapy or radiation treatments a child might receive for cancer.

Also, parents should keep in mind that not all children who fail the newborn screening will turn out to have abnormal hearing after all. A newborn with normal hearing may fail the first screening due to debris in the ear canal, fluid in the middle ear, or movement or crying during the test. This is why more than one test is done when a baby does not pass the screening in the hospital. After a second screening, if the baby still does not pass, additional testing is performed that gives more information about the degree and type of hearing loss.

LISTEN UP

Newborn screening is great! But not all children with hearing loss acquire their hearing loss at or before birth. A number of conditions cause hearing loss after birth or cause a mild loss to get worse with time. It's very important to remember that even if a baby passes screening, hearing should always be tested again before beginning speech/language therapy or entering any kind of special education program.

As a result of early intervention, many children with hearing loss are able to learn to communicate as well as other children their age by the time they enter school, where their language ability is important to academic achievement. We describe treatment or intervention for hearing loss in children in Chapter 15, but first the hearing loss must be identified. Newborn hearing screening is only the first step.

Warning Signs of Possible Hearing Loss

Because a child might pass newborn screening but still have a hearing loss or lose hearing later, parents should know the signs of hearing loss in children. Following are some things to look for.

In early infancy:

- The baby does not startle to loud sounds.
- The baby does not wake up to loud sounds.

In older infants:

- The baby does not search for or locate sounds he or she should hear.
- The baby is not soothed by sounds such as speech or music.

- The baby does not use his or her voice or make a variety of speech sounds.

- Close to a year of age, the baby is not imitating speech sounds.

In toddlers:

- The child is more than a year old but does not understand simple spoken language such as "Where are your shoes?" or "Where's mommy?" or "Show me the kitty."

- The child has not started to say words between 12 and 18 months of age, especially if he or she also appears not to understand simple spoken language.

- The child is not putting two words together by 2 years of age ("Daddy go," "doggie bark").

- The child responds inconsistently to sounds and speech, sometimes appearing to understand and sometimes not.

In preschoolers:

- The child does not seem to know or use as many words in a sentence as other children the same age.

- The child's speech is difficult to understand.

- The child responds inconsistently to sounds and speech, sometimes appearing to understand and sometimes not.

In preschool and school-age children:

- The child does not pay attention in class.

- The child has difficulty understanding spoken directions or other information.

A parent can perform a "subjective" test when a child is engaged in a quiet activity. When the baby's back is turned to you, ask a simple question in a normal conversational loudness level from about 6 feet away. No response or an inappropriate answer could be a sign that the child is not hearing well.

Remember that if a child has otitis media (fluid in the ear), there may be some hearing loss until the fluid in the middle ear goes away.

LISTEN UP

If a doctor or teacher recommends speech therapy, a hearing test should be performed. There is no sense in spending time working on production of sounds that the child cannot hear!

Testing Hearing in Children

Since young infants cannot be trained to respond to sound in the way older children or adults do, several tests of hearing are used that don't require a direct response from the child. We talked about some of these in Chapter 2, but in addition, the following hearing tests may be conducted on children.

Auditory brainstem response (ABR) measures the brainwave or nerve patterns sounds generate. For this test, it's usually best if the baby or very young child is sleeping. When ABR is used in newborn screening, the sound is presented at a single soft level. If a response is seen, the baby passes the screen. In the more complete ABR testing, sounds are used that give more specific information about what frequencies (pitches) the child can hear and at what levels. This information can be used for fitting a hearing aid.

Auditory steady state response (ASSR) measures a different type of nerve potential than ABR but gives similar information that we can use to estimate an audiogram.

Otoacoustic emissions (OAE) testing uses a very small microphone placed in the ear canal to measure the activity of the inner ear in response to a sound introduced into the ear canal by a very small speaker. When OAE testing is used as the screening test, the baby passes if a large emission is found. If not, the baby goes on for more testing. When OAEs are used as part of a diagnostic battery of tests, presence or absence of OAEs is used together with ABR (and often together with ASSR) to obtain more complete information about the type (conductive, sensorineural, or mixed) and degree of hearing loss (how well or poorly the baby hears and at what frequencies).

ABR, ASSR, and OAEs are the most informative procedures available for babies in the first six to eight months of life. The results of these tests allow the audiologist to move ahead right away with hearing aids if a hearing loss is found.

Tympanometry and acoustic reflex testing are used in children as well as adults. Abnormalities on tympanometry may indicate fluid in the middle ear or a problem with the eardrum or ossicles.

Behavioral observation audiometry is performed with very young infants in a quiet sound booth testing chamber. The audiologist looks for any signs, such as movement, eye blinks, or making sounds, that indicate the baby is responding to speech and sounds of different frequencies and at different intensity levels or loudness. Behavioral testing becomes more specific and more reliable once the child is able to sit up and turn toward the source of a sound. Once the child has reached this stage of development (six to eight months of age), the audiologist uses a procedure called visual reinforcement audiometry (VRA). The child is seated on a parent's lap or in a high chair. Sounds are presented through earphones (one ear at a time) or speakers, and as the child begins to turn toward the sound, the audiologist turns on a lighted or animated toy. Once the child learns there is a reward for responding to the sound, he usually will turn repeatedly when the audiologist presents sounds at different frequencies. Using VRA, the audiologist can obtain thresholds—the softest sound the child responds to—for each frequency, in each ear, and plot them on an audiogram form.

Between the ages of 2½ and 3, most children can learn to perform a conditioned play task or play audiometry. The child holds a block or similar toy and waits for a sound; when he or she hears it, the child drops the block into a bucket or puts a peg into a pegboard. The audiologist presents softer and softer sounds until the child no longer responds. Using play audiometry and earphones or headphones, the audiologist can obtain a complete audiogram for each ear.

Speech perception testing can be performed as soon as the child develops speech and language skills and is able to cooperate by pointing to pictures or repeating words. Especially with children who have hearing loss, speech understanding is an important part of hearing testing because it is not possible to tell from the audiogram alone how clear or unclear speech sounds to a child. Two children with identical audiometric thresholds may have very different abilities to make sense of what they hear. Speech perception scores contribute to how the audiologist chooses and sets hearing aids or cochlear implants.

How Does Hearing Loss Affect a Child?

Generally, the more hearing loss a child has, the more it affects the child's ability to learn to talk, to develop social skills, and to succeed in school. The following table shows the ages at which a normal-hearing child is expected to show certain communication behaviors. Keep this in mind when considering the impact of hearing loss on speech and language development.

Development of Communication Behaviors (adapted from www. betterhearing.org)

Age	Communication Behavior
5 months	Turns toward source of moderate and soft sounds
6 months	Recognizes familiar voices; does "vocal play" with parents
9 months	Demonstrates understanding of simple words
10 months	Babbles by stringing together multiple, single-syllable speech sounds
12 months	Produces one or more real, recognizable spoken words
18 months	Understands simple phrases; gets, puts, or handles familiar objects on spoken request; points to body parts on request; speaks vocabulary of 20 to 50 words and short phrases
24 months	Speaks vocabulary of 200 to 300 words; speaks in simple sentences; most speech is understandable, even to adults who do not see the toddler regularly; sits and listens to read-aloud story books
3–5 years	Uses spoken language constantly to express wants, reveal emotions, give information, and ask questions; understands nearly all that is said; vocabulary grows rapidly: 1,000 to 2,000 words; produces complex and meaningful sentences; all speech sounds are clear and understandable by 5 years

Mild Hearing Loss

A child with mild hearing loss may or may not have normal-sounding speech but can certainly be expected to have difficulty hearing and understanding in noisy environments, in situations in which the speaker is more than a few feet away, or when the speaker's face is not clearly visible. Classrooms, playgrounds, and cafeterias are by nature noisy environments, and teachers may not always be facing the class or be close to the child. Kids with mild hearing loss will have at least some degree of trouble in school. Because they may be unaware of subtle conversational clues, they may seem inappropriate or awkward and are often mislabeled as having attention or behavior problems.

HAVE YOU HEARD?

A child with mild hearing loss—even as little as 16 to 25 dB of loss—can miss up to 10 percent of a speech signal when the teacher is more than 3 feet away.

Sometimes parents resist the idea of hearing aids for their child with mild loss because the problem may not be very obvious. However, it's important to understand that with even a mild hearing loss, a child is working harder to focus and pay attention than children with normal hearing. At the very least, a child with such loss who does not get a hearing aid should be tested frequently to determine whether the hearing loss is stable or could be getting worse. Close attention should be paid to the child's progress in school. Because teachers and classroom aides often assist children in primary grades, an older child may begin to struggle as the demands on his or her listening abilities become greater. Also, a child with a mild hearing loss may miss parts of the typical fast-paced peer interactions (ever listen to a group of kids talking?) which could have some impact on socialization and self-concept.

Moderate Hearing Loss

Children with moderate hearing loss are unable to hear soft conversation. They can hear speech when it's louder than usual or when they are very close to the speaker, but they won't be able to hear and understand the typical teacher's voice in the classroom. They'll also miss a lot of the normal conversation going on around them and hear just bits and pieces of speech, leading to misunderstandings. The child may be accused of "hearing when he or she wants to," of daydreaming, or of not paying attention, which can affect self-esteem.

Also, as a result of missing conversation, a child may be delayed in developing the ability to express him- or herself through speech, as well as have problems with speech production. A child with a moderate hearing loss might experience difficulty learning early reading skills based on letter-sound associations. However, with early fitting and consistent use of hearing aids and with auditory and speech/language therapy, most children with moderate hearing loss can learn to speak well and attend regular schools.

Severe Hearing Loss

Children with severe hearing loss are unable to hear even loud conversation or most sounds around them. Without immediate intervention—fitting of hearing aids and intensive therapy—these children will not develop spoken language skills. The greater the delay in intervention, the less likely they will be able to catch up to the level of their peers as hearing will not be normal even with hearing aids. But children with severe loss will be helped greatly both by hearing aids and by use of visual cues (see Chapter 19). Many children with severe hearing loss do develop age-appropriate spoken language skills and attend regular school. There are also special classrooms for children with hearing loss. Children with severe loss will probably need additional services in school, such as regular monitoring by a Deaf and Hard of Hearing educator and an FM system (see more on this later). Older children may need a note-taker or caption service.

Profound Hearing Loss

Children with profound hearing loss may have at least a little residual hearing, but usually they won't be able to hear or understand normal conversation even with powerful hearing aids. Strong hearing aids may let them hear some of the speech sounds, but usually children with profound loss still can't hear high frequencies. Unfortunately, many consonant sounds are comprised of high frequencies, for example, the sounds represented by the letters *s, f, th, p,* and *t.* It's very difficult to understand speech without hearing these sounds. Even if the speech is loud enough to be detected, someone with a profound hearing loss cannot easily tell the difference between words such as *cat/fat/pat/sat* or *hot/shot/thought.* In conversational speech, these sounds are even harder to distinguish. For children with a profound hearing loss from a young age, oral language skills—the ability to express themselves verbally through speech and understand the verbal expressions of others—are very delayed. And the child's own speech is usually very difficult for others to understand.

HAVE YOU HEARD?

Although there are exceptions, most hearing losses are worse in the high frequencies. So how important are high frequencies? Very! Without them, we can't understand English, and children with severe high-frequency hearing loss have difficulty learning to speak correctly. Think about personalized license plates. What if we put only vowels on the license plate: I A AE. Can you figure out what that license plate says? Not without consonants, you can't. But what if we use only consonants for the same license plate? DCK ND JN. If you say it out loud, you can pretty easily figure it's "Dick and Jane." Now, imagine what it's like not to hear those consonant sounds. It's next to impossible to understand what people are saying if you can't hear consonants, and it's nearly impossible to learn to produce sounds you can't hear.

For children who do not get enough benefit from hearing aids to develop oral language and where learning to listen and speak is the goal, a cochlear implant may be an option (see Chapter 18). Some children with profound hearing loss and minimal or no benefit from hearing aids might communicate best through use of sign language in classrooms specifically for children learning sign language or in regular classes with a sign language interpreter.

Hearing Loss in One Ear

Many children with varying degrees of unilateral hearing loss (loss in only one ear) succeed in school and in the workplace with little handicap. But numerous studies have shown that unilateral loss can have negative effects on educational achievement. In fact, studies have found that children with unilateral hearing loss are 10 times as likely to be held back at least one grade compared to children with normal hearing. Children with unilateral loss have a hard time telling where a sound is coming from and greater difficulty understanding speech in noisy environments. And they may have difficulty detecting or understanding soft speech from the side of the poor hearing ear, especially in a group discussion. In particular, children who may already be having difficulty in school because of learning disabilities, language delay, recurrent fluid in the ear, or attention deficits may be more greatly affected by unilateral loss.

For even greater detail on the effects of hearing loss of differing degrees in children, Appendix D provides a parents' guide to the relationship of hearing loss to listening and learning needs.

True Stories

Addressing hearing loss in children is so important, but not much can be done unless we recognize that there is a loss. Our case files are full of stories about children whose hearing loss was not diagnosed or not taken seriously enough at the youngest possible age. Here are just a few stories about finding hearing loss in young children.

Parents Are Right!

Before universal newborn screening, many deaf babies were not identified for months or even years. But in many cases, the parents had expressed their suspicions of hearing loss to their physicians for many months only to be told that babies couldn't be tested until they were older. Sometimes the doctor even suggested that the parents were just worry-warts.

Steven was born before newborn screening programs were available. Although he seemed to respond to his parents' voices, he was the soundest sleeper ever. His parents began to worry that maybe he was responding to them more because he could see them than because he could hear them. When they tried to test him at home, they became even more suspicious; but they were still unsure—and hoping for the best. Their doctor said that all first-time parents were afraid their kids weren't "normal" and told them to just relax and enjoy him as he would develop in his own time. By the time Steven was 19 months old, he had not begun to say his first words (and didn't seem to understand any words, either). His parents were frantic. One day, they were at a community parade and a fire engine went by, sirens blaring. Steven remained asleep in his stroller. The next day, his mother called an audiologist and scheduled an appointment. Steven was severely deaf and most likely had been since birth!

Anna was born when newborn screening was just getting started, and her birth hospital did not yet offer it. She was a healthy newborn who went home from the hospital with her mother. But over the next few days, the mother began to suspect that Anna did not hear. This mother had three other children and knew Anna was not responding to sound as her other new babies had. She contacted her pediatrician, who attempted to calm her fears by saying it was impossible to tell at this early stage. Fortunately, the mother knew this not to be the case and demanded a referral to an audiologist. Anna was tested with ABR and OAEs. She was profoundly deaf.

These cases are similar but different. Steven got his first hearing aids at the age of almost 2 years and struggled with his oral language development. Anna received her first hearing aids at the age of 5 weeks, and with the help of cochlear implants provided at age 1, she is now entering regular kindergarten with very normal speech and language for her age.

Temporary Hearing Loss Is Still Hearing Loss

Emily was a child with almost constant middle ear fluid for the first two and a half years of her life. Her vocabulary was obviously less developed than most other children her age, and she was very difficult to understand. She was treated with antibiotics; when the fluid went away, it wasn't for long. Her family physician didn't seem to want to recommend more aggressive treatment, but her parents finally consulted an ear specialist who decided she should have tubes placed in her eardrums (see Chapter 6) so that the fluid could not build up. Emily's father worked the late shift. So Emily slept late in the morning and went to bed after Dad got home. Mother and child would watch *The Tonight Show* while they waited for him. Within three weeks of receiving the tubes in her ears, Emily uttered her first very intelligible sentence: "Here's Johnny!"

Everybody Needs a Test

Newborn screening is meant for the benefit of a newborn baby, but it can sometimes benefit other family members as well.

Jacob was screened at birth and did not pass. When follow-up testing showed moderate sensorineural hearing loss in both ears, he was fitted with hearing aids immediately. Because hearing loss often runs in families, it was recommended that Jacob's older brothers and sisters be tested as well. His parents were shocked to discover that two of their other four children also had mild to moderate hearing loss. None of these older children had been screened at birth and, except for the oldest two whose hearing was normal, they were under age five so hadn't yet been screened at school. When the two other children received hearing aids, the parents noted an improvement in their speech development and attention span within a very short time.

So She Passed Newborn Hearing Screening

Lisa passed her newborn hearing screening and by age 18 months was beginning to say words and even a few short sentences. But by age 2, she had not progressed in her language, and her behavior began to be quite odd. She didn't interact with her parents the way she used to, and she didn't respond to them as much when they talked, read, or sang to her. Because she had passed the hearing test at birth, all assumed her hearing continued to be normal. Her pediatrician feared she might be showing signs of autism and referred her to a program for autistic children. Fortunately, her very observant teacher suspected that she was not hearing very well and referred Lisa to an audiologist for more testing. It turned out that Lisa had a moderate to severe sensorineural hearing loss. A CT scan showed that she had an inner ear malformation that often causes progressive hearing loss. Fitted with hearing aids, Lisa began to respond to sound again. Her speech and language development progressed, as did her desire to interact and play with her parents.

The Least You Need to Know

- Because there are many causes of hearing loss in children, parents should become familiar with the warning signs.
- Hearing tests for newborns are available and are valid; don't let anyone tell you that babies can't be tested.

- As children learn most of their words and grammar by overhearing what people around them are saying, a hearing loss can have a huge impact on the development of speech and language.
- Trust your instincts; if you think your child is not hearing normally, demand an evaluation.
- If your child has several episodes of fluid in the ear, see an ear specialist and have an audiologist test his or her hearing.
- If your child has mild hearing loss, don't be fooled into thinking that no help is needed.

Treatment of Hearing Loss in Children

15

In This Chapter

- Hearing aids and other devices for children
- Ways to improve hearing and understanding in the classroom
- Types of therapy and training to improve listening
- Ways to help a child with a hearing loss

You've been told your child has a hearing loss. So now what? Many families clearly remember the day they were told their child was hearing impaired but don't recall being told what they could do about it. They say they felt abandoned and left to make too many decisions on their own. Their audiologists usually remember the initial evaluation differently and are surprised to find that parents feel they were not given enough information.

Most likely, the facts lie between the two perspectives. Parents might be too shocked by the news (or confirmation of their suspicions) to be able to understand much more information that day. Audiologists may talk too fast or provide too much or not enough detail to parents who are still adjusting to the diagnosis. So we hope this chapter will be useful to parents who are still learning what they can do for their child with hearing loss.

Although many of the same things that cause hearing loss in adults can also affect children, in this chapter, we focus on how children with hearing loss can be helped with hearing devices, education, and therapy. We also give you some helpful hints on how to communicate most effectively with your child.

Professional Intervention—Earlier Is Better

One national study by the Better Hearing Institute found that only about 12 percent of young people with hearing loss in the United States receive the help they need. We have discussed how important early identification of hearing loss is because of the impact that even mild hearing loss can have on development of speech and language, on social skills, and on educational success. But early identification must be followed by early intervention. A baby whose hearing loss is discovered through newborn hearing screening can be fitted with hearing aids right away and enrolled in an early intervention program well before the age of six months.

Hearing Aids

Hearing aids, often referred to as *amplification*, can help children with all degrees and types of hearing loss. These types of hearing aids are described more fully in Chapter 16, where we explain their use in adults.

DEFINITION

Amplification is another term sometimes used for hearing aids. In this context, amplification means increasing the volume of sound.

Infants and young children with hearing loss are most often fitted with behind-the-ear (BTE) style hearing aids. In-the-ear (ITE) styles, which are much smaller, are rarely a good choice for a young child as they pose a swallowing hazard and don't work well for more than mild hearing loss in very small ears. In-the-ear styles also usually lack some of the features that are important for young children, such as a direct audio input that allows hookup of an FM system (assistive listening device; see below) to the hearing aid. And the outer casing of an ITE aid must be changed frequently as the child's ears grow.

However, ITE styles may be okay for some school-aged children. The child's preferences may go into the decision regarding what style hearing aid to use, but we must also consider the size of the ear canal. A completely in-the-canal style may not be possible to make for a very small canal, and it may not fit completely in the canal. We must also consider the degree of hearing loss and the features of the hearing aid that would most help the child.

Happily, behind-the-ear hearing aids are available in very small cases for mild to moderate loss and in much smaller cases for severe and profound loss than were available only a few years ago. And hearing aids come in colors to match a child's skin or in bright colors such as pink, blue, red, purple, or yellow. They can be decorated with flower, animal print, sports, or other colorful stickers. The custom-made *earmolds* that connect the hearing aids to the child's ears also come in clear material or in any conceivable color, with glitter, multicolor swirls, stripes, or spots.

 DEFINITION

Earmolds are formed pieces of silicone, vinyl, or other soft materials created from impressions of the individual hearing aid user's ears. An earmold fits snugly into the ear, connects to the behind-the-ear hearing aid by a small tube, and delivers the sound from the aid to the ear.

Hearing aids usually last three to four years, and earmolds must be replaced more frequently, especially for rapidly growing babies. So we need to consider the life of the hearing aid and earmold when selecting colors. Plain beige or brown hearing aids may well last into the years when the child herself might really want pink. And children who will soon be preteens might prefer hearing aids and earmolds that are less visible; parents themselves may prefer less visible colors; or preteens may even choose outrageous combinations of colors and designs to make a fashion statement! Encouraging the child to love and want to wear the hearing aids is important, even if the choices are not exactly what the parents have in mind. Young infants and children require flexible, adjustable amplification. No single hearing aid works for all hearing losses, but modern digital technology allows for one model to be adjustable to many different degrees and configurations of hearing loss. Initial settings of any hearing aid need to be changed as a child grows physically and as more complete audiometric information is available over time. Flexible amplification can also address a child's changing needs if hearing levels fluctuate. Changes in hearing loss could happen because the hearing loss is progressive or because the child has episodes of otitis media that reduce hearing until the condition resolves.

No hearing-aid technology is made exclusively for children, as the same technology used for adults is beneficial for children as well. But some companies do focus on children by offering a wide variety of colors and accessories that are most useful for babies and young children. These accessories include devices that help secure the aids to the child in case he or she is inclined to take them off (and perhaps throw them!), battery testers, and listening stethoscopes. With a stethoscope, parents can listen to the hearing aids and know if they sound scratchy, work intermittently, or seem softer than usual. If they do, the parent can contact the audiologist and arrange for the aids to be repaired. "Kid kits" supplied by child-friendly hearing aid companies usually include toys or coloring books for the children and information books for parents and teachers.

> **SOUND ADVICE**
>
> Children lose hearing aids! Many products are available to help with this prob-
> lem, including devices to attach the aids to the child's clothing and colorful
> covers that serve both to help keep the hearing aids clean and dry and to make
> them show up better than beige or brown when they are lying on the ground
> or in a child's cluttered room.
>
> It's also a good idea to have insurance coverage for hearing aid loss. The manu-
> facturer of the hearing aids offers coverage for repairs, for loss, and for damage
> for a limited period of time. Often, coverage for repairs is longer than coverage
> for loss and damage. The manufacturer may also offer the opportunity to
> extend this coverage. If not, there are insurance companies that do cover loss
> and damage after the manufacturer's warranty expires. Ask your audiologist.

For infants and young children with atresia or other serious middle ear abnormalities, use of an earmold inserted into the ear canal may be impossible. Either a conventional bone conduction hearing aid or a bone-anchored hearing appliance (Baha) can provide sound to the inner ear by vibration through the bones of the head. The Baha processor may be worn with a soft retention band by children of any age, and the surgical Baha procedure may be an option for children five years old and older (see Chapter 16).

Cochlear Implants

For children with severe and profound hearing losses, a hearing aid may not be of much benefit. In such cases, a *cochlear implant* might provide better access to sound. Cochlear implants have been approved for use in children by the United States Food and Drug Administration for nearly 20 years. Unlike a hearing aid, a cochlear implant does not present amplified sounds to the ear. Instead, electrodes are surgically placed into the inner ear (cochlea), and an external device converts sound to an electrical signal, transmitting it through the skin to an implanted receiver and then on to the inner ear. In Chapter 18, where we describe cochlear implants in detail, you'll find a description of the evaluation process and the benefits and risks that might be expected for children.

DEFINITION

A **cochlear implant** is a surgically implanted device that electrically stimulates the hearing nerve to provide sound to severely and profoundly deaf people who cannot benefit significantly from a hearing aid. Children as young as 12 months are candidates for the implants.

Mixed Hearing Loss

It's possible for children to have conditions that cause both sensorineural and conductive hearing loss. Any combination of middle ear and cochlear or nerve abnormalities can cause mixed hearing loss, such as a problem in the cochlea plus a hole in the eardrum or a problem in the cochlea plus a problem with the movement or shape of the ossicles. Children with sensorineural loss can also have fluid in the middle ear or otitis media, which may be brief and occasional or frequent, long lasting, or chronic. The conductive part of the hearing loss is likely to be medically treatable (see chapters in Part 2). For the sensorineural part, the child would need hearing aids. But be aware that the child's hearing aids need to be programmed and reprogrammed, depending on the degree of the hearing loss during the time of the conductive loss and the success of the treatment for it.

Hearing Loss in One Ear

A conventional hearing aid is not likely to help profound unilateral (one-sided) loss because of the degree of impairment and also because some children with one normal-hearing ear find the amplified sound from the ear with a hearing loss to be uncomfortable or unclear. But if a child has a less-than-profound hearing loss and some ability to understand speech in the impaired ear, a hearing aid may help.

Some adults with one-sided loss find CROS hearing aids, which route sound from the impaired ear to the other ear, beneficial. But they are not usually recommended for children. The Baha device, another option for adults, may provide some promise for children with unilateral loss (see Chapter 16). But at this time, the device that provides the clearest benefit in the classroom to children with unilateral hearing loss is the FM system, in any of its many configurations (see next section).

In the Classroom

Every person with hearing loss, even if he or she uses hearing aids or cochlear implants, will have more difficulty hearing and understanding speech in a noisy environment than in a quiet one. Of course, we all have this problem, but it is magnified for the hearing-impaired. The classroom is certainly one of these noisy environments. Children tend to be noisy by nature—talking to each other, rattling papers, shuffling feet. And the nature of the room itself is likely to make matters worse. Hard surfaces such as tile floors, blackboards, and uncovered windows all cause sound to bounce throughout the room. Heaters and air conditioners may be loud. The classroom may be located near a busy street where traffic noise can be heard. Chair legs may scrape against hard floors. Some of these issues can be improved with wall and window coverings, acoustical tiles on the ceilings, and sound-absorbing materials (such as tennis balls) on the bottoms of chair legs. While these measures all help, they can't compensate for students themselves making noise or for teachers with soft voices who may not always face the class.

Children in noisy environments may not even be aware they are missing or misunderstanding information! Or they may be embarrassed to call attention to themselves by telling the teacher that they're not following the class discussion very well. In Chapter 17 we describe assistive listening devices referred to as FM systems. The teacher or talker uses a microphone and a small transmitter. Typically, the microphone is worn on the lapel or around the neck and the transmitter is worn on a belt or in a pocket. The student may have personal receivers attached directly to his or her hearing aids or cochlear implant speech processors, or there might be a small speaker on the student's desk or table. Some schools have a system in place that projects the FM signal through speakers all over the classroom, called a soundfield system. FM systems allow the student to hear the teacher's voice through the receiver regardless of where the teacher is standing or facing in the classroom (face not visible, back turned, or strolling the aisles of the room). Such a system reduces the effects of noise in the room and allows the hearing-impaired child to make the most effective use of hearing aids or cochlear implants.

SOUND ADVICE

FM systems can also be useful during extra-curricular activities such as sports, dance class, religious services, or riding in the car. For example, what if you're driving and your hearing-impaired child is sitting in the back seat? You could wear the FM transmitter and microphone, and the child sitting in the backseat could wear the receiver. No more excuses about how he or she didn't hear your instructions!

FM systems do not have to be connected to a hearing aid or cochlear implant. They can also benefit children with minimal hearing loss, fluctuating hearing loss (including from otitis media), learning disabilities, attention deficit disorders, and unilateral hearing loss.

Therapy and Auditory Training

When children are diagnosed with hearing loss, they almost always benefit from one-on-one therapy with a person who specializes in working with deaf and hard-of-hearing children. The greater the hearing loss, the greater is the need for therapy. This therapy can take many forms and may be provided by a variety of specialists, so it's important for parents to learn about all the communication options open to them and have a good understanding of the choices before selecting a program for their child.

Parents need to consider what makes the best sense for their child's level of hearing, what types of programs are likely to help the child reach the parents' goals, and what is workable in view of the needs of other family members. For example, if a family wants a cochlear implant for their profoundly deaf child, the surgery should be done during the optimal period most likely to bring spoken language success. A child with profound hearing loss whose parents are not interested in pursuing a cochlear implant may be best served by a sign language program. If this is the choice, it will be essential for all members of the family to learn sign language as well, not only to communicate effectively with the deaf child but also to be models of complex language. Children with mild to moderate hearing loss may need less intensive intervention. But they will need some special assistance to ensure that they can make the most of their hearing aids, develop language at the level that's right for their age, and learn good speech habits.

Children can obtain educational services and therapy to help them learn language from a variety of sources. Laws require public schools to provide or arrange for early intervention services for children with hearing loss, even if they are infants, and to provide special services as needed throughout a child's public school life.

HAVE YOU HEARD?

The Individuals with Disabilities Education Act (IDEA, 1997) is a law ensuring services to children with disabilities throughout the nation. IDEA governs how states and public agencies provide early intervention, special education, and related services to eligible infants, toddlers, children, and youth with disabilities. The law requires children with hearing loss to have a therapy and education plan created specifically for the individual child. The Individual Family Service Plan (IFSP) is the legal document that lists services that will be provided to a child who is under age three. The Individual Education Plan (IEP) is the legal document that lists services that an older child is to receive. These services are decided upon by a team that consists of teachers, therapists, and—very importantly—parents.

Private services are also available from licensed, certified *speech language pathologists*, certified *auditory-verbal therapists*, and teachers of the deaf who may provide therapy or extra-curricular programs to encourage spoken or signed language development. An essential key to success is that the therapist be highly qualified, knowledgeable, and experienced in working with children who are deaf or hard-of-hearing.

DEFINITION

A **speech language pathologist** (also called speech pathologist or speech therapist) is a person with a clinical license or professional certification that allows him or her to assess, diagnose, treat, and help to prevent disorders related to speech, language, cognitive-communication (brain damage, stroke), voice, swallowing, and fluency (e.g., stuttering).

An **auditory-verbal therapist** is usually a speech language pathologist, teacher of the deaf, or audiologist who has special training and certification to work with hearing-impaired children on listening skills for the development of spoken language.

Training for Listening

Parents who want to emphasize learning to understand and use spoken language can choose from two basic approaches: the auditory-verbal and the oral or auditory-oral.

The auditory-verbal (AV) approach focuses on listening and learning much as normal-hearing children do. For children to learn spoken language through this method, early detection and intervention are important. Children must have at least some remaining hearing and be able to hear many of the sounds of conversational speech with hearing aids, or they must be using cochlear implants.

An important part of auditory-verbal therapy is parental involvement, as the parent learns during the individual AV therapy sessions how to follow up at home and continue the listening activities. Parents who choose this approach must be strongly involved in working with their hearing-impaired child at home. Also, a goal of this therapy is for the child to succeed in *mainstream* education, as placement in a mainstream classroom also helps to provide normal language models for the child to imitate and from which to learn.

> **DEFINITION**
>
> A **mainstream** education is one in which children attend school or classes
> with their same-aged, normal-hearing peers. Children with hearing loss can
> be mainstreamed for all or part of their school day, attend some mainstream
> classes and other special education classes during each day, or be "reverse
> mainstreamed," where some of the children in the class have hearing loss and
> some do not.

The oral, or auditory-oral, approach uses many of the same methods as the auditory-verbal approach, but it may also place emphasis on use of visual cues such as speechreading and natural gestures. The oral approach is often used in classes that are specifically for deaf and hard-of-hearing children where spoken language is the goal. In this setting, listening and speaking are a main focus of daily classroom instruction. Many children who receive oral classroom education in preschool are able to enter mainstream kindergarten or be partially (and later fully) mainstreamed for certain subjects once they go to elementary school.

In both the AV and the oral approaches, sign language is not used and may be strongly discouraged.

Using Vision and Hand Signals

Some children with severe or profound hearing loss may not have enough benefit from hearing aids to develop spoken language effectively, and their parents may not choose for the child to undergo surgery for placement of a cochlear implant. These children usually are able to develop language skills through the use of one of several types of sign language. Many Deaf people consider American Sign Language (ASL) their native language (see Margin Note). ASL is a completely visual language system with its own grammatical structure, which is different from the structure of English. There is no written form of ASL. For children who have little hearing and not much benefit from amplification, ASL provides a language system. It allows communication with other ASL users and learning in classes taught by teachers using sign language. Because ASL does not translate directly into English, it is difficult to speak English and sign at the same time.

> **HAVE YOU HEARD?**
>
> Many profoundly deaf people who use sign language for communication con-
> sider themselves members of "Deaf culture," a social movement that considers
> deafness to be another form of human experience but not a disability. When
> used to have cultural meaning, the word *deaf* is often capitalized and referred
> to when speaking as "big *D* Deaf."

Other forms of sign language have been developed that use the grammar of English. These include Manually Coded English and Signing Exact English (SEE). Often these kinds of sign language are used in what are called Total Communication (TC) programs, in which both spoken and manual (sign) languages are used. Some studies suggest that sign language that follows the grammatical structure of English can improve the ability of deaf children to learn to read and write in English.

Cued speech is a different means of using hand signals to improve communication. Cued speech uses hand signals placed near the lips to help clarify the many sounds that are not visible through speechreading. Some families find it very effective when the child is not wearing his or her hearing aids or implant processors (such as in the bath, in the pool, or when the listening device malfunctions). A limitation of cued speech is that while the child's family and close friends may learn to cue, very few other people are familiar with it.

Hints for Helping a Child with Hearing Loss

If your child has a hearing loss and wears a hearing aid or cochlear implant, there are additional things you should do to maximize your child's benefit and chances of success.

Understand Your Child's Hearing Loss

Have your audiologist explain how to read the audiogram and give you some guidance as to what speech sounds and environmental sounds your child can and cannot hear, with or without hearing aids. If you're present in the test booth during testing, you'll be able to hear the level at which your child responds to sounds of different frequencies and to hear how well he or she understands words and sentences. This information can give you a better understanding of what kind of help your child needs in therapy sessions and what difficulties the child might encounter in the classroom.

Keep the Hearing Aids On

Keeping hearing aids on young babies can be challenging because they grow so fast that earmolds don't fit well for very long. Poor-fitting earmolds create feedback, that whistling sound you hear when a microphone is too close to a speaker or sometimes in older people who wear hearing aids. Feedback is rarely the fault of the hearing aid itself, but rather the fit of the mold. The more powerful the hearing aid, the more feedback occurs. Earmolds must be remade frequently in young babies. It's less of a problem once the baby can sit up and less of a problem still once rapid growth slows down.

SOUND ADVICE

When a baby wearing a hearing aid is lying with his or her ear up against padding in a carrier or being cuddled in your arms, feedback from the hearing aid is often worse. So when you are holding or feeding your baby, you may want to turn off the hearing aid that is up against you. Leave on the one that is aiming outward, and switch when you change sides.

Older babies and toddlers fitted with hearing aids for the first time know how to reach up and take them off. Use a firm and friendly approach; let your child know that the hearing aids go on when you say so and come off only when you say so. Soon the child will be more willing to wear the aids, recognizing that hearing is better with them on.

Talk to the School

If your child is in a regular classroom setting, talk with the teachers to help them understand what your child's hearing loss means for his or her ability to follow instructions, understand lecture material, or socialize with friends. Offer to go over tomorrow's material, and review today's material, with your child at home. Give the teacher suggestions on how to communicate most effectively with your child: get the child's attention first and speak face to face whenever possible. Encourage the teacher to use the FM system if it has been recommended for your child.

If your child begins to wear hearing aids after starting school or goes to a new school or class where no other children are using hearing aids, take the opportunity to educate the class. An older child may wish to do this by giving a presentation about hearing loss and hearing aids or cochlear implants, but you may wish to make this kind of presentation for your younger child. Explain hearing loss and how the hearing aid or implant works on a child-friendly level. Many hearing aid manufacturers provide toys, booklets, and pictures that you can use for this kind of project.

Talk to Other Parents

It helps to talk to other parents. When you first become aware that your child has a hearing loss, it's tremendously distressing. If you've never had hearing loss in your family, you are probably unfamiliar with what this means for your child and his or her future and what it requires of you as a family. Don't try to do everything all by yourself. Talking with professionals is essential to have the correct information, but talking with other families helps you get a picture of how you can deal effectively with the unexpected changes in your life that hearing loss may bring. If your child is enrolled in an educational program that includes a parent group, you ought to participate. But there are also parent groups online and through organizations for families of children with hearing loss.

Talk to Your Child

Remember that children learn to talk more by overhearing others talk than by having you teach them individual words and phrases. Keep in mind that children with any degree of hearing loss have more trouble hearing at a distance or understanding in noise, which makes that overhearing more difficult. You can improve communication by following these simple suggestions:

- Get the child's attention first and talk face to face.

- Turn off the TV, the running water, the dishwasher or other noisy appliances, and put your barking dog outside while you talk to your child.

- If you're not sure the child understood you, don't ask whether he or she heard you because children often say "yes." Instead, ask *what* the child heard you say.

- If you need to repeat, it may help to simplify your language or break directions down into smaller units. But don't keep everything you say too simple! Children need examples of complex language.

Read to a hearing-impaired child often, even if he or she is too young to understand. Sing songs to and with the child. While doing chores together such as making beds, running the bath, buckling into car seats, or buying groceries, talk out loud about what you are doing and use descriptive language. Ask questions and help the child devise answers. If you're getting her dressed, talk about the pretty red sweater and shiny new shoes. If you're playing with him, make talking about the activities part of the game. Expand on simple statements she may make; for instance, if she says,

"Mommy ball!" you could say "Yes, there is a big blue ball! I see it! It has white stripes on it!" Point out sounds in his environment: the running bathwater, a ringing telephone, the radio, the dog barking. Children with hearing loss may need more direct teaching, but incidental learning that all children accomplish simply by listening is equally important. So make your household a language-rich place for your child.

True Stories

As you read in this chapter, there are many ways to help a child who has a hearing loss. Often, the parents must make decisions about what might be the best treatment or therapy options for their child. Every child and every family is different, but following are a few examples of the many, many children with hearing loss we've seen in our clinic and what course of action their parents decided to follow.

Families Help Families

Diana and Steve were stunned to learn that their new baby Sara had moderate hearing loss. Although still struggling with disbelief, they did go ahead with the hearing aid fitting. The hearing aids were a nuisance. They were difficult to keep in; they whistled when Diana or Steve held Sara; and they were a constant reminder that there was a problem. They found it easiest to ignore the hearing loss most of the time because they couldn't see any clear evidence of it in the young baby's behavior. But with some gentle urging, their audiologist persuaded them to enroll Sara in the local Early Start program, and they began to attend the program's parent meetings as well. There, meeting families much like themselves, they began to see how important it was to keep Sara's hearing aids on and to participate in the therapy provided in Early Start. Perhaps most important, they began to accept Sara's hearing loss as a manageable condition. They saw they had plenty of company as parents in this situation and both wished they had gone sooner. Now they are enthusiastic participants in the group, helping other new parents who are going through the same difficult experiences.

To Sign or Not to Sign?

Jake was born with profound hearing loss into a large and close family of normal-hearing parents and relatives. While his parents were more than willing to learn sign language, they felt Jake would have more options in life if he were able to hear and that it would be easier for them as a family if they all communicated by speaking with one another, so they elected to provide Jake with a cochlear implant for each ear when he was 13 months old. With frequent and regular therapy and much support at home, Jake was able to go to kindergarten with hearing children his own age.

Melissa, also deaf, began using hearing aids and signing with her parents at a young age. When she was three, her parents decided on a cochlear implant for her, but she struggled with the development of her listening and speaking skills. Although she did make some progress, by the time she was ready for kindergarten, her ability to speak was still well behind other kids her age. She entered a Total Communication program where the primary mode of communication was sign language. The teachers also used their voices. She received speech/language therapy at school and therapy from a speech-language pathologist after school two days per week. Melissa's signing skills improved rapidly, and her listening and speaking continued to improve slowly but steadily. Now in junior high, Melissa communicates primarily through sign language at school and with many of her friends. But at home she talks with her family and neighbors and with other hearing people when she is out in her community.

Ryan was also born with profound hearing loss. He received little benefit from hearing aids even though his parents were careful about having him wear them. Ryan's mother was deaf from birth and communicated using ASL; Ryan's father was a hearing child of deaf parents. He grew up using both Sign and speech to communicate. Comfortable with deafness and with Sign as an extremely effective mode of communication, the parents communicated with their son through both Sign and speech. They chose to enroll him in a program for deaf children where ASL was taught as the main method of communication. There—and with their help at home—he thrived, both academically and socially.

A Tale of Two Cochlear Implants

Janie was born with a profound hearing loss in one ear and normal hearing in the other. She functioned essentially like a normal-hearing person, developing age-appropriate speech and language and achieving high grades in mainstream classes. At age 14, she was in a bad automobile accident and suffered a temporal bone skull fracture which caused her to lose all the hearing in her previously normal ear. A month after her accident, Janie received a cochlear implant. With the help of an auditory therapist, she was able to learn to listen and understand with her cochlear implant very quickly.

Juan initially had a different experience. He was born with normal hearing, but when he was a junior in high school, he suddenly developed a profound hearing loss in both ears due to a medical condition. His parents were eager to proceed with a cochlear implant, but Juan was afraid of the surgical procedure, and he didn't really want to wear the external equipment. If his parents attempted to force him to undergo surgery right away, he would probably have simply refused to use the device. Instead, his audiologist helped him contact several other implant users his age, one of whom was Janie. Within a month, Juan was ready to proceed with cochlear implantation and has been a remarkably successful user of this technology.

The Least You Need to Know

- If your child has hearing loss that is not medically treatable, hearing aids and/or cochlear implants and expert therapy can help; the earlier, the better.
- No one educational or communication method is right for all children.
- Make use of an FM system to help your child in the classroom and in other noisy situations.
- Parent education is important, too; it helps you understand your child's needs.
- Deaf children can grow up to lead normal lives; the key is language development, whether through hearing and speaking or through sign language.

Help for Hearing Loss

5

Everyone is familiar with what a hearing aid is—or are you? This is an area that has improved vastly in just the last few years. Actually using an aid takes a little getting used to, so we explore the technology, the different types, and their use. If a hearing aid can't help you, several surgically implanted devices are available. We also describe the many types of assistive listening devices that can help anyone with hearing loss. And finally, we talk about how to cope, whether you have hearing loss or whether you're communicating with someone who has hearing loss.

Hearing Aids and How They Work

16

In This Chapter

- Determining the best hearing aid for you
- The many types of hearing aids and available features
- Adjusting to a hearing aid for the first time
- The cost of hearing aids
- Caring for your hearing aids

In 2009, the National Institutes of Health held a working group meeting on accessible and affordable hearing health care for adults with mild to moderate hearing loss. They reported that hearing loss is the third most prevalent chronic health condition in seniors, yet fewer than 20 percent who require treatment seek help. Most people who do use hearing aids lived more than 10 years with their hearing impairment and waited until it had progressed to moderate to severe levels before seeking a hearing aid. And these people are not just seniors.

More than 18 million adults in the United States of working age (ages 18 to 64) are estimated to have some degree of hearing loss, and many of these people would benefit from a hearing aid. In Chapter 20, we talk in detail about the consequences of hearing loss. But if you have a hearing loss, you're already familiar with some of the many problems that can accompany this sensory impairment. So are you using a hearing aid?

What is a hearing aid? In simple terms, it's a microphone, an amplifier, a speaker, and a power supply. Fortunately, advances in technology have enabled us to take those components and miniaturize them into something that can be worn on or in the ear with a very tiny battery as the power supply. Hearing aids have changed dramatically in the past 10 years, with new technology options and improved performance and wearability.

In the previous chapter, we discussed the use of hearing aids in children but promised more detail about the aids themselves, their use, and care. So in this chapter, we describe the various types of hearing aids for adults, including conventional aids and recently developed implantable hearing aids. We talk about the many special features now available, the cost, and the care. We also provide you with many suggestions on how to adapt to and learn to use a hearing aid if you're a first-time hearing aid user.

Hearing Aid Evaluation/Consultation

Federal regulations prohibit a hearing aid sale unless the buyer has first received a medical evaluation from a physician. If you're at least 18 years old and are aware of the recommendation to receive a medical exam, you can sign a waiver to forego it, but we don't think this is a good idea unless you've previously seen an ear doctor, because it's possible that you have a treatable form of hearing loss or a problem that might interfere with use of the aids. An otolaryngologist, audiologist, or a certified hearing aid specialist can dispense (fit and sell you) hearing aids, which should be custom-fitted to your ear and hearing needs. Hearing aids purchased by mail order typically can't be custom-fitted.

> **HAVE YOU HEARD?**
>
> President Ronald Reagan was known as "The Great Communicator." He understood that good communication was more important than hiding a hearing problem and was the first president to acknowledge needing hearing aids. He was fitted with hearing aids in 1983 and put hearing loss in the national spotlight with wide media coverage. If a president of the United States was willing to wear hearing aids, certainly you can, too!

The hearing aid evaluation usually takes about an hour. In addition to evaluating your hearing, the professional should help you understand hearing devices and what you might need for the best hearing results. This includes discussing the hearing test and how your degree of hearing loss will affect your ability to communicate, the different styles of hearing aids, and the appropriate styles for you. Many factors go into determining which style of hearing aid might be best for you. These factors include the following:

- Degree and type of hearing loss

- Shape of the ear canal and its tendency for skin or moisture problems

- Manual dexterity (one's ability to handle small items)

- Lifestyle (activities you participate in and their physical environments)

- Cosmetic concerns

- Listening needs (e.g., telephone use) and environments (theaters or music halls, large family gatherings)

After the consultation is complete, a detailed prescription for hearing aids can be made. If you decide to purchase hearing aids, it's common to expect at least two visits for fitting, follow-up measurements, counseling, and possible design changes.

One major question to resolve is whether to use one or two hearing aids. The most common causes of hearing loss—age-related and noise-related—typically produce hearing loss levels that are similar in both ears (binaural, see Chapter 1). Binaural hearing aids allow you to have balanced hearing, with speech perceived equally loud in both ears, to localize sounds and to hear better in noise. When using hearing aids, there is another advantage. Using two aids results in a significant increase in the perceived loudness of sound due to a phenomenon called binaural summation. That is, there's an additive effect on loudness; you can reduce the volume setting for each ear and still have the sound be loud enough. This, in turn, lessens the impact of background noise.

Types of Hearing Aids

Hearing aids have the basic function of increasing the loudness of sound for the hearing-impaired listener, or amplification. Human-made devices for doing this date back hundreds of years. Online, you can find pictures of all kinds of interesting devices used to filter out noise by directing the sound of choice straight into the ear using a tube or trumpet. People have used versions of ear trumpets, including animal horns, seashells, and, later, metals, for thousands of years.

HAVE YOU HEARD?

Royalty often had special thrones and chairs built to allow visitors to the court to speak quietly yet maintain a respectful distance from both hearing and deaf royals. The speaker would kneel before the throne and speak into openings in the arms of the chair. A small tube connected to a resonator in the throne's arms, and wings conveyed the sound to the royal ear.

Electric hearing aids first became commercially available in about 1901, with the first wearable models in the 1930s and 1940s. Jumping way ahead, digital processing hearing aids became available in the 1990s. Until then, hearing aids used analog processing, simply amplifying the continuous sound wave. Now, most hearing aids are digital and offer a wide variety of advanced technology features. Sound comes into the microphone in analog sound waves. Then a small computer chip digitizes or converts it into digital form. Digitization changes the incoming sound into millions of small units, called digits. While the sound is in this stage, the computer chip inside the hearing aid can process or alter the incoming sound and even determine which of the incoming sounds are speech sounds and which sounds are random noise. The hearing aid then attempts to reduce unwanted noise and enhances speech. All this is done within microseconds!

Conventional Hearing Aids

We categorize hearing aid type primarily by where the device is worn, and here we define the major types of hearing aids. In Appendix F, we provide a more detailed look at the various features offered with digital hearing aids.

Behind-the-ear (BTE): A BTE hearing aid hooks over the top of the ear and rests behind the ear. It attaches to a custom-made earmold that brings the amplified sound from the hearing aid into the ear and is appropriate for any degree of hearing loss, from mild to profound. This type might be required when medical conditions of the external auditory canal make you unable to use other hearing aid types.

A relatively new type of BTE instrument is referred to as open fit because the ear canal is left open and not totally blocked by an earmold. It consists of a small BTE connected to a very thin tube, which is attached to a small dome inside the ear. The advantage of an open fit is that you'll be able to use your natural hearing as well as the increased volume provided by the hearing aid for those frequencies where you have a loss. This style of hearing aid is generally appropriate only for people with mild to moderate hearing losses.

In-the-ear (ITE): An ITE hearing aid is all one piece that's custom-molded to fit entirely in the concha (bowl) of your ear. ITEs are easy to manipulate if you have poor vision or manual dexterity problems. ITEs are appropriate for mild to severe hearing loss and may even fit some profound losses.

One of the most common problems people have with ITE hearing aids is the fit because the ear canal can change size over time and these hearing aids are usually meant to fit very snuggly within the ear canal to prevent *feedback*. This high squealing sound is what you hear when a hearing aid that's turned on is placed in your hand, and you don't want feedback when wearing the aid.

> **DEFINITION**
>
> **Feedback** is the squealing sound produced by a hearing aid when amplified sound leaks out of the ear and is forced back into the microphone a second time. The result is an overload of the amplifier and a tell-tale whistling.

In-the-canal (ITC): An ITC hearing aid is also made using a mold of the ear and is all one piece. It's similar to an ITE but is smaller, filling only the outer portion of the ear canal. An ITC hearing aid is suitable for mild to moderate losses if you have an adequate-size ear canal and no moisture or skin problems of the ear. New technology is now even allowing this type of aid to be fit on some people with severe losses.

Completely-in-the-canal (CIC): A CIC hearing aid is similar to an ITC aid but fits deeper into the ear canal to provide maximum cosmetic appeal. It's the smallest hearing aid available and takes advantage of the ear's natural resonance and shape. However, it does require good manual dexterity, a normal outer ear canal, and no medical conditions that would prevent its use. It is appropriate for mild to moderate losses, although, as with some of the other small hearing aid styles, stronger circuits are allowing CIC aids to be fit on some people with severe losses.

Contralateral routing of offside signal (CROS) hearing aids: A CROS aid is recommended for people with single-sided deafness. With a CROS, you wear two hearing aids, one on the "dead" ear and one on the "good" ear. The hearing aids are then connected, either through a cord or wirelessly. The purpose of wearing a hearing aid on the deaf ear is to collect the sounds on that side of the head and deliver them to the opposite ear where hearing is good. By doing this, sounds normally missed on the deaf side can be heard in the good ear. However, because you are hearing the sounds only in one ear, you still won't be able to localize or tell the direction of the sound source.

Bone Conduction Hearing Devices

People with sensorineural hearing loss use most of the hearing aids because conductive hearing loss is often medically or surgically treatable. But there are cases of conductive hearing loss where use of a conventional hearing aid isn't possible. Aural atresia, the congenital absence or closure of the external ear canal, can sometimes be surgically repaired when a child is older (see Chapter 3). But in the meantime, it's important for the child to receive sound, particularly if the atresia exists on both sides. A special type of hearing aid, called a bone conduction hearing aid, serves this purpose. Like any hearing aid, a bone conduction aid has a microphone to pick up sounds and a processor to amplify the sounds. But rather than playing the amplified sound back to the ear, as in a conventional hearing aid, it transmits the signal to an oscillator. The oscillator vibrates against the skull, causing the fluids of the inner ear to move. From there, the usual hearing process continues. A bone conduction aid is usually worn using a headband which can make it uncomfortable because the oscillator must fit tightly against the skull. The sound quality may also be poor because the skin acts as a barrier to the sound.

HAVE YOU HEARD?

Normal-hearing people sometimes use bone conduction hearing devices when they work in occupations where they must cover their ears for quite a few hours a day. This is particularly common among marine biologists, professional scuba divers, and even avid swimmers whose gear interferes with normal hearing.

To overcome some of the disadvantages of bone conduction aids, a new type of bone conduction device, called a bone anchored hearing system or bone conduction implant, has been developed. This device is primarily for a person with conductive or mixed loss hearing impairment or unilateral deafness. It consists of a surgically implanted titanium post, an external abutment or base that connects directly to the post, and a sound processor. The sound processor fits onto the abutment and transmits sound vibrations to the titanium implant. This vibrates the skull, which gets the fluids in the cochlea to move.

The first available of these devices was the Baha. The newest (July 2009) version of that system sold by Cochlear is called the Baha BP100. It uses automatic digital signal processing that adapts to the user's sound environment and can be used with other lifestyle accessories such as iPods and Bluetooth adapters. A more recently FDA-approved bone anchored hearing system is the Oticon Ponto, which also makes use of digital hearing aid technology. Because of the direct conduction to the skull without the skin barrier, bone conduction hearing systems offer significantly better sound quality than that of a traditional bone conduction hearing aid and don't require wearing a headband. A Baha device, including surgical placement, costs approximately $7,000 to $8,000. The Ponto will probably cost a similar amount. Currently, another bone conducting device is in development (by Sonitus) that will transmit vibrations to the inner ear via a sound processor attached to a tooth!

Implantable Hearing Aids

With a conventional hearing aid, a speaker or earmold delivers the amplified and filtered sound to the ear canal. But for some people, this process isn't effective or isn't practical. Chronic otitis externa, canal exostoses, or frequent earwax impactions might make it difficult for an individual to wear hearing aids (Chapter 3). Also, a person with very narrow or sensitive ear canals can find wearing a hearing aid quite uncomfortable. A more severe hearing loss requires a tighter fit of the aid or earmold, and there's a greater chance for feedback to occur.

If feedback or comfort issues can't be resolved, the individual can't get the necessary amount of amplification . But now some implantable hearing aids are available either commercially or in clinical trials that are either partially or completely embedded in the skull, in the ear canal, or in the middle ear. Unlike cochlear implants, which electrically stimulate the auditory nerve (see Chapter 18), implantable hearing aids work through the mechanical function of the middle ear, just like conventional aids ultimately do.

Implantable hearing aids do involve surgical risks, including possible facial nerve injury, cerebrospinal fluid leak, damage to middle ear structures, skin complications, or infection around the implant site. Insurance does not typically cover them, and because they have metal in them, they might interfere with your ability to have an MRI unless the device is removed. But the idea of an effective hearing aid that can't be seen and doesn't need to be frequently taken on and off is very appealing. Continued research and development of these devices may make them the wave of the future! Talk with your otologist about whether your hearing loss qualifies you for any of the currently available devices.

Special Features

Hearing aids can be configured with a number of special features to improve your ability to hear and function in your specific environment. We list many of these features and on what types of hearing aids they're available in Appendix F. Most digital aids automatically control volume but do also have a user-operated control. Some of these aids have volume-learning circuits. As you adjust the volume in different circumstances, the hearing aid "learns" your volume preferences and adapts automatically the next time you're in that situation. A program switch might also be added to a hearing aid to allow you to choose different listening programs for different listening situations. Telephone use is enhanced by the addition of a telecoil, or T-coil, which allows you to hear speech through the telephone much more clearly. Recently, many hearing aids are being equipped with Bluetooth technology to allow direct transmission from a cell phone right into your hearing aid. In Chapter 17 we discuss assistive listening devices and how they might work in conjunction with certain hearing aid features.

Digital hearing aids come in different levels of technology, which is what largely determines price rather than the style of hearing aid—that is, a BTE, an ITE, and so on. All the aids from a particular manufacturer might use the same base chip, with the top-of-the-line products having all the advanced features while the mid-level or basic products have a less-featured version of the advanced chip. Here are some of the features now available:

Multiple memories/listening programs: Two to four programs in an aid allow you to maximize hearing in different listening situations. You might use one program in a quiet situation, another program to control noise in a restaurant, and another for music or theater listening. You can change programs using switches directly on the hearing aid or by a small, hand-held remote control. Believe it or not, some hearing aids are actually able to determine the best setting or program based on what they detect. The program settings automatically toggle between one another based on the hearing environment, and you don't even need to push a button. Higher-end digital aids provide even more programs.

SOUND ADVICE

If you've tried a hearing aid for your hearing loss from Ménière's disease but found that sometimes it seemed too loud and sometimes not loud enough (because your hearing fluctuates), or you've never tried a hearing aid, consider an aid with a multiple listening program feature. The audiologist can reprogram the aid if your hearing needs change.

Directional microphones: Directional microphones (two or three microphones placed strategically on the hearing aid) greatly improve the ability of hearing aid wearers to hear in background noise. A directional microphone focuses the hearing aid to hear in one direction, generally in front of you. The effect is a dramatic reduction in the amount of surrounding noise the aid picks up behind you. But certain listening situations can be more complex because noise might be coming from all directions. Advanced digital hearing aids are able to use technology to adapt constantly and to focus the microphones on different sound source locations.

Multiple channels: Think of your hearing loss as a picture. If you were using a digital camera to capture this image, you'd want to have lots of pixels for better resolution and to capture the small details of the image. Hearing aid channels (also called bands or handles) act like pixels, allowing the hearing aid to be digitally matched to the valleys and troughs of your audiogram (see Chapter 2).

Hearing loss affects everyone differently. For example, some people have a flat hearing loss—the ability to hear all frequencies (low, middle, and high) has been affected equally. Others might have a sloping hearing loss—thresholds for the high frequencies are much poorer than those for the low frequencies. The number of channels on a hearing aid provides flexibility in fitting the aid to one's particular hearing loss. This feature is important for people who need to hear in challenging or noisy environments.

Noise reduction: Noise reduction, or suppression, is accomplished during the sound-processing phase in hearing aids with a noise-reduction feature. The digital hearing aid analyzes the characteristics of the incoming sound and decides whether the sound is speechlike or appears to be random noise. If the sound has the characteristics of speech, it's amplified. If it seems to be noise, it's reduced or suppressed. One type of noise suppression controls loud bursts of noise to protect the ear. Another focuses on ongoing noise, to suppress it and allow better perception of speech in noise. Most hearing aids have some type of noise reduction strategy, but the higher the technology, the more sophisticated the noise reduction. If you're frequently exposed to noisy environments such as business meetings, restaurants, lecture halls, or places of worship, you might want to consider a more advanced noise reduction strategy. If you spend the majority of your time in quiet settings, you might choose a more basic noise reduction feature.

Feedback suppression: In the past, the only way to guard against feedback was to be sure the hearing aid or earmold fit tightly in the ear so no amplified sound could escape. But new technology in digital hearing aids can suppress feedback through various electronic means, including a sound cancellation effect. As a result of this type of circuitry, hearing aids can now be fit with much more power and in a more open or non-occluding manner and still produce little or no feedback.

HAVE YOU HEARD?

If you wear bilateral hearing aids, you can get them with a feature that allows them to communicate with each other! They read the sound environment, and each aid sets its parameters to work together to maximize noise reduction and enhance speech.

Using a Hearing Aid for the First Time

Your age, the severity of your hearing loss, and your acceptance of the need for the aid strongly influence your reaction to using amplification. The type and degree of your hearing loss also plays a role in the benefits you gain from hearing aids. People with a conductive hearing loss can expect maximum benefits from a hearing aid because discrimination ability is not greatly affected by that type of hearing loss. Just making the sound louder does the trick. With a conductive hearing loss, you should be able to adjust easily to a hearing aid.

With a sensorineural hearing loss such as age-related or noise-induced hearing loss, adjusting satisfactorily to a hearing aid can be more difficult. People with sensorineural loss will often say, "I hear, but I can't always understand what I hear." Certainly speech must be loud enough to hear before you can understand. A hearing aid amplifies sounds. But just making speech louder does not necessarily lead to improvement in discrimination, because the hearing nerve has become less sensitive to the acoustic differences of speech sounds. With amplification, however, some sounds of speech can be heard and understood more easily than with unaided hearing. And if you can hear some of the sounds, your brain will be better able to fill in the gaps and make a word intelligible.

The major problem for a new hearing aid user in adjusting to the hearing aid is noise. But the many innovations in hearing aid technology and fitting have made it easier for new hearing aid users to live with noise. Changes in circuitry of hearing aids, specially designed earmolds, and highly adjustable or programmable aids have greatly eased the initial learning process.

Whatever your hearing impairment, it's important to follow a planned program of learning to use the hearing aid. The ease or difficulty of hearing will vary depending on the loudness of background noises, the distance you are from the source of sounds, the clarity of speech or of music, and the lighting (which can enhance or interfere with speechreading). We discuss speechreading and many other things you and your family or friends can do to improve your ability to communicate in Chapters 19 and 20. Here, we provide some recommendations for learning to use a hearing aid effectively.

- Use the hearing aid at first in your own home. Your hearing aid amplifies noise as well as it amplifies music or speech, so background noise might disturb you. Concentrate on listening for all the normal household sounds, and try to identify each sound you hear. Once you can identify background noises, such as the hum of the refrigerator or the slamming of doors, they'll tend to be less annoying and distracting to you because they won't seem like just noise.

- Wear the hearing aid only as long as you're comfortable with it. If you're tired after using the aid for an hour or two, take it off. Let the way you feel be your guide, but over a period of several weeks, gradually lengthen the amount of time you wear it.

- Start by listening to just one other person—a spouse, neighbor, or friend. Talk about familiar topics; use common expressions, names, or a series of numbers for practice purposes. After a few days of practice with one person in a quiet environment, try a different listening exercise. Turn on the radio or television and, with this auditory distraction, try to understand your companion's speech.

- Don't strain to catch every word. Listening carefully and concentrating on what's being said is important, but don't worry if you miss an occasional word. Normal-hearing people miss words or parts of sentences and unconsciously fill in with the thought expressed. Do keep your eyes on the face of the speaker; speechreading is an important supplement to the hearing aid.

- Don't be discouraged by the interference of background noises. Normal-hearing people are aware of background noises, too, but have learned to push them out of conscious awareness. As you learn to discriminate between noise and speech and to identify various background sounds, you'll be able to ignore extraneous noises.

- Practice locating the source of sound. Determining the direction from which a sound came can be difficult with hearing aids. One exercise to develop directional perception is to relax in a chair, keep your eyes closed, and have someone speak to you from different places in the room. Attempt to locate the speaker's position just through the sound of his or her voice.

- Increase your tolerance for loud sounds. New hearing aid users tend to set the volume too low for effective listening. Over time, you can increase your tolerance for sound. While listening to one speaker or to radio or television in your own home, gradually turn up the volume of your hearing aid until the sound is very loud. When it's uncomfortable, very slowly turn the volume down. After some practice, you'll find that your comfort level has increased considerably. If your hearing aid has automatic volume control, you should find yourself using the manual control less and less.

- Practice learning to discriminate different speech sounds. Prepare a list of words that differ in one sound only (For example: *food/mood*, *ball/all*, *see/she*, *feel/peel*, *could/good*, *gown/down*). Have a helper pronounce these words slowly and distinctly. Watch the lip movements closely while you carefully listen for the differences in similar pairs of words. Then try to discriminate the words by listening alone. A good exercise in listening is to have someone read aloud from a magazine or newspaper while you follow along with your own copy of the reading material. At irregular intervals, your reader should stop and have you repeat the last word read.

- Gradually extend the number of people you talk with at one time. Start at home first. You'll find that it's more difficult to carry on a conversation with three or four people than it is to talk with one. Concentrate mainly on the individual who's doing the most talking.

- Gradually increase the number of situations in which you use your hearing aid. After you've adjusted to background noise in your own home and to conversation with several people at once, you'll be ready to extend the use of your aid to public places. Dining out can be difficult, so eat your first meal in public in a quiet restaurant with carpeted floors. (In Chapter 20, we discuss restaurant listening.). As your tolerance for noise increases, you'll find it easier to be in more noisy environments.

- Take part in an organized course in speechreading, as it will help you in general communication with others (see Chapter 19). Online courses are available. Although it has many limitations, speechreading combined with a hearing aid is often more satisfactory than either alone.

- Use the telephone. If your hearing loss is not especially severe, you'll probably be able, with a little practice, to use your hearing aid with the telephone. Place the receiver end of the telephone next to the microphone of the hearing aid. In some hearing aids, a telecoil is built into the aid (see Chapter 17), and the cordless portion of the telephone is placed in contact with the case of the aid. Getting used to the placement of the telephone and getting used to listening in this manner requires practice. Have a friend call you at a certain time each day for several days to practice.

Adjusting satisfactorily to a hearing aid requires practice, even with using these commonsense steps. Don't expect perfection. Different people learn at different rates. Some, perhaps because of the severity of their loss or because of the nature of the hearing impairment, might require many weeks to learn to use the aid. Others will be wearing an aid without any great difficulty within a few hours. The prime objective in wearing a hearing aid is to have more normal communications in everyday life. To achieve this, speechreading is almost always required, so speechreading rehabilitation should accompany your practice training in using the hearing aid (see Chapter 19).

The Cost of Hearing Aids, and Who Pays

You need to be prepared for the cost of hearing devices. In 2004, the hearing industry's national survey found that the average price of a hearing aid was $1,369. A more recent industry survey found a price range per aid between $1,182 and $2,876, while a recent consumer survey showed consumers spending $1,800 to $6,800 for a pair of hearing aids. The style, type of technology, and local market all influence the hearing aid cost. Financing is often available, depending on the individual dispenser. The table in Appendix F shows the approximate price range for hearing aids with different features.

Usually, the price that a hearing health-care provider quotes you includes professional services (testing, fitting, and follow-up care, usually for at least one year) as well as the hearing aid itself. It's usual practice, and required by law in some states, to provide a trial period for you to be sure the hearing aid is the right one for you. You typically will have at least 30 days in which to return the aid for a different one or a refund. Watch out for excessive, nonrefundable fees, such as a high restocking fee, and be skeptical of free hearing tests. As you would for any major purchase, ask questions before you buy.

LISTEN UP

Hearing devices that cost less than $100, often called "starter aids," only do some amplification of the low frequencies and are not very useful for most types of hearing loss. They've been shown to have a great deal of input noise and could potentially damage residual hearing from the excessive noise amplification.

Low-cost hearing aids are available only on the Internet or through newspaper or magazine ads, all of which you should consider suspect. And remember, your hearing aids need to be custom-fitted, which isn't likely to happen if you don't get a complete hearing aid evaluation and buy from a licensed hearing aid dispenser. However, some mid-range ($100 to $500) devices could be helpful at least as a starter device for someone with a mild to moderate, high-frequency or flat sensorineural hearing loss.

You will also usually need additional supplies, such as batteries, cleaning kits, and drying kits, which the dispensing professional should review with you. Hearing aids are electronic devices, so understand that although reliability is very good, the technology continues to improve. Your dispenser can tell you how often your aid requires routine maintenance. It's also recommended that you reassess your hearing aid every four to five years. This doesn't mean you'll need to buy a new hearing aid, but you should at least determine if new hearing aids are warranted.

Unfortunately, many private insurance policies don't cover the cost of hearing testing or hearing aids. Medicare Part B covers some of the services, such as the hearing tests and some professional services, but won't pay for the hearing aids. If you're a veteran with a documented service-connected hearing loss or a disability rating of 10 percent or more, you might be eligible for hearing aids from the Veterans Administration. There is currently—as of 2009—a legislative bill under consideration in the United States Congress to provide a tax credit on the purchase of hearing aids. The Hearing Aid Assistance Tax Credit Act would provide a $500 tax credit per hearing aid available once every five years. Let's hope that by the time you read this, it will have become law! If not, contact your representative in Congress.

Caring for Your Hearing Aid

Your hearing aid dispenser should teach you proper insertion techniques for your hearing aid or earmold. This usually involves a slight twist to get the hearing aid to fit properly into the ear canal because of the canal's curved *s* shape. You might need to wiggle the hearing aid slightly to ensure the proper fit. An improperly fitted hearing aid can result in discomfort and eventually skin breakdown in the ear canal, which can lead to infection. Wearing a hearing aid should not be painful.

Occasionally, the skin around the hearing aid gets dry. In this case, you can apply a tiny amount of mineral oil or baby oil to the ear canal, but use only a very small amount. Excess baby oil can damage your hearing aid! Applying oil might also be helpful if you are just starting to use a hearing aid and it seems like a tight fit. Your hearing aid dispenser can also provide you with a lubricant used to make hearing aid insertion easier.

Your dispenser should also give you instructions on how to care for your aid. Here are a few things to remember: try not to drop it; keep it dry and away from direct heat; when not in use, keep it in a case. Use a clean, dry tissue to wipe the aid, never a damp cloth or other cleaner. If you're getting feedback, check for earwax in the aid or the earmold and take out and reinsert the aid or earmold to be sure it was in correctly.

The Least You Need to Know

- An evaluation by a licensed professional is necessary to determine what type of hearing aid is best for you.
- There are many styles of hearing aid, from tiny completely-in-the-canal styles to those worn behind the ear.
- Modern hearing aids offer many technological features, including automatic noise reduction and programs for use in different listening situations.
- A first-time hearing aid user should follow a planned program to get used to wearing, using, and caring for a hearing aid.
- Hearing aids are expensive and not usually covered by insurance, but they provide great benefits and improve the quality of users' lives.

Assistive Listening Devices

In This Chapter

- Devices that can help in everyday situations
- Using a telephone, either with sound or through visual means
- Listening in the home: television, radio, music
- Listening in a group setting or in a large area
- Alerting and signaling devices: doorbell, fire alarm, baby crying, alarm clock
- Places to purchase assistive listening devices

A hearing aid (or cochlear implant) may not provide the best solution to a hearing-related problem in many everyday situations. For example, if you have only a mild hearing loss and little or no problem in a quiet office or one-on-one communication, you might feel little need for a hearing aid. Yet you might not be able to function well in a noisy business luncheon or conference setting. What if you get uncomfortable feedback (see Chapter 16) when trying to use your hearing aid with a landline phone that isn't Bluetooth compatible? Maybe you successfully use hearing aids during the day but can't hear the alarm clock in the morning. Or perhaps you are concerned about hearing your baby crying at night when you're not wearing your hearing aid. A wide variety of products are available to help in these kinds of situations. As a category, these are called assistive listening devices or ALDs.

You probably think of ALDs as flashing lights that provide a visual signal for a doorbell, smoke alarm, or the telephone. Yes, these are among the available devices. But today there are many devices to help people with mild to moderate hearing loss, as well as severe to profound loss. Relatively new technologies, such as Bluetooth, are not aimed at the hearing-impaired but can be used effectively to overcome some of the problems associated with hearing loss. Many of these technologies can work in conjunction with digital hearing aids.

In this chapter, we tell you about these other devices that may help you with telephone communication, listening to the radio or television in your home, and listening in meetings, conferences, places of worship, or the theater. Alerting or alarm devices are also available. And did you know you can get a special pet, a "hearing dog," to help with problems you might otherwise encounter because of your hearing loss?

Telephone Devices

The telephone is the primary means we use to communicate with people not in our immediate voice range. Even for those with normal hearing, the signal produced by most telephones is not 100 percent intelligible. If you have a hearing loss, not only is the speech signal over the telephone less intelligible, but you also can't make use of the visual cues that are so helpful in face-to-face communication (see Chapter 19). People with a hearing loss that prevents effective use of the telephone may feel especially isolated. But today, many devices are available to assist telephone communication, even if you have a significant hearing loss.

Amplifiers and Amplified Phones

Telephone amplifiers are designed for hearing-impaired people who don't use a hearing aid or who wish to have additional aided amplification. These include portable amplifiers, volume control handsets, and modular amplifiers. Lightweight portable amplifiers can be carried in the pocket or purse and clip directly over the telephone receiver. These are battery operated and convenient if you travel or use a number of different telephones. For your primary phone at home or at work, you can get a volume control handset—a standard telephone receiver equipped with a thumb-operated wheel that adjusts the loudness of incoming messages. These are available from your phone company. A modular amplifier can be installed easily on any standard desk set modular (jack-style) telephone. The loudness is adjusted with a volume control, and no batteries are required.

SOUND ADVICE

Check with your local phone company or state services. Many states provide free telecommunications equipment and services to people certified by a doctor or an audiologist as having difficulty using the telephone. California, for example, has a state-mandated program, under governance of the California Public Utilities Commission. Equipment and some network services are available at no charge to eligible consumers.

You can also purchase special telephones that provide "sound shaping" technology, phones designed to improve clarity rather than just amplifying sound. In some makes, the earpiece has been designed for ease of use with hearing aids. Such phones range in price from less than $50 to about $250, depending on the features you want. You can even get an amplified cell phone (priced around $250). One phone, priced around $500, has remote control and clarity speakerphone features.

Standard telephone amplifiers can work with your hearing aid in two ways: acoustically or inductively. For acoustic coupling, you simply hold the amplifier up to the microphone of your hearing aid. This works well if you have a completely-in-the-canal (CIC) type of aid (see Chapter 16). But with larger types of hearing aids, putting the phone or a phone amplifier near the hearing aid can produce annoying feedback. To avoid this problem and to give you a better signal to noise ratio, many hearing aids provide a telephone or "T" switch. When the switch is moved into the "T" position, the microphone becomes nonoperative and the induction coil (telecoil) inside the hearing aid is activated. A telecoil is a small coil of wire around a core that induces an electric current in the coil when it's in the presence of a changing magnetic field. Placing the telephone receiver near the hearing aid allows direct induction of the telephone conversation into your hearing aid without the interference of background noises from the environment.

Some newer models of hearing aids have an automatic, or touchless, telecoil that turns itself on when it detects the telephone. This requires having a telephone that is hearing aid compatible (HAC), but this shouldn't be a problem because legislative action in 1991 mandated that all land-line phones sold in the United States be hearing aid compatible. Today, a number of cell phone manufacturers also make cell phones that are compatible with hearing aids. The Better Hearing Institute has posted a list at their website (www.betterhearing.org) of those models of cell phones that are most compatible with hearing aids. New technologies allow hearing aid users to connect wirelessly to a cell phone as well as to MP3 players or Bluetooth devices.

If you use hearing aids on both ears and have better speech understanding when listening with two ears, you can get a portable, battery-powered acoustic-to-magnetic adaptor that attaches to the earpiece of a telephone handset. This device changes the sound from the telephone into electromagnetic energy that a hearing aid telecoil can pick up. A special cord (called a silhouette inductor) can be plugged into the device to go to your nonphone ear so you can make use of two hearing aid telecoils at the same time.

LISTEN UP

Other sources of electromagnetic signals besides the telephone can interfere with the performance of your hearing aid telecoil. This is especially likely to occur in the workplace where computer monitors, fluorescent lights, and electrical panels can cause a humming sound when you turn on your telecoil. Sometimes just moving will lessen the interference.

Some special telephones with built-in technology for the hearing impaired allow you to connect a direct audio input (DAI) cord or an induction device such as the silhouette inductor (worn behind the ear) or a neckloop inductor (worn around the neck). These induction devices pick up the electronic signal from the telephone (or other sound sources) and convert the signal to electromagnetic energy your hearing aid telecoil can receive. Similarly, a cochlear implant can be directly connected to one of these phones.

Visual Technology

If you have a profound hearing loss, you may not be able to use telephone amplifiers or even hearing aids with telecoils for long-distance communications. If you're young, with nimble fingers and good eyesight, you can use an inexpensive cell phone and text-messaging to send messages to anyone else with a cell phone that can receive text messages (and most cell phones now do). Or you can make use of the instant message function of most personal computers, which allows two or more people to read and write text messages to each other via their computers. Of course, there is also e-mail when immediacy is not an issue. Pagers are now popular among business workgroups. Modern pagers allow users to send and receive fairly lengthy text messages. And a number of smartphones now on the market list instant messaging among their capabilities.

Devices are also designed specifically to be used by people whose hearing loss prevents them from using standard telephones. These are usually referred to as TTYs, which stands for text telephone yoke or teletypewriter, or TDDs—telecommunication device for the deaf. TTYs don't require any special telephone equipment or installation other than the TTY device itself. You can buy a TTY all-in-one telephone or a TTY device with an acoustic coupler cradle into which you put the handset of your regular telephone. The message from the other party is displayed for you to read on a small LCD screen. These devices range in price from less than $40 up to more than $700, again depending on the features. Feature choices include an answering machine, amplified volume if there is a phone handset, or a flashing light to announce ringing. Some have printing capabilities, and some TTYs have the capability to connect to cordless phones and cell phones.

To use a TTY, either the person you are calling must also have a TTY machine or you use a telecommunications relay service (TRS), an operator service that allows people who are deaf or hearing-impaired (as well as the speech-disabled or deaf blind) to place calls to standard telephone users. In the United States and in many other countries, relay service is provided free of charge. It's paid for on a state-by-state basis using a small surcharge on all phone bills. The state uses this surcharge money, usually only a few cents a month per phone bill, to contract with a relay service, which provides relay operators (also called communication assistants). The relay operator can voice your texted message to the person you are calling and type the response back to you.

If you can't understand over-the-voice telephone even with amplification but do want to talk directly to the other party, you can use a system called voice carry over (VCO). VCO, also referred to as "read and talk," allows people who can't hear on the phone but have good speech to use a phone. For VCO, you dial a relay operator (often 711) from a special VCO phone (for example, a TTY with built-in phone handset). The relay operator connects you to the person you're calling. You speak in your normal voice, but when the other person speaks, the relay operator types out what that person says.

HAVE YOU HEARD?

Now, relay also provides IP-relay (Internet protocol relay), which allows you to make relay calls from any computer connected to the Internet. You connect to a relay service operator using a chat-like window in your browser. Most of these services don't require any special computer software. Like other forms of Internet long-distance communication, IP-relay calls are free because they use the Internet and not the phone system for long distance. Modern technology has made it possible to use almost any generic connected device to use a relay service, such as a personal computer, laptop, mobile phone, personal digital assistant, or other device capable of using the connection methods provided by an IP-relay provider.

Home Listening

A major problem for someone with a hearing loss is listening to TV at a comfortable loudness without bothering normal-hearing family members. And, of course, there's the problem of impaired understanding. This is made worse by the fact that much of the speech and other sounds during a TV show may be coming from characters or objects that are out of visual range during part or all of the scene. Of course, radio and music always lack a visual element. As we noted for telephone usage, this removes the helpful visual information you get in direct face-to-face communication.

Television Viewing

There are both inexpensive and expensive devices, hard-wired and wireless, to solve these problems, with or without hearing aids. Hard-wired devices use an actual electrical wire or cord to transmit sound. We've already mentioned silhouette and neckloop inductors. If you wear a hearing aid with a telecoil, you can plug these devices into a sound source. This is more commonly used for a personal device such as a CD player rather than television because you are tethered to the sound source, with freedom of movement limited by the length of the cord. Earphones and loud-speakers are inexpensive devices you can plug into the television set and place next to or on your ear. You control the volume independently of the volume control on the television.

Two types of wireless systems are better suited to the television listening problem. An infrared system is the more expensive option, but the one with the highest fidelity. It's used in many theaters, auditoriums, and classrooms but is also available for home use. The system requires a transmitter that is plugged into the electrical wall outlet and placed on the television set with its microphone positioned to pick up sound from the television speaker(s). This transmitter converts sound signals into infrared waves (invisible light beams). The receiver, which may be in the form of a wireless headset or a body receiver for use with a hearing aid, converts the infrared waves into amplified sound. The television is set at a volume comfortable for family and friends who are watching with you (or who are nearby trying to concentrate on something else!). The infrared system transmitter transmits the television signal to your receiver, which you adjust to your desired volume.

More than one receiver can be used with one transmitter, each having individual volume controls. Powered by rechargeable batteries, the receiver can be coupled to headphones or to hearing aids using an inductor device or with a direct audio input cord to a behind-the-ear hearing aid. Unlike FM systems, which we discuss later, infrared energy stays confined within the walls of a room if privacy or security are a concern. These systems for home use start at about $70 and range upward to several hundred dollars. Such devices also are compatible in many theaters and other public buildings that use 95 KHz infrared systems.

Another type of wireless system available for home use is the audio loop (or induction) system. The transmitter is a loop of wire connected to the output jack of the television or other sound source, strung around the room, and then connected to the input jack of the same sound source. It's essentially a room-sized version of the neckloop inductor, and the receiver is your hearing aid telecoil. These systems for small areas, such as your home, can cost several hundred dollars. They are also commonly used in large public facilities.

Finally, we mention closed-captioning television, which allows text display of spoken dialogue. All televisions with screens of at least 13 inches diagonal measurement must have built-in captioning. This is a menu item option that you probably currently have available on your television set and can turn on or off as necessary.

Radio, Music, MP3 Players

For this category of listening, hard-wired devices are probably the easiest solution. If you wear a behind-the-ear hearing aid, you can successfully enjoy a stereo signal with your CD player by making use of a direct audio input (DAI) connection. That is, you plug one end of a two-ear DAI cord into the device and the other ends into your hearing aids. You can similarly plug into a PC or laptop computer, home stereo, or other sound source. Smaller hearing aids don't have DAI connections, but you can use the neckloop or silhouette inductors. Either of these devices can be plugged into a CD player or other audio source, and your hearing aid telecoil can receive the signal. The advantages are that you can set your volume while not bothering those around you and you get a direct signal without room reverberation or background noise interference.

Listening in Groups or Large Areas

If you are hearing impaired, you have undoubtedly found that you have difficulty hearing and understanding in the presence of background noise. Listening in group situations, whether socially or at work, can be affected by noise interference, room reverberation, and the distance between you and the talker. Because many theaters, auditoriums, places of worship, and classrooms may be wired for infrared sound or audio loop transmission, these systems can often work directly with your hearing aid, your own silhouette or neck loop inductor, or you can ask to borrow the proper receiver device at the public venue. Another type of wireless system used in these larger settings is FM transmission (see Chapter 15).

A personal FM system allows you to place a microphone near the speaker in a group, board meeting, or conference. The wireless microphone/transmitter is placed near the desired audio source and focused to allow that source to feed sound directly into your hearing device. For example, if you're attending a meeting or lecture, you could put the wireless transmitter on the lectern and transmit sound directly to the receiving device you're wearing while sitting anywhere in the audience. The transmitter picks up the sound from a microphone placed near the talker (or loud speaker) and sends the signal by radio waves to a receiver that has been tuned to the same frequency as the FM transmitter. (These devices typically use one of 40 channels in the 216 MHZ band).

If you wear a BTE hearing aid that has a DAI, you can plug a tiny FM receiver directly into your hearing aid. Newer BTE FM receivers plug into the bottom of any brand of BTE hearing aid that has DAI capability. Body-worn styles of FM receivers are also available for use with all types of hearing aids. If you have only a mild loss or wear a completely-in-the-canal hearing aid, you can use the FM receiver with earphones. With other types of hearing aids, you can use inductive coupling, as we've previously described, as long as your hearing aid is set to telecoil mode. There are also some hearing aids with integrated or built-in FM reception.

A newer type of FM transmitter is sleek and hand-held. You can point it at the talker, place it on a tabletop, or have the speaker wear it. These transmitters have a built-in microphone that picks up sound from all directions. When used in public facilities, the FM microphone/transmitter is built into the overall sound system. You're provided with an FM receiver that connects to your hearing aid or to a headset if you don't wear a hearing aid. Or you might be able to use your own FM receiver if you personally own a system.

 HAVE YOU HEARD?

The Americans with Disabilities Act (ADA) mandates that large area wireless sound systems be installed in movie theaters, state and local government buildings, schools, and in other public facilities. These might use infrared, induction loop, or FM technology.

FM systems are probably the most versatile of the listening technologies because they are portable and can be used anywhere—indoors or outdoors. The transmitters can also be plugged into the jack of a home entertainment system, telephone, computer, or any other sound-generating device. FM transmitters can even link to cell phones equipped with Bluetooth technology. We didn't mention them for home use only because they are a more expensive option than the others for that purpose, with prices in the $300 to $1000 range for many of the FM systems. But you can probably think of many one-on-one communication situations in which such a system could be extremely helpful. In a restaurant or in a car, where you want to be able to hear one person easily, you could give that person the microphone of your FM system. If you're giving a lecture or running a meeting or participating in a small group discussion, your microphone could be passed to the person in the audience with a question or to the current speaker in a group.

One other method of making speech more available to those with a hearing loss deserves mention: changing the spoken word to readable text. We've already noted the availability of closed captioning on your television set. Captioning and computer-assisted realtime transcription (CART) are also sometimes used in large venues. Computerized speech recognition, which allows a computer to change a spoken message into a word-processed document, has greatly improved in recent years and is frequently used by doctors dictating their patient reports as well as in other fields in which programs with specialized vocabularies have been developed.

Alerting and Signaling Devices

With even a mild hearing loss, you may be having difficulty hearing certain alerting or warning signals, such as the telephone, the doorbell, alarm clock, or smoke detector. One solution might be simply to amplify the problem signal. A different approach is to substitute another sound that you can more easily hear. Hearing impairment often affects primarily the high frequencies. So, for example, you can request from your telephone company an 805Hz (low tone) bell on your telephone or substitute a buzzer for the doorbell.

A variety of alerting devices are available today to address most of the common problems related to the inability to hear signal or warning sounds in the home, in school, in the workplace, or even while traveling or during recreation. These devices alert you to the source of the sound visually or through vibration. Depending on the system, either a microphone or an electrical connection is used to pick up the sound signal and send it to you through either hardwired or wireless transmission in a form you can detect.

One alternative for home use is to attach a system that activates a flashing light when the telephone or the doorbell rings. If you live in a small apartment, you might just need a device that plugs into one of your lamps. For a larger house, you can get a system that triggers flashing lamps in every room when the doorbell chimes, the telephone rings, or the fire alarm sounds. You can get smoke/fire, carbon monoxide, and telephone signalers that both produce a very loud sound and continuously emit a strobe light when activated. Some of the systems available today make use of coded flashing lights to tell you what sound event has occurred (for example, five flashes for the doorbell as opposed to one flash for every time the phone rings). Rather than flashing lights, you might prefer a body-worn pager that vibrates and displays a number corresponding to the sound source. Simple phone amplifier and strobe light devices can cost less than $50; an entire alert system may be about $200.

Do you need to be sure that you wake up in time for the day's activities? You can purchase alarm clocks that provide adjustable, louder-than-normal volume and tone alarms so you can choose a frequency of sound that you can hear. A bedside lamp, a strobe light, a buzzer, or a bed vibrator can be attached to an electrical alarm clock. The clock activates the alarm signal, which in turn causes the light to flash, the buzzer to sound, or the vibrator to move the bed frame. If you're a heavy sleeper, some alarm clocks beep, flash a lamp or a strobe light, and shake the bed all at the same time. For daytime alarm clock use, you can get a watch with a vibrating alarm signal ($40 to $60). Combination alarm clocks with amplification, light, and shaker are available for $50 to $85; a travel alarm with shaker might be as little as $30.

Several instruments are available to monitor smoke detectors or the cry of the baby from another room. An electronic switch can be installed to convert such specific sounds into visual or vibratory stimuli seen or felt throughout the home. Several companies make a baby sound monitor that you can purchase to work in conjunction with their alert systems for an additional $50.

HAVE YOU HEARD?

What if your doctor has a hearing loss? Can he or she really hear your heartbeat or breathing through that stethoscope? Guess what. There are special stethoscopes and stethoscope amplifiers available for use by medical personnel with hearing loss.

Hearing Dogs

You're probably familiar with the concept of service dogs for the blind. In fact, many programs also train service dogs for the deaf. These dogs (and the programs that provide them) are usually referred to as "hearing dogs." A hearing dog may be helpful to an adult with a severe or profound hearing loss who lives alone. The dogs are not trained as guard dogs but are trained to alert you to specific sounds, such as alarm clocks, doorbells and knocks on the door, ringing telephones, a baby's cry, or a smoke alarm. Once placed with a deaf partner, the dogs usually learn to respond to additional sounds that might be important to you in your home, such as the microwave, tea kettle, washer/dryer, or other sounds.

In public places, a hearing dog provides an increased awareness of the environment. Although they aren't usually specifically trained to alert to sounds such as sirens or horns, they will react to sound just like all dogs do. You can get a sense of events happening in your surroundings by paying attention to your hearing dog when the dog turns to look at something it hears.

Some charitable organizations provide hearing dogs free of charge, other than perhaps a small application fee. Others charge a portion of the costs of training the dog (according to one site, this cost is about $20,000). In addition, some of the programs require you to attend a several-day training program to learn to work with your dog before the program sends it home with you. You can find out about hearing dog programs, their costs, and the requirements you must meet by doing an Internet search for "hearing dogs" or "dogs for the deaf" or other similar search terms.

How Do I Get Assistive Listening Devices?

Because ALDs have not typically been covered by public or private health plans and are not easily available in mainstream retail stores, you may not have previously been aware of the broad range of devices available to help with your hearing problems. Where can you find the devices you need? We suggest that you first start by consulting with your hearing health-care professional. Many offices sell some of the more commonly used devices, particularly those developed for use with hearing aids. Even if your otolaryngologist, audiologist, or hearing aid dispenser doesn't sell any ALDs, they can help you determine what types of devices might be best suited to your needs.

Of course, in the modern era, you can find everything on the Internet. Some browsing might help you think about the possibilities, or it might be overwhelming. In Appendix B, we provide a list of ALD companies and dealers recommended by the American Speech-Language-Hearing Association. ASHA also points out centers across the country where you can examine the types of assistive listening devices available to determine which products to purchase. To locate loaner devices and device demonstrations, they suggest visiting the National Assistive Technology

Technical Assistance Partnership (NATTAP) website (see Appendix B) and select from the state contact list.

True Stories

We've told you about a wide variety of ALDs. Here are just a few examples of how some of these devices have helped other people overcome problems related to their hearing losses.

I See What You're Saying

Bess, who is 85 years old, lives on the East Coast and has a daughter who lives on the West Coast. They used to talk on the telephone every few days so they could remain close in spirit though living far apart. Bess's hearing had deteriorated, and she used hearing aids on both ears. Even though the aids had telecoils and she had an amplified phone, she was finding it harder and harder to understand speech over the phone. One day when her daughter called, she thought she was a solicitor and actually hung up the phone! Although she had always been very social and had many friends, Bess was starting to feel quite isolated by her lack of ability to use the telephone. Her daughter did some research and suggested that Bess consider trying a VCO telephone using a free relay service. After all, Bess's vision was still good and she could read. Now when they converse, Bess speaks into the phone like always, but the relay operator types her daughter's responses so that Bess can read them and fill in anything she wasn't able to get through hearing.

Wired—No, Wireless

A 15-year-old girl, Elise, who wore bilateral hearing aids, was unhappy because when she used her iPod, she had to wear it in only one ear and leave the other ear free to be able to hear her friends and the environment. But new technology came to the rescue. She was fitted with digital hearing aids with built-in inductive technology (telecoils) and also purchased an external control unit that can receive Bluetooth signals from cell phones or any other device that uses Bluetooth technology. It had plug-in capability for her iPod (or any other MP3 player). The external unit, a small medallion-looking device that Elise can wear around her neck, picks up the Bluetooth signal or the direct plugged-in signal and transmits it directly to the hearing aids. Now, Elise has the option to hear only her iPod or to have the iPod and her hearing aids on simultaneously.

Speak into the Microphone

Robert is a very active 62-year-old businessman with severe high-frequency hearing loss. He wears bilateral digital hearing aids and hears fairly well with them, but he wanted to improve his ability to hear in challenging listening situations such as meetings, lectures, plays, and family gatherings. He was fitted with an FM system that helps reduce the signal-to-noise ratio in these difficult listening environments. Now, when Robert has a meeting or lecture, he puts the small transmitter on the podium or on the table. He can also hand it to family members to speak into at gatherings or in a noisy restaurant. The FM signal carries the voice of the speaker directly into the receiver attached to his hearing aids. Robert can hear and communicate more effectively with this device and has been happy to be able to use it in difficult listening situations.

When Gordon Met Sally

Gordon and Sally recently celebrated their forty-fifth wedding anniversary. Since tying the knot when they were in their early 20s, they've done everything together—well, almost everything. For the past year or so, especially since Gordon's retirement, they've been separated by the television. Gordon has a family history of hearing loss and has for the last year needed the volume on the television to be up; way, way up, if you ask Sally. It's so loud for her that she goes to another room to watch her own television, even though she and Gordon are viewing the same program! Neither of them liked the separation, but trying to watch television together was causing them to argue. Luckily, a recent visit to a friend's home brought them back together. They learned of a system that could allow Gordon to listen through headset earphones at a volume he could understand, while allowing Sally to sit in the same room watching the program at a volume she controlled and that was comfortable for her. They purchased such an infrared ALD and now happily sit right next to each other to watch their favorite shows.

The Least You Need to Know

- Many assistive devices are available to help with the everyday problems caused by even mild hearing loss.
- Portable telephone amplifiers, amplified phones, and visual technology allow you to use telephone communication regardless of hearing level.

- Most or all states provide a free telephone relay service for the hearing impaired.

- Infrared, induction, and FM wireless systems are available for help in home listening situations and are mandated to be available in large public facilities.

- A wide variety of relatively inexpensive devices exists to help alert you to sound signals in the home you might not be able to hear.

Restoring Hearing to the Deaf

In This Chapter

- A cochlear implant restores hearing in profound deafness
- Eligibility for a cochlear implant and the required evaluation
- Cochlear implant surgery and its risks
- Device fitting and hearing performance from an implant
- Future directions in cochlear implantation
- The auditory brainstem implant

For most people with sensorineural hearing loss, hearing aids amplify sounds enough to provide good speech understanding and communication. But some people have such severe hearing loss in both ears that speech discrimination is not possible, even with the most powerful hearing aids. Sometimes, this hearing loss is caused by one of the many inner ear diseases we've described in previous chapters. Also, remember that approximately 1 to 3 in 1,000 newborns is born profoundly deaf, and most of these children can't benefit from hearing aids. This means that as many as 200,000 children in the United States might be in need of hearing help beyond hearing aids.

Over many years, treatment for profound hearing loss has evolved from a concept to the current state—a true bionic ear. The technology uses electrical current to bypass damaged or missing portions of the inner ear. The device to stimulate remaining hearing nerve fibers is called a cochlear implant (CI). It's cousin, the auditory brainstem implant (ABI), bypasses even the hearing nerve and stimulates the next center up on the path to the brain. Electrical stimulation has been used in medicine since the 1800s, and by the late 1800s, a new field developed called electro-otiatrics. However, by the turn of the twentieth century, it had died out. Now, in the twenty-first century, the idea of using electrical stimulation in medicine is widespread.

In this chapter, we discuss the two types of electrical stimulation devices used to restore some hearing to the deaf: cochlear implants and auditory brainstem implants. We explain how they work, who might be a candidate for each device, the surgical procedures, and what results to expect.

Some History of Cochlear Implants

In 1957, a patient brought a newspaper article to the attention of Dr. William House, who is now considered the "father of neurotology." It described how French scientists had directly stimulated the auditory nerve in two deaf patients using an implanted wire electrode, enabling the patients to hear sounds. Dr. House began studying this as a possible treatment to restore hearing to the deaf, and he and then others implanted several experimental devices in deaf volunteers in the early 1960s. This work was highly controversial, and many people, including some scientists, opposed it. Beyond the concern about safety, many people didn't believe that a limited number of electrodes could in any way replace the more than 15,000 hair cells that normal-hearing people have. Nevertheless, the potential value of cochlear implants for people with profound hearing loss was an exciting prospect.

HAVE YOU HEARD?

Auditory sensation as a result of putting electric current into the ear dates back at least to Volta, an Italian physicist and the inventor of electrochemical cells (you and I call them batteries!). In 1800, he inserted metal rods in each of his ears and attached them to a circuit containing 30 or 40 of his newly developed batteries. He is said to have reported hearing a sound "as of viscous [thick] liquid boiling." He didn't repeat that experiment!

Developments in microsurgical techniques and continued research on implantable materials led Dr. House to implant three deaf adults in 1969 and 1970. In 1973, a wearable stimulator was completed and one of these deaf volunteers was able to take it home and hear outside of the laboratory for the first time. Eventually, larger-scale clinical trials began, including a trial for children beginning in 1980. The 3M Company joined Dr. House and his group in further developing this first commercial cochlear implant.

In November 1984, the United States Food and Drug Administration (FDA) formally approved the 3M Cochlear Implant System/House Design for use in adults. In a press conference announcing this decision, the FDA noted that this was the first time a medical device had been approved that partially restored one of the five major senses. Since then, there's been widespread development of cochlear implants, and the technology has benefited greatly from improved signal processing and miniaturization techniques. Now, there are a number of different manufacturers with models commercially available in the United States (see the following sections). These devices use multiple electrodes, fit all on the head, and have complex processing strategies.

An estimated nearly 190,000 adults and children all over the world have cochlear implants. This includes 41,500 adults and 25,500 children in the United States. Some famous people have had this surgery, including a Miss America, a national radio talk show host, and a former professional football player.

How a Cochlear Implant Works

A cochlear implant is an electronic device that is partially implanted surgically into the cochlea, the hearing organ of the inner ear. A microphone, processor, and transmitter are worn externally.

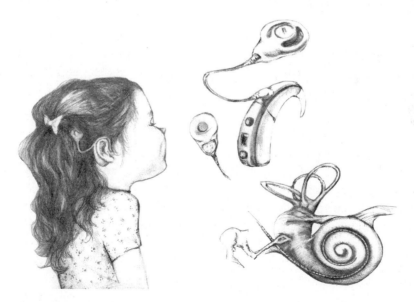

The external and internal cochlear implant components appear here, including the electrode in the cochlea, in a child.

From *Clinical Management of Children with Cochlear Implants* by Laurie S. Eisenberg. Copyright © 2009 Plural Publishing, Inc. All rights reserved. Used with permission.

Cochlear implants detect sound through an ear-level microphone that sends the sound to a wearable sound processor, which converts sounds to tiny digital impulses. The newest sound processors are small enough to fit behind your ear. Different devices use different processing schemes. The electronic impulses from the processor are then sent to a half-dollar size coil worn behind the ear and positioned over the implanted receiver. The coil sends the signal through the skin to the implanted receiver. The receiver and the electrodes that attach to it have been surgically placed.

From the implant receiver, the sound impulses (in the form of electrical signals) are delivered to tiny electrodes placed inside the cochlea (inner ear). These signals carry information about the frequency and loudness of speech and other sounds. The electrical current flows through these electrodes and bypasses the missing hair cells by directly stimulating the cells of the auditory nerve. Once the auditory nerve is stimulated, it carries the message to the cortex of the brain where it is interpreted as sound.

Who Is a Candidate?

If you have a severe to profound sensorineural hearing loss in both ears and don't get much benefit from hearing aids, you might be a candidate for a cochlear implant. This means a hearing loss in both ears of greater than 70 dB and poor speech discrimination (less than 50 percent correct on a sentence recognition test) in the better-hearing ear. To determine whether you are a candidate, you'll need a complete evaluation, including hearing tests and a CT or MRI scan of the ear.

Children as young as 12 months of age can receive a cochlear implant, usually after a 3- to 6-month trial with hearing aids in both ears and intensive auditory training. It's important to ensure that hearing aids can't provide the child the same amount of benefit as an implant. The same implant device used for adults is used in children, because the cochlea is adult size at birth. The middle ear space is smaller in children and will grow as they get older. The wires that connect the internal receiver to the electrodes in the cochlea can be coiled up at the time of surgery and will stretch out as the child grows. On the other end of the age spectrum, adults as old as 90 (a "young," healthy 90) have had implant surgery! Regardless of age, a patient must be medically fit to undergo the surgical procedure.

A complete otologic examination is performed to confirm the diagnosis of your hearing loss and make sure that it's the type of hearing loss that might benefit from a cochlear implant. The CT or MRI scan can identify partial or complete bony blockage of the cochlea, congenital inner ear malformations, and the position of surgical landmarks. It must be possible to insert an electrode system into the cochlea. Either an absent cochlea or an absent auditory nerve is an absolute contraindication to having a cochlear implant, but these situations are rare.

Pure-tone and speech hearing tests are performed (see Chapter 2). Extensive testing is done to determine how well you do with appropriately fitted hearing aids. If your hearing performance is better with hearing aids than that of the average person with a cochlear implant, you'll be advised to continue using hearing aids rather than having surgery for an implant. Children will also have speech and language testing.

Just as important as the audiological criteria, you must have appropriate motivation, psychological fitness, and willingness to participate in the device programming and rehabilitation program. This means making a time commitment of three to four visits during the first year for the necessary rehabilitation process. For children, parents must have appropriate expectations, and the child must have proper support both at home and at school.

SOUND ADVICE

Adults and children older than about age 3 are likely to receive the most benefit from a cochlear implant if they acquired their profound deafness after developing speech and language and are implanted within a few years of the onset of deafness.

People who do best with cochlear implants are those who want to be part of the hearing world and who have the support of friends and family. Children who can be enrolled in an educational program that stresses auditory and oral language development are likely to get more benefit from their implant.

Device Choice and Cost

There are currently three cochlear implant manufacturers in the United States: Cochlear Corporation, Advanced Bionics Corporation, and Med-El Corporation. Each has specific FDA-approved indications for the use of their particular device. The choice of which implant to get can depend on your (or your child's) age, hearing thresholds, preference, and availability of a particular device or devices from the implant center you decide to use. There are other manufacturers of cochlear implants outside of the United States. The external components—the microphone and processor—of all currently available cochlear implants are similar in size, and all the devices require a similar surgical procedure.

The implant, the surgery, and the device setting and training that happen after surgery are estimated to cost $60,000 to $70,000. Of course, you won't necessarily pay all these costs. How much you pay depends to a large degree on your insurance coverage. Medicare, Medicaid, and private insurance may cover most, if not all, of the costs. Today, the majority of private health plans, including HMOs, provide benefits for the procedure and related services. Your cost might depend on the amount of your deductible or your eligibility for Medicare or Medicaid.

As of 2009, Medicare provides coverage for about two thirds of total costs for obtaining a cochlear implant. The coverage for the surgery can be reimbursed under either Part A or Part B of Medicare. This depends partly on whether the surgery is performed on an inpatient or outpatient basis. Part B also pays for long-term postoperative care and maintenance.

All states now either fully or partially reimburse the hospital for the cost of an implant for people eligible under the guidelines of each state's Medicaid program. A prior authorization request is required. For children, this request can't be denied under the Early and Periodic Screening, Diagnosis, and Treatment (EPSDT) Program. Similar coverage is available for adults under the Americans with Disabilities Act (ADA). In either case, you must be eligible for Medicaid coverage to apply for benefits under the EPSDT or ADA.

HAVE YOU HEARD?

According to economists who study the costs of disease, all services, special education, and other expenses related to deafness for a child born deaf or who becomes deaf before the age of 3 years will add up to about $1,020,000 over a lifetime, assuming the child remains deaf. For a child who becomes deaf between the ages of 3 and 17, the lifetime cost estimate is $919,000 per person. For adults, when deafness occurs during a person's working career, the estimated cost over a lifetime is $453,000. (These costs might be reduced by a cochlear implant.)

All cochlear implant external devices currently have a three-year warranty, which doesn't include cables or batteries. The manufacturers offer extended maintenance contracts at the end of the warranty period, or users can purchase extensions from specialized insurance companies for about $300 to $400 per year. Keep in mind that there will be ongoing costs associated with cochlear implantation over the long term.

Cochlear Implant Surgery

One person's cochlear implant surgery may differ slightly from another's, depending on the surgeon's preferences. Surgery is done using general anesthesia, but it can be performed as an outpatient procedure or may require a night in the hospital. The surgery usually takes from 1½ to 2½ hours for one ear. An incision is made in the skin behind the ear, and a mastoidectomy is performed. This includes drilling out some of the mastoid bone to reach the middle ear and the cochlea through what is called the facial recess, a small, triangle-shaped space between the ear canal and the facial nerve. (You'll recall from Chapter 1 that the facial nerve, which provides sensation and movement to the muscles of the face, runs through the middle ear space.)

For adults, a "seat" or depression for the internal receiver of the implant is then drilled. For children, a space or "pocket" is created between the scalp and the bony skull for the receiver. Next, a hole is drilled into the cochlea. Then the implanted part of the device is inserted under the skin and muscle, and the internal receiver is placed into the drilled depression or pocket. The electrode bundle is then carefully inserted into the cochlea, and the incision is closed using buried surgical sutures (no need to remove them) and steristrips (narrow pieces of paper tape) over the incision. A gauze dressing is kept on overnight and removed the following day.

If you are a candidate for bilateral cochlear implants (implants on both sides), some surgeons perform the implantation surgery for both ears at the same time. Some people get a cochlear implant in one ear and then later choose to have the other side implanted as well. You can find the possible advantages of binaural hearing (hearing from both ears) in Chapter 1.

Risks and Complications of Cochlear Implantation

The risks and complications of cochlear implant surgery are similar to those of surgery for chronic ear infection (Chapter 5), which can include the risks of general anesthesia, infection of the incision, and meningitis. There is a risk of loss of residual hearing in the ear. Also, there's a possibility that the device won't work or that you may fail to hear sound even though the implant device is working. Infection around the implanted device could lead to the need to remove and later replace the device.

Over the long term, the skin overlying the internal coil could become irritated from being pressed between the magnets on the inside and outside. This occasionally results in a breakdown of the skin so that the internal coil is exposed to possible infection, a complication that can usually be resolved with treatment. In a small number of people, the internal coil has to be removed, but it can be replaced after the skin heals.

LISTEN UP

The cochlear implant internal receiver contains a magnet. So someone with a cochlear implant can't have an MRI scan unless the implanted magnet is removed first (the magnet can be removed without removing the receiver coil and electrodes). The strong magnet used by an MRI machine can attract magnetic metal objects nearby and cause them to fly across the room! You can find stories and even pictures online of wheelchairs, gurneys, gas tanks, and other equipment jammed inside MRI scanners whose powerful magnets yanked them from hospital workers. In one case, a police officer's pistol flew out of his holster and discharged toward a wall when it hit the magnet. Such a magnetic field might be able to pull a metal object inside the human body enough to move it or damage it or the surrounding tissues.

Turning On the Cochlear Implant and Rehabilitation

The cochlear implant sound processor must be specially fitted for you, and audiologists trained in programming (often called "mapping") these devices usually do this. It involves measuring your sensitivity and comfort levels to the electronic impulses as well as other sound qualities such as pitch. The audiologist uses your responses to customize your implant system specifically so that sound is as clear and comfortable as possible.

Depending on the implant center, initial stimulation and programming usually occurs about three to five weeks after surgery, when the surgical incision has healed. In our center, the first visit occurs over a two-day period. Each appointment is one to two hours long. Initial stimulation levels are set, and you're instructed in the use of the device. Another one- to two-hour visit occurs two weeks later. Additional check and adjustment visits occur during the first year, and then you'll be scheduled for return visits every one to two years.

It's important for both adults and children to practice with their devices. For children, we strongly suggest auditory verbal therapy to help them learn to listen (see Chapter 15). For either you or your child, playing games with your family that require hearing can be a fun form of rehabilitation. You can also apply many of the suggestions we made for first-time hearing aid users in Chapter 16 to people with cochlear implants. In addition, some software programs—usually available free from the cochlear implant manufacturer—can assist implant users with training themselves to use their implant better.

LISTEN UP

Your cochlear implant can set off airport screening devices, even without the external equipment, so your implant center will give you a card explaining your implant. Show this to the security agents right away or tell them about your implant. But given the current rules, you'll probably still have to undergo the one-on-one wand screening.

Also be aware that electrostatic discharge can affect the processor programming and require a return to the clinic for resetting your implant. In children, sliding down a plastic slide is one thing that can sometimes cause this problem although improved shielding in the device has lessened the risk of this.

What to Expect from a Cochlear Implant

Many factors can affect how well you might hear with a cochlear implant. Nearly all implant patients will have hearing thresholds in a range that allows them to detect many environmental sounds and the sounds of speech. But not everyone will be able to identify all these sounds or understand 100 percent of speech just by listening. Some factors that can affect results with the cochlear implant include your age when you became deaf, the length of time you were deaf before receiving an implant, and whether you were able to use hearing aids for some of that time before losing all of your hearing. Adults and children who were able to acquire some speech and language before becoming deaf (postlingual deafness) will usually do better than those who were born deaf or who became deaf so early that they had not yet acquired these skills (prelingual deafness).

Expectations for Adults

Modern cochlear implants can provide very high levels of sound recognition. Quite remarkably, some people are able to communicate on the telephone the very first day their sound processor is fitted. Others take longer to work up to being able to understand sentences well, particularly in noise. Still others can't understand a person speaking to them on the telephone very well but might be able to use the speaker-phone option. Finally, some people benefit greatly from being able to hear sounds in the environment, including warnings, and can communicate better while also using lipreading, but are not able to understand much speech just by listening alone.

Expectations for Children

Children with cochlear implants still require intensive family, school, and specialist (audiologist, speech pathologist, psychologist) effort to develop speech and oral language skills (see Chapter 15). If implanted young (less than age two or three), many children can be mainstreamed in school. Ongoing speech therapy and individual attention are still likely to be necessary. Children implanted at an older age and who have been deaf since they were young are likely to perform less well.

Bilateral Implantation

There is some evidence, especially in children, that hearing performance is better with two cochlear implants than with just one. The benefit of two ears for sound localization and hearing speech in noise can be seen in the test performance of people with cochlear implants, just like these advantages are found in normal hearing. However, some doctors and scientists feel that the gains achieved by implanting both ears aren't great enough to justify the added cost and use of health-care resources.

The Future of Cochlear Implantation

Cochlear implants have advanced in many ways since their introduction. Devices continue to become smaller, more technologically complex, and implanted through smaller incisions. Candidacy criteria have also expanded, and children as young as 12 months of age are currently candidates for cochlear implants. Some children younger than 12 months are being implanted in special clinical studies. In several areas, current research is leading to the next steps in the use of cochlear implants as a treatment for deafness.

Implanting People with More Hearing

Now that both doctors and patients have had many years of experience with cochlear implants and the implants have been shown to be safe and effective, use of the implants is expanding. People with some remaining hearing in one ear and poor hearing in the other ear are receiving cochlear implants in the bad ear. They then can use a hearing aid on their better ear at the same time as their cochlear implant. Remember the advantages of having two hearing ears!

An FDA-approved clinical trial is also currently examining the usefulness of cochlear implantation in ears with some remaining low-frequency hearing. The device being studied uses a shorter electrode to preserve any hearing that is still present in the ear prior to implantation. With this hybrid device, you would use the implant to restore hearing in those frequencies where normal hearing has been lost (usually the high frequencies) and also use a hearing aid to take advantage of the low-frequency hearing that you had remaining before implantation. In other words, you would wear both a hearing aid and a hybrid cochlear implant on the same ear.

Totally Implantable Cochlear Implants?

Earlier cochlear implants used a sound processor about the size of a pack of cigarettes, with cords hanging from the external transmitter on the head to the processor worn somewhere on the body. First, the boxes got slimmer and smaller; now, current devices use a small all-on-the-head processor worn something like an over-the-ear hearing aid. An external magnet is still used to keep the transmitter in place immediately over the implanted receiver coil. As we noted earlier, this has the potential to cause irritation of the skin overlying the internal coil. Also, current implant technology requires both frequent recharging of the external processor and the need to surgically remove the internal coil magnet if an MRI scan is necessary.

For all these reasons, researchers are trying to develop a totally implantable cochlear implant device that would not require the use of an external processor or magnet. This would allow MRI scanning and avoid an external processor. Periodic charging of the device could occur transcutaneously (through the skin) using a special charger device. However, figuring out where to place the microphone is still a problem. If it's placed under the skin, there's the potential that your own speech or the sound of brushing your hair will be too loud! But it might be possible to place it on or near the eardrum.

Auditory Brainstem Implants

A cochlear implant works by stimulating remaining auditory nerve fibers. But what if disease or tumor removal leaves you with no functioning auditory nerve? You would not be a candidate for a cochlear implant. The auditory brainstem implant (ABI) was developed to restore some hearing to people in this situation. In most cases, these are people with neurofibromatosis type II (NF2) who have tumors in both ears (see Chapter 11). As a result of the tumors or their surgical removal, hearing is lost and the hearing nerves are destroyed. The ABI bypasses even the damaged hearing nerves by placing electrodes in the next center up the pathway to the brain, the cochlear nucleus complex in the brainstem.

HAVE YOU HEARD?

Dr. William House and his neurosurgeon colleague, Dr. William Hitselberger, placed the first ABI device in 1979. A woman with NF2 who was undergoing removal of her second tumor volunteered to have the experimental procedure (the tumor removal would otherwise have left her deaf in both ears). She was able to hear sounds and wore this device for many years.

Like cochlear implants, the ABI continued to develop and a cochlear implant device manufacturer began to work with the House Ear Institute on developing a commercially available device. The Nucleus multi-channel ABI received FDA approval for clinical use in October 2000. A newer version of the device is now available; it consists of an implanted component and an externally worn component, similar to a cochlear implant. The implanted receiver-stimulator is attached to an electrode array composed of 21 platinum disks mounted on silicone and mesh.

The external components are similar to a cochlear implant. Unlike the cochlear implant device, however, there is no magnet in the internal receiver. Instead, the external transmitter coil is held in place using double-sided tape or a disc glued to the head and to which the external transmitter coil can attach. This is important because people with NF2 may continue to develop tumors in various areas of the body and need to undergo regular MRI monitoring.

The ABI is usually placed at the time of surgical removal of an acoustic tumor. It can be placed during the first tumor removal to give you time to adjust to the sound before losing all the hearing in your other ear. The tumor is removed using the translabyrinthine approach (see Chapter 11). After removal of the tumor, the ABI electrode array is placed completely within the cochlear nucleus, and tests for electrical auditory responses are performed. These tests are helpful in determining whether you'll be able to hear sounds from the device.

Initial device stimulation usually occurs four to eight weeks after implantation. The overall hearing ability of people who have received ABIs is generally similar to that of people with earlier simple cochlear implants. Eighty-five percent of people who have received an ABI do have auditory sensations. When combined with lipreading cues, most people with an ABI have improved sentence understanding at three to six months after initial stimulation. They also hear environmental sounds and can understand words when a limited set (such as multiple choice) is presented. But you shouldn't expect to be able to understand much speech just by listening alone.

The ABI device is also being used in Europe in people who don't have NF2 but who aren't candidates for a cochlear implant. This includes people with extensive bone growth in the cochlea prohibiting insertion of electrodes or an absent or damaged cochlear nerve. Early results indicate that some of these people are able to understand speech at a level comparable to successful cochlear implant users, including the ability to converse on the telephone.

True Stories

In Chapter 15 we provided some true stories of children and cochlear implants. Here we highlight a few stories about adults who were (or were not) candidates for a cochlear implant or an auditory brainstem implant.

Off to Hear the World

A 73-year-old man, Max, had had very poor hearing for some years but got by with hearing aids. Unfortunately, during a hospitalization for kidney problems, he experienced a sudden further hearing loss that left him deaf. He became very depressed over his inability to hear and communicate well and refused to join his wife in any social activities. A complete otologic and audiological evaluation confirmed that he was profoundly deaf and a suitable candidate for a cochlear implant, so Max underwent surgical placement of the device and four weeks later returned to the implant center to have the sound processor fitted. Within a few months, he was able to score 100 percent on sentence testing. His whole countenance changed. Now Max and his wife are planning international trips together.

Parents Aren't Always Right

Sam, 36 years old, visited the office with his mother. Sam had been deaf since birth, the specific cause unknown. He attempted to use hearing aids through grade school but refused to wear them in high school because he felt they really didn't help him. He was educated in a "total communication" setting (see Chapter 15) and relied primarily on sign language to communicate. At the office visit, the otologist communicated through a sign language translator and learned that Sam's mother was the one interested in a cochlear implant for her son. Sam himself was not really interested. The doctor explained to Sam's mother that people with an early age of onset of deafness and a long duration of deafness, especially those who rely on sign language, usually don't do very well with a cochlear implant. Even if they get the device, they usually become nonusers. The doctor agreed with Sam that he shouldn't receive a cochlear implant.

One More Time

Judy was in her late 20s when she had a large acoustic tumor removed from her left ear, leaving the ear with no hearing. A few years later, a small tumor on the right side caused her to go deaf. She became something of a recluse until several years later when she became one of a small number of people who have had a tumor removed but are still able to have a cochlear implant. This was possible because her auditory nerve remained intact after tumor removal. Nearly 15 years later, when she began having facial pain, it was suspected that she had another tumor on her right hearing nerve pressing on the facial nerve. At that time, in order to have an MRI, the cochlear implant had to be removed. When the MRI showed another tumor and Judy was diagnosed with NF2, she was sent to our institution to have the tumor removed and an auditory brainstem implant placed. At first stimulation, Judy described voices as sounding like Donald Duck (a common comment), but with time and practice, voices started to sound much more like she'd remembered.

Shave and a Haircut

A college-age man with NF2 came to have removal of his first tumor and placement of an ABI. When he asked the surgeon if his entire head would have to be shaved, he was reassured that no, only a little hair behind the ear would have to come off. To that he responded, "uh-oh." Apparently, all his fraternity brothers had shaved their whole heads to show their support for him! Of course, the surgeon agreed to give him a complete shave job, no extra charge.

The Least You Need to Know

- A cochlear implant is a surgically implanted device that uses electrical stimulation to provide hearing to a deaf ear.
- Children as young as 12 months and adults of any age with profound hearing loss may be candidates for an implant.
- Medicare, Medicaid, and most private insurers usually cover part of the cost of a cochlear implant.
- Many people with cochlear implants understand speech just by listening (no lipreading) and can use the telephone.
- Children implanted at an early age may acquire near age-appropriate speech and language skills.
- The auditory brainstem implant can provide some hearing to those who are deaf from removal of tumors in both ears.

Communicating Effectively

In This Chapter

- Use of visual cues from a speaker's face
- Some limitations of speechreading
- Making the sounds of speech
- Using the rhythm and context of conversation
- Stage-manage the situation to improve communication
- Help the speaker help you

If you have a hearing loss, you can do several things to help make yourself a better communicator. By knowing and practicing these things, you can be more comfortable in your ability to handle communicating with your friends, family, and even strangers.

Whatever the means of acquiring the skill of using visual clues to understand speech, it is essential to improving your ability to understand a conversation. Viewing the face of the speaker and learning to use visual cues to help understand speech is helpful to all hearing-impaired people. So in this chapter, we provide you with some insights about what you can do to improve your ability to understand and be understood. We give you hints for improving your communication abilities, including how you can stage-manage the communication situation to make things easier for yourself and how you can help the speaker be a more effective communicator.

Vision and hearing complement each other in understanding speech. But none of these helpful hints are intended to replace hearing. If you have a hearing loss, you need to get treatment and use hearing aids or other hearing devices. Fortunately, many of the sounds that are most difficult for people with hearing loss to hear—high-frequency speech sounds—are the easiest to see on the lips. And some of the sounds that are hardest to tell apart visually are the easiest to hear.

Speechreading

It's not uncommon for a person with impaired hearing to say "I can't hear a thing without my glasses." This expression is a sure indication that he or she relies heavily on *speechreading*.

DEFINITION

Speechreading is the use of visual clues from the lips, facial movements, and gestures of the speaker to understand speech. It is more than just lipreading. Some sounds cannot be seen on the lips, and many different words may look the same on the lips. A speechreader makes use of all visual cues, not just lip movements.

Many people use speechreading without really knowing they're doing it. Over the years, the listener with a hearing impairment unconsciously learns to use visual clues of speech from the lips and facial expressions of the speaker. In fact, most of us, even normal-hearing people, make use of visual clues in understanding speech. If you've ever been in a noisy restaurant or bar, you know it seems even harder to hear when you can't see the person who's talking! That's because you're missing those visual clues.

Speechreading is a skill that enables someone with a hearing loss to better understand conversation by attentively observing the person talking. All of us, whether we have a hearing impairment or not, use the sense of sight as well as the sense of hearing in ordinary conversation. We find it easier to understand if we can watch the speaker's facial expressions, lip movements, and hand and body movements or gestures. Facial expressions and gestures can tell us whether the speaker is making a statement, asking a question, or ordering us to leave the room. A study of the fundamentals of speechreading makes conversation less of an effort and more pleasant for both the speaker and the listener.

Speechreading Has its Limitations

First, understand that many factors make speechreading difficult. When the distance between the speakers is great or when you have poor lighting or impaired vision, you may not be able to see the speaker's lips clearly enough to speechread adequately. Some people have beards, hold their hands over their mouths, or smoke as they talk, making speechreading difficult if not impossible. And don't expect ever to speechread a ventriloquist!

The hearing-impaired listener must recognize characteristics of the English language (assuming you are trying to speechread someone speaking English). Many sounds and many words look the same on the lips even when they sound quite different. Look into your mirror, and say each of the following groups of sounds (as represented by the letters) and words:

f, v

p, b, m

beet, meet

shoe, chew

few, view

Each pair or group of sounds and words looks the same on the lips.

From the context of the sentence, the speechreader must determine which word is being used, just as the normal-hearing person must depend upon the context to tell which of two or more words that sound the same are being used. For example, in the sentence, "The boy has a vacant stare in his eye," *boy* sounds the same as *buoy*; *stare* sounds the same as *stair*; and *eye* the same as *I*, but the listener has no difficulty selecting the words intended and understanding the meaning conveyed from the context.

The hard-of-hearing person should be aware that it's impossible to see certain words on the lips and that he or she continually needs to fill in gaps in words and in sentences. Look in your mirror again, and say the sounds represented by the following letters: *k, g, n, l, t*. It's impossible to see these sounds on the lips because they're formed in the mouth and at the back of the throat. Only about 40 percent of all sounds in the English language are visible on the lips, and one estimate is that the speechreader could not expect to receive more than 10 to 25 percent of the information one can get about speech by using hearing. Because of the difficulties presented by sounds, we encourage the speechreader to follow the context or thought of what is being said rather than try to lipread each word.

The Sounds of Speech

We can't see the sounds and words produced in the back of the mouth (for example, the word *key* or *hay*). We can't see the vibrations of the vocal cords that make a difference in sounds represented by *b* versus *p* or the opening of the nasal passage that makes a difference between sounds represented by *b* and *m*. All of this makes speechreading difficult.

HAVE YOU HEARD?

HAL joins MI5: An online news report (www.i711.com; May 30, 2007) said, "Big Brother is now doing our job. The British government, perhaps no longer interested in its stiff upper lip, instead wants to read other people's lips." This and other sites reported in 2007 that lipreading technology would be added to some of the approximately 4 million surveillance cameras in Great Britain in order to identify terrorists and criminals by watching what everyone says. Automated lipreading systems apparently already exist but are inaccurate and require good lighting and nonmoving heads (just like humans!). A computer vision expert and colleagues in England have been given funding to further develop this lipreading technology. When the system finds someone speaking certain key words or sentences, an alert message would automatically be sent so police or security agents could be sent to the scene to question the individual.

It might be helpful to discuss how speech sounds are produced and what makes one sound different from another. A phoneme is the smallest segment of sound that forms a meaningful difference between utterances. This is not the same as the alphabet. In English, for example, there are at least 44 different phonemes, according to the *International Phonetic Alphabet*—20 vowel sounds and 24 consonant sounds, even though we have only 26 letters in the written English alphabet. The *k* sound in both *kite* and *cat* is the same phoneme, even though we spell it using different letters of the alphabet. And then there are sounds produced by letter combinations, such as *ch* and *th*.

DEFINITION

The **International Phonetic Alphabet** (IPA) is a system of phonetic notation based on the Latin alphabet. It was devised by the International Phonetic Association (beginning in 1886) as a standardized way to represent in writing the sounds of spoken language. The general principle of the IPA is to provide one symbol for each distinctive sound. It is used to transcribe speech by foreign language students and teachers, linguists, speech pathologists and therapists, singers, actors, lexicographers, and translators.

Vowels are "open" sounds and are determined by what sound frequencies have the most energy when the sound is made. Usually the two different frequencies occurring with the most energy in a vowel are what defines it (these are called formants). We classify consonants, on the other hand, based on three characteristics: manner of production, place of production, and voicing.

Manner of production refers to how the sound is produced. First, we have plosives or "stops," an exploding sound in which we build up the pressure and then get a sudden burst of air coming out like an explosion. Examples of plosives include the sounds of

b, *p*, *d*, *t*, *g*, and *k*. Another manner of production is the nasal in which there is a resonating of the air in the nose passage. A structure opens and closes the nasal cavity. This
includes the sounds represented by *m*, *n*, and *ng*. Say these sounds, and you almost feel
them in your nose. Next, we have fricatives, which are blowing sounds with friction
such as the sounds represented by *v*, *f*, *z*, *s* and *h*. Then there are affricates, which are
a combination of plosive and fricative such as the sounds represented by *ch* and *j*. And
finally, there are several others, including liquids (involving the sounds represented by *l*
and *r*) and semi-vowels (involving the sounds represented by *w* and *y*).

Place of production is where in the mouth and throat the sound is made. These might
include the lips (labial), the tongue (lingua), the teeth (dental), the bump behind
the front upper teeth (alveolar ridge), the roof of the mouth (hard palate), the vocal
cords (glottal), and combinations of these. For example, there are bilabials—both lips
involved—such as in the sounds of *b* and *p* (which are also plosives; so guess what—
these sounds are called bilabial plosives) and *m* (a bilabial nasal). In labiodental sounds
both the lips and teeth are involved, such as when we make the sounds represented by
v and *f*. Lingua-palatal sounds made by the tongue and hard palate include fricatives
such as *z* and *s* and affricates such as *ch* and *j*. The velar place of production uses
the back of the tongue and the roof of the mouth and produces plosives such as the
sounds represented by *g* and *k* and the nasal *ng*. In English, the one sound produced
just at the vocal chords (glottal) is the *h* sound.

HAVE YOU HEARD?

The five most frequently occurring consonants in spoken English (*t, n, s, d,* and *l*)
are produced at the same place in the mouth and look no different on the lips.
Also, the sound represented by *y* looks no different from these consonants.

Then presidential candidate George H.W. Bush famously once said, "Read my
lips: no new taxes." If we were to read his lips, he might just as well have said
any of the following:

- Do new nukes.
- You sue Texas.
- So do ducks.
- … Add your own phrase here!

The third characteristic of a speech sound is voicing. A sound is voiced if the vocal
chords are actually vibrating when the sound is produced. If they are not vibrating,
the sound is voiceless. Just because a sound can be heard doesn't mean it is voiced.
Place your hand on the front of your throat while saying "ah," and you can feel the

vibrations of the vocal chords. Now produce a soft, hissing "sss" sound. You can hear this, but there is no vibration of the vocal chords. Voicing is an important distinction. For example, the sounds for *b* and *p* are both bilabial plosives, but they differ in voicing—the *b* is voiced and the *p* is voiceless. Unfortunately, you can't see voicing when trying to speechread. *Bay* and *pay* look the same, even though we know they sound different. The same thing is true for the sounds represented by *v* and *f*. The *v* is voiced and the *f* is voiceless. But they are both labiodental fricatives and look the same on the lips.

The Rhythm of Conversation

The speechreader is also helped by being keenly aware of the rhythm of conversation. A change in rhythm is a definite aid to use in understanding what's being said. Pauses between words and between sentences, stress, and intonation all affect what the speechreader sees and should convey different meanings.

Say the following sentences in a mirror, or have someone speak them to you. Note the differences in the meaning even though the sentences contain the same words.

Yes, I heard you tell him.

Yes, I heard you. Tell him.

Yes, I heard. You tell him.

Did you notice that the sentences look different on the lips because of the differences in pauses and in stress?

Pay Attention to the Situation

To master speechreading, one must become acquainted with the setting of a given situation. For instance, if invited to a gathering, the hearing-impaired person should find out as much as possible about the occasion to get a background for speechreading. Who will be present? What are the names of some of the persons who are likely to attend? What are the interests of this particular group? What are they most likely to discuss as a group or individually?

If the impaired listener is alert to the situation, speechreading will be easier—even when the situation is unplanned or unexpected. If a motorcycle police officer approaches after you have gone through a red light, you should obviously know what is likely to be said. Similarly, you can anticipate the remarks of a salesperson behind the counter or of a repairman who has arrived to repair the television or the washing machine. When you join a group of people who are already talking, ask a friend what the discussion is about.

It is frequently said that people with impaired hearing have an "extra mile to go." It's certainly true in the sense that they need to be forever on the alert for what is going on.

Teaching Yourself

Books on the subject of hearing loss may be available at the public libraries, but unfortunately, a person can't read one of these books and become a speechreader. With the help of family and friends, however, the person can practice the lessons in speechreading contained in some of these books. Video courses on speechreading are also available for purchase online (a Google search for "speechreading" led to more than 140,000 hits!). Professional help can then be supplemented with help from the family. Also, television may offer a limited way to practice lipreading at home. Turn down the volume, and watch the lips, facial expressions, and gestures to interpret what is being said. Check the correctness of your interpretation with a member of the family. You'll also notice how difficult this can be since the speaker may frequently be off camera or have his or her back to the camera!

One study found that deaf adults who lost their hearing after acquiring language (postlingual) did significantly better on a test of speechreading than did normal-hearing adults—and women did better than men. This tells us that practice and experience using vision for reception of speech is important and can make a difference.

HAVE YOU HEARD?

In spite of the difficulty of speechreading, a few rare deaf people could read lips so well that they were recruited by the FBI! One such real-life story was made into a TV show. *Sue Thomas: F.B. Eye* was inspired by the true story of Sue Thomas, who although profoundly deaf from the age of 18 months, overcame significant obstacles to work surveillance for the FBI.

Get Help from a Professional

The person who is learning to speechread, learning to use a hearing aid, or both should have the help of a professional trained to teach these skills. This help is usually available from a number of different institutions. Or your neighborhood school may be able to direct you to the services of a teacher trained in these special skills who might provide private tutoring.

Most speech and hearing clinics at universities and colleges offer speechreading help or referral to such help. The adult division of the Board of Education in most large cities sponsors speechreading classes for adults. In some large cities, the Veterans Administration provides classes in speechreading and auditory training for veterans.

You should realize that hearing-impaired individuals differ greatly in their ability to speechread. However, be assured that many studies have shown that the ability to speechread is not related to intelligence! Some of the differences may be related to the degree of hearing loss and how much a person has depended on hearing rather than visual clues. But speechreading is a very difficult thing, even under the best of circumstances, and you should not expect it to solve communication problems completely.

More Ways to Help Yourself

If you have a hearing loss, you can do much to improve your communication abilities in addition to learning to speechread. If you follow these suggestions, you'll find communicating and relating to others much easier in spite of a hearing problem. Always remember that the success of your auditory rehabilitation largely depends on you, your attitude, and your acceptance of your problem.

The Invisible Handicap

People in general are sensitive toward those with a physical handicap. But a hearing person is faced with a number of problems when meeting someone who has a hearing impairment. First, this handicap is invisible—there is no prior warning of the condition. If you meet someone in a wheelchair, you know immediately that that person has a disability. You may try not to pay any attention to the wheelchair so as to not hurt his or her feelings, or you may hold open a door or in other ways help the disabled individual.

Even if the hearing-impaired person is openly wearing a hearing aid or cochlear implant and the hearing person recognizes the nature of these devices, most hearing people have little experience talking to people who have a significant hearing loss. But hearing loss can so greatly affect communication that the problem cannot be ignored. One is immediately faced with the problem of how to communicate with the hearing-impaired individual.

Because of this, it's important you let others know you have a hearing problem. This can lessen the uncertainty others have, make them less concerned about hurting your feelings, and perhaps even lead to a discussion of hearing impairment sooner than might otherwise occur.

SOUND ADVICE

These days, so many people use Bluetooth earpieces for their cell phones, iPods, and MP3 players that we may not even notice or recognize that a device such as a hearing aid or cochlear implant is being used for hearing loss. This "lost in the crowd" feeling might be nice when you are walking down the street, but if you are trying to communicate, you must tell people you have a hearing loss.

The education of the public is your responsibility. You can't help others understand your problem if you conceal it from them. Do not hide the fact that you wear a hearing aid or that you depend on speechreading to understand conversation. By letting others know about your problem, you can make communication easier for you. It's only through mutual acceptance and through understanding of the problems of people with impaired hearing that the "outsider" can be expected to adjust to the needs of the speechreader. Without this understanding, the outsider may unintentionally add to the communication difficulty of the hearing-impaired person.

Relax

Make every effort to relax. Don't strain either to hear or to see speech. Strain causes tension and makes speechreading much more difficult. A combination of hearing and seeing, under relaxed conditions, enables people with impaired hearing to understand most speakers much better.

Do not expect to understand every word in a conversation, but follow along with the speaker. As you become familiar with the rhythm of the speech, key words will emerge, and you'll be able to understand the complete thought.

Be determined to master speechreading. Make a hobby of it. It will help in every conversation. Knowing you have this skill can help you relax.

Stage-Manage the Situation

Try to stage-manage the situation to your advantage. Lighting is important. Avoid facing a bright light, such as the sun outside or a bright window while inside, and avoid having a shadow on the speaker's face. Six feet is an ideal separation from the speaker; at this distance you can readily observe the speaker's lip movements, facial expressions, and gestures.

To the degree that you have control of it, try to reduce background or other noise. If you're in someone's home, ask the person you're visiting to turn down the radio, television, or music that's playing. In your own home or car, adjust the base and treble switches (lower the base and increase the treble) to emphasize the higher-frequency sounds, which will better help you hear consonant sounds in speech from the music or radio. It's the consonants that often create the most difficulty for people with hearing loss, because they usually give distinct meaning to a word.

Anticipate difficult listening situations, and make plans to minimize their effects. For example, if you're dining out with family or friends, suggest going at a time not likely to be busy and therefore noisy. With a business associate, recommend a restaurant you know is relatively quiet—for example, one with carpeting, plants, and sound-absorbent materials on the tables and walls. These days, you may be able to learn about the restaurant's menu online before going, making discussions about everyone's meal choices and communication with the waiter more effective. Try to choose a seat at the table farthest from the noisy kitchen or other likely sources of noise, such as the bar. If you're seated near a brightly lit window, sit with your back to it so you can reduce glare in your eyes and have a good view of the faces of the others.

Show an Interest in Conversation

Maintain an active interest in people and events. If you keep up with national affairs and events in your community and your close social circle, you'll be able to follow discussions much better. Remember that speechreading is easier if you can make use of context.

Conversation is a two-way affair. Don't monopolize a conversation in an attempt to direct and control it. On the other hand, don't let it pass by without participating. Take an active and interested part whenever possible. A friendly, sympathetic interest in other people and in their problems can do much to smooth one's own path.

Be particular about your speech. A hearing impairment of long duration may bring about changes in volume as well as in *articulation* and voice quality. A pleasant, well-modulated voice is a great asset. You will find people more likely to have a long conversation with you if you can correct problems you may have with your speaking voice, particularly volume problems.

Help the Speaker to Be Clear

If you understand at least part of what a speaker is saying, but don't get it all, don't say, "Huh?" or "What did you say?" Instead, say something such as, "I know you're talking about a new restaurant, but I didn't get where you said it's located." In this way, the talker doesn't have to repeat everything he or she just said.

Determine why you are having difficulty with a particular speaker, and then make specific requests. Does the speaker have a soft voice? Rather than constantly asking him to repeat, ask him to speak a little bit louder. Or if the speaker is talking too fast, say, "Please slow down a bit so I can keep up with what you're saying!" If the speaker has turned away from you while talking, use a specific request such as, "Please face toward me when you speak so I can speechread." If someone is talking with a hand over her mouth, say, "Could you please put your hand down so I can see your lips?" These requests will help the speaker understand that there are things that improve communication other than just repeating over and over again. Always use positive and polite words when you need help from your communication partner, such as "Could you please speak a bit louder?"

Bluffing or pretending to understand will usually be exposed sooner or later, sometimes with very embarrassing results. By nodding or indicating agreement with an "uh-huh," you might later find that you've made a commitment you can't or don't want to keep. Or you could end up saying something completely inappropriate, such as, "that's nice," when someone has actually just related bad news. If you have the slightest doubt that you understood a message correctly, confirm the details with the talker. It could save you some embarrassment or complications later.

HAVE YOU HEARD?

Speechreading in real life and in fiction:

True story: Soccer fans might remember this event from 2006. After the World Cup finals, France's Zinedine Zidane delivered a head butt to the chest of Italian Marco Materazzi. Afterward, neither man would discuss what was said. According to news reports, various groups hired lip readers to view the tape to determine what the two athletes actually said to each other. Interestingly, the BBC radio and BBC television stations who both called in experts got different answers about what was said. But that's not surprising, given what you now know about speechreading!

In the movies: We mentioned HAL earlier. Remember the chilling scene in *2001: A Space Odyssey* when HAL (the intelligent computer) tells Dave that, despite all the precautions taken, he knows—because he can read lips—that Dave was planning to disconnect him?

On TV: *Seinfeld* aired an episode in 1993 titled "The Lip Reader." Jerry sees an attractive woman calling lines at a tennis match and asks her out. He discovers she is deaf (played by Marlee Matlin, the well-known deaf actress) but able to read lips. George wants Jerry's girlfriend to read the lips of his ex-girlfriend to find out what she's saying about him at a party. While she is reading the lips, Kramer does the translation from sign language, making mistakes that force George into an embarrassing situation.

The Least You Need to Know

- If you have a hearing impairment, you will benefit from at least attempting to master speechreading.
- Many words look alike on the lips, so follow the thought of what is being said; don't expect to lipread each word.
- Pay attention to the rhythm of conversation—the pauses between words and the stress.
- Use all possible visual clues.
- Take charge of your listening environment in regard to lighting, background noise, and position to maximize successful communication.
- Don't let your hearing impairment be an invisible handicap; let others know you have a hearing loss.

The Impact of Hearing Loss

20

In This Chapter

- Hearing loss affects many aspects of a person's life
- Hearing loss also affects family members and friends
- Hearing loss can affect getting or keeping a job and overall earning power
- Family and friends can work to improve communication

Hearing is one of a human's two major distance senses. The other, vision, is directional and can focus only on the area immediately in front of you (although children and students do often feel that mothers and teachers have an ability to see behind their backs!). Hearing encompasses all directions at once, persists even during sleep, and keeps you in continual contact with your environment. Sound is one of nature's surest signs of activity. Your hearing scans the background at all times and calls your attention to changes.

Clearly, hearing has been important to human survival. Hearing provides some of our first contacts with the world outside of the womb, even while we're still in the womb. At birth, the cochlea is the only organ that is already full size. Through hearing, we get most of our warnings of threats to safety. Hearing also provides an auditory background to daily living as we hear the tick of a clock, distant traffic noises, and vague murmurs from people in other rooms or outside without consciously realizing it. This helps maintain a feeling of being part of a living world. And, of course, hearing provides a means for understanding communication by spoken language.

This chapter is really for those of you who have family members or friends with a hearing loss, whether mild or profound. Its aim is to give you a better understanding of the consequences of hearing loss. We hope to broaden your thinking about how we use our hearing in everyday life and help you recognize the wide variety of problems someone with a hearing loss might experience. The chapter also provides some helpful hints and specific information on a speaking style that can make you a better communicator to someone with hearing loss. If you are the person with a hearing loss, you may recognize yourself in some of our discussions and realize you're not alone in experiencing these things.

Impact of Hearing Loss on the Individual

A study at House Ear Institute identified eight major themes related to the impact of hearing loss based on hundreds of interviews with profoundly deaf patients who once had hearing and lost it. Issues and concerns patients and their family members talked about generally fell into these categories:

- Sense of safety

- Emotional reactions

- Nature of interpersonal relationships

- Social activities

- Sense of isolation

- Communication problems

- Employment

- Involvement with hobbies/recreational activities

Although that study involved people with profound deafness, the areas of life impacted are relevant to people with any degree of hearing loss. So let's look at some of these areas.

Communication

Most of us recognize hearing loss in another person when that person doesn't respond, or doesn't respond appropriately, to something we say. If you're the person with the hearing loss, you may not even realize when you misunderstand what is said. For most of us, hearing is critical to effective, in-person communication. Yes, these days you can always use e-mail, but when someone is in the same room with you, speaking and listening is our natural communication method.

And what if you can't just pick up the telephone and make an appointment, or what if you miss the appointment because you misunderstood the date or time over the phone? Hearing loss, even a moderate uncorrected hearing loss, can negatively impact a person's ability to communicate easily and effectively. The frustration for both the hearing-impaired person and for his or her friends and family can be considerable.

Besides just the daily getting and giving of information, the ability to communicate and ease of communication are key factors in interpersonal relationships. Experts say that healthy communication is an important factor in a successful marriage, and hearing loss that interferes with communication ability can hurt a marriage. One study found, after interviewing a large number of people over the age of 55 with hearing loss, that 44 percent felt their relationship with their partner, friends, or family had suffered because they couldn't hear properly. In another similar study, 48 percent of respondents felt their marriage had suffered because of their spouse's hearing loss.

HAVE YOU HEARD?

Helen Keller, who was both deaf and blind, once said that blindness cuts you off from things, but deafness cuts you off from people.

In a large study, the Better Hearing Institute (BHI) found the quality of interpersonal relationships between an individual and his or her family, including things such as arguments, tenseness, and criticism, as well as interpersonal warmth in relationships, declined as hearing loss increased. Lack of effective communication undoubtedly plays a big role in this. In Chapter 19, we discussed what a person with a hearing loss can do to try to improve communication, so in this chapter, we give family and friends suggestions for what they can do to improve the communication ability of their hearing-impaired friend or loved one.

Quality of Life

Studies have found that hearing loss is associated with these side effects: embarrassment, fatigue, irritability, tension and stress, anger, avoidance of social activities, withdrawal from social situations, depression, negativism, danger to personal safety, rejection by others, reduced general health, loneliness, social isolation, less alertness to the environment, impaired memory, less adaptability to learning new tasks, paranoia, reduced coping skills, and reduced overall psychological health. Of course, these effects differ depending on the degree of loss and the individual, but it's important to understand the widespread effects hearing loss can have on one's quality of life.

Inability to communicate effectively is a major factor affecting quality of life, but realize that in the course of day-to-day living, much information about what's happening comes from sounds other than speech. At the extreme end of hearing loss, deafened adults tell about experiences such as vacuuming the rugs only to find that the vacuum cleaner wasn't even plugged in; leaving the garbage disposal running; grinding the ignition in the car, unable to tell the motor was already running; and, of course, not hearing someone at the door or the phone ringing. These may be inconveniences, but they can add to a hearing-impaired person's feelings of incompetence, lowered self-confidence or self-worth, anxiety, or a sense of having lost control over life events.

A number of studies have compared people with hearing loss who use hearing aids to others with similar levels of hearing loss who don't use hearing aids. Hearing aid wearers had higher self-concepts, significant improvements compared to unaided hearing loss in emotional and social effects of hearing handicap as well as improvements in cognitive functioning and depression. Even functional health status improved. In a very large study reported by BHI and done in conjunction with the National Council on the Aging, hearing aid wearers were more likely to engage in activities involving other people. They were less likely to be tense, insecure, unstable, nervous, discontented, and temperamental, and less likely to display negative emotions or traits.

In fact, for all levels of hearing loss, the hearing aid wearers displayed higher self-concepts, showed fewer emotional and social deficits because of hearing loss, functioned at a higher cognitive level, and struggled less with depression. The top three areas of improvement for those using hearing aids compared to nonwearers were relationships at home, feelings about self, and life overall. This research provided strong evidence for the value of hearing aids in improving the quality of life of people with hearing loss of all levels from mild to severe. The flip side of the study is to show the significant impact that uncorrected hearing loss has on so many aspects of quality of life.

The Impact of Hearing Loss on Significant Others

A psychologist who worked with our institution once wrote that illness is a social event as well as a biological one. Its impact extends beyond the victim and adversely affects the lives of people with close ties to the patient. This is certainly true of hearing loss. It isn't unusual for you to feel anxiety, panic, depression, and anger when a loved one suffers a serious hearing loss. Of course, you fear most for the safety and welfare of your family member, but his or her loss often means that new and perhaps heavy burdens fall on the shoulders of you and other family members or close friends.

Further, significant hearing loss can be devastating because it's so disruptive to communication. When a key member of the household—a husband, wife, or parent—is unable to communicate effectively, the burden of making phone calls for appointments, arranging social gatherings, or handling financial affairs often falls to others who previously didn't have those responsibilities. Because these and other new tasks imposed upon you can disrupt your life, your concern for your hearing-impaired loved one can be mixed with feelings of resentment at how your own life is affected.

Sometimes children who grow up with a hearing-impaired parent don't realize until they're older that their household might be different from that of other children. For example, one of the doctors of our group who grew up with a hearing-impaired father recalls that none of his friends wanted to ride with him in the family car. His parents always purchased cars with low-end factory radios and no other sound system. His father couldn't hear conversation in the car if music was playing, so a good sound system was not something his parents would have appreciated or even used. Imagine what it would be like, as a teenager, to have to communicate your emotions in a loud voice, regardless of what those emotions are.

When he first brought a girlfriend home from college, he realized some other differences. While eating dinner, nobody spoke, which was normal in his household. Because his father couldn't hear with the rattling of plates and other table noise, they waited until after dinner to have family conversation. But because of the silence, the girl thought his parents didn't like her.

One of our deaf patients commented on how prior to getting her cochlear implant, she'd never been able to have a conversation with her son while she was driving him in the car. She also noted the emotional burden that her children bore; they were sensitive to store clerks who looked at her like she was stupid when she didn't respond the way they expected. The children also had to wake themselves up for school because she couldn't hear an alarm.

Socio-Economic Consequences of Hearing Loss

For those who are still in the workforce, uncorrected hearing loss can have a negative impact on overall job effectiveness, extending into promotion opportunities and perhaps lifelong earning power. Workplace communication is critical to both job performance and getting a job in the first place. Employers rank excellent listening skills high as a desirable job attribute.

LISTEN UP

You may think that to look young for a prospective employer you can't be seen wearing a hearing aid. In fact, you're much more likely to be perceived as old and less capable if you are unable to be an effective listener.

Household income is found to be related to the level of hearing loss. The difference in earnings between mild and profound hearing loss is many thousands of dollars a year, although the income drop is primarily for those with severe to profound hearing loss. And the difference in income based on hearing level is greater for those who don't wear hearing aids. People with hearing loss are less likely to be working and, if working, are likely to have a lower income than hearing adults of working age. These differences are likely to be greater in harder economic times because people with disabilities are more vulnerable to the impacts of economic downturns.

Practical Suggestions for Family and Friends

Someone with a hearing loss must actually stop, look, and listen to hear and understand speech, so understanding some of the aspects of hearing impairment can prepare you to communicate more effectively with your friends or family members who have a hearing loss. You can do some easy things to make communicating easier for a hearing-impaired person and avoid things that can otherwise make communication more difficult.

Relatives of the hearing-impaired often say, "Oh, he hears when he wants to hear." Sometimes a person is able to hear and understand without apparent difficulty. However, this "selective hearing" is often the result of an ideal listening situation in which communication was taking place at a short distance with a clear speaker and with no background noise. Attempts to communicate in noise or with poor speech patterns or from another room in the house often end in failure.

A person with a hearing loss expends an enormous amount of energy trying to sift out the important clues of speech, as attending to the task of hearing requires concentration. To listen for long periods of time can be quite a strain, and a hearing-impaired person may tire more easily than other listeners. Realize that this may be why he or she wants to go home earlier than you do from parties, family dinners, or other group activities. Remember that hearing impairment is a complex handicap. You can ease the task of adjusting to this handicap by remembering a few simple rules. Get the hearing-impaired person's attention, enunciate clearly, and speak loudly enough. Don't speak rapidly. Above all, be patient, and treat the hearing-impaired person with dignity and respect.

Position Yourself

All hearing-impaired people need to be able to view the face of the speaker because the visual cues from the speaker's expression and from the lips greatly aid in understanding. To be sure the hearing-impaired person can see your face:

- Wait until the person can see you before speaking.

- Touch the person to get his or her attention.

- Position yourself four to six feet away when speaking.

- Don't speak from another room or while walking away.

SOUND ADVICE

Do not startle the hearing-impaired person by suddenly touching or poking him when he is unaware of your presence in the room. Someone could get hurt! Conversely, if you hear something you must respond to, such as the telephone or doorbell, remember that the person you're speaking with may not have heard it. Don't just disappear, leaving her to wonder why you're walking away. Tell her why you're leaving the room.

Don't speak directly into the person's ear, as this distorts the message and hides visual clues. Also, don't sit or stand with your back to a window, because the glare makes it difficult to see your face. Covering your mouth, chewing gum, or sucking on a pipe during a conversation also deprives the impaired listener of valuable visual information.

Don't forget that most hearing-impaired people can hear something, especially if they use hearing aids or a cochlear implant. Although most people have hearing loss that is similar in both ears, occasionally the loss is distinctly greater on one side than the other, or they wear an aid on only one side. If you know which ear hears better, stand toward that side. If you don't know, ask.

Also, a large distance separating the speaker and the listener—upstairs to downstairs, down a long hall, or from one room to another—adversely affects hearing and eliminates any possibility of speechreading. One of us knows a husband who always complains that when his wife walks in front of him, he can't hear her. But the wife complains that he walks too slowly and that's why she always ends up in front of him. One solution is for the wife to slow down and turn around when she says something she wants her husband to understand. Otherwise, enjoy the outdoors and forget the conversation!

Preferential seating can also make a big difference. At home, many people have a favorite seat at the dinner table or in a chair in the den from which to watch television. It's always hard to change old habits, but it might be necessary to change the seating arrangements so that family members are in position to be talking to the hearing-impaired person's better-hearing ear. Similarly, preferential seating should take into account things that will make speechreading easier and reduce background noise.

Speech Patterns

Poor speech habits interfere with the speechreading of the listener and also introduce distorted speech sounds. So, too, does overly precise lip movements or exaggerated mouthing. Studies have actually found that simply asking a person to speak more clearly results in approximately a 20 percent increase in how much hearing-impaired listeners understand.

You can speak more clearly to a hearing-impaired person by remembering some relatively simple points. A very loud voice further amplified by a hearing aid becomes distressing and sometimes painful to the hearing aid user. If a person seems to hear but not to understand, shouting does not help matters. It just further distorts the sound as well as the lip movements. However, speaking slightly louder than usual may be of benefit. Also don't drop the loudness of your voice at the end of a sentence. Because the hearing-impaired listener does not understand all the sounds even when they are properly uttered, faulty enunciation further reduces understanding. Remember your mother's scolding: "Don't speak with food in your mouth!" Then, it was a matter of etiquette; now, it's a matter of understanding.

SOUND ADVICE

Maybe you have a regional accent with which your hearing-impaired listener is not familiar. Well, you can't help that. But beware of using colloquialisms—words or phrases specific to your local lingo. In other words: don't be a Soprano—bada bing!

Rapid speech is very difficult for someone with a hearing loss to understand. Because spoken words last only a fraction of a moment, the brain must quickly identify each group of sounds in a word and assign meaning. If groups of sounds (that is, words) are run together or if any single sound is distorted or omitted by fast speaking, then the listener's understanding is affected. The listener has only a short time to identify each word. Frequently, the hard-of-hearing give the wrong answer to a question not because they don't know the answer but because they have misinterpreted the question. One way to help your listener keep up with you is to pause at meaningful places in a sentence. The pauses shouldn't disrupt the natural flow of conversation, but they should be long enough to give your listener a chance to process what is said before moving on to the next important bit of information in the sentence.

Speech Clues

Because a hearing-impaired listener loses or misinterprets the meanings of many words, the speaker can be helpful by offering as many clues as possible to establish the meaning of a conversation. Using several different words to express the same thought provides additional clues to the context. For example, instead of saying, "Would you like to see the paper?" you may say, "*The Gazette;* would you like to read the newspaper?" You'll notice that the loss of some of the more important words is less critical when other words indicate the same idea. However, the misinterpretation of a single word, such as *paper* in the first sentence, results in a complete breakdown in communication.

Also remember to give clues about changes in the conversation topic. Perhaps even say, "I'm changing the topic now" or simply, "new topic." When giving directions or making important arrangements, ask if the person is clear on the directions by saying something such as, "Did that make sense?"

Be Prepared

When accompanying a hearing-impaired person to an event that is likely to be a difficult listening situation, think of ways ahead of time to minimize communication problems. For example, if you're going to a lecture or speaking event, arrive early and get a good seat. Talk beforehand about the lecture topic as a way of anticipating what the lecturer will say.

If you are hosting a social event and know that someone attending has a hearing loss, strategize about how you might reduce problem situations. Choose a relatively quiet restaurant, or ask to have a private, carpeted room for your event. Ask the restaurant to turn down the music, and do the same if the event is in your home. The efforts you take to plan for a noise-free event will probably benefit all your guests. Reducing competing sounds can improve understanding tremendously for a hearing-impaired person. This is one of the single most important actions you can take to improve someone's hearing.

For a dinner party in your home, arrange the seating so that anyone with a hearing loss can interact easily with other guests. At the dinner table, use preferential seating by placing your hearing-impaired person near those he's most likely to want to talk with. Although candlelight might be nice for setting a mood, it doesn't work well for the hearing impaired.

At a party or any social get-together, joke telling is often a frustrating experience for people with a hearing loss. Not catching clever words in the joke or missing the punch line itself can mean missing out on the joke. Be sensitive to this, and when someone tells a joke, repeat the major points to the person, if necessary, so he can participate in the laughter.

Restaurants

For many people, eating out is an important part of their quality of life, whether as a regular activity or reserved for special occasions. In either case, you can help make it a more pleasant experience for your hearing-impaired friend or family member. In fact, even if you have normal hearing, you've probably been frustrated while trying to converse in a noisy restaurant.

A number of features identify whether a restaurant is a good—or poor—listening environment. Restaurants with poor listening environments have these characteristics:

- Crowded tables that mean more conversations compete to be heard.

- High ceilings and hard surfaces, such as glass walls, that cause sounds to amplify or echo.

- An open kitchen or open bar that allows noise to be transmitted to the seating area.

- Hardwood floors and tile floors that cause sounds to echo. The bigger the seating area or room, the more noise is transmitted.

In contrast, restaurants with good listening environments have these characteristics:

- Multiple small seating areas that are divided by solid walls. This breaks up the amount of sound transmission and ensures that the seating area is separated from the kitchen.

- High-back booths that facilitate communication by blocking other people's conversations and by "containing" your conversation sounds.

- Carpeted floors that absorb sound.

- Low ceilings that prevent transmission of sounds from other tables and from other areas of the restaurant.

Some restaurants offer outside seating areas. Outside seating near the street allows background street noise to interfere with communication. But a large outdoor space can provide a calming environment that also separates multiple conversations. Because many restaurants have music playing, request a table away from the speakers. Or if you're comfortable with being direct, ask that the music level be lowered. But do this in a way that does not embarrass the hearing-impaired person.

The actual seating location around the table is important. The hearing-impaired person should sit with his or her back to the wall. This prevents sound from coming from behind and competing with conversation and also allows the hearing-impaired person to see the wait staff as they approach the table. And as we noted in Chapter 19, windows behind the hearing-impaired person both reduce possible glare and highlight other speakers' faces to aid in speechreading.

If you have more than four people in your dining group, ask for a round table. It's easier to see people on all sides with a round table, and this allows the person with a hearing loss to see the faces of whomever might be talking. And remember preferential seating. If your hearing-impaired dining companion has better hearing in one ear, seat her or him with that ear toward the more important speaker in the group if there is one.

SOUND ADVICE

For the hearing-impaired person: if "back against the wall" seating is not available, you may be able to tell what's going on behind you by watching the eyes of your friends or family across the table. Most people follow moving objects with their eyes when someone is approaching the table. This can alert you that someone (presumably the waiter or waitress) is coming up behind you. Of course, it can also be very distracting if your eating companions are people watching or letting their eyes wander all over the place!

Going to See the Doctor, Banker, Lawyer

Because most professionals, including doctors, have no idea what it means to be deaf or significantly hearing impaired, you can help a hearing-impaired person by accompanying him or her to health-care appointments as well as to the bank and lawyer's office. It's not that most people with a hearing loss are not or do not want to be independent, but there are situations in which it might be more than just embarrassing if communication isn't good. Your family member or friend might feel sensitive about having you involved in his or her private business, so respect his or her intelligence. You are there to facilitate communication, not necessarily advise. A companion who is aware of the difficulties a hearing-impaired person might experience in conversation involving important medical or legal jargon can play a significant role in making such appointments run smoothly.

Assure your friend or loved one that you want to go along only to help when needed and will generally "keep your mouth shut" unless advice is requested. If you realize the hearing-impaired person might not understand something the professional is saying (even though he or she is nodding in agreement), you can repeat the instructions or information, rewording or giving clues as we described earlier. You might ask the professional to write down any suggestions or information in lay terms so the patient or client can take them home to reread.

When confronted with a professional who seems to have no idea about how to talk to a hearing-impaired person, provide tidbits of instruction without being offensive. Most professionals are delighted to have a family member present who can assist with communication. However, be sure the professional talks to the hearing-impaired person, not to you. Common problems you may have to discuss with professionals include the following:

- The tendency to talk too loud.
- Facial hair that distorts lips and inhibits speechreading (full beards with moustaches covering thin lips). Of course, you can't expect him to shave right there and then, but being aware of the problem may make him more patient!
- Use of highly technical language not broken down into concrete terms.
- Turning away from the listener when speaking.
- Treating the hearing-impaired person as if deafness means a lack of intelligence.

True Stories

In this chapter, we use the "true stories" section to share with you some of the things our patients or their family members have told us that have happened because of hearing losses. Some of these are humorous misunderstandings of speech, but they could just as well have had serious consequences. Others illustrate some of the very real problems of daily life caused by hearing loss.

- My deaf mother-in-law was visiting a specialist because of a thyroid tumor. The doctor proceeded to examine her without giving any instructions. He grabbed her tongue with gauze; thrust her head back, preventing her from seeing his face for speechreading; and proceeded to look down her throat, asking her to say "ahhhhhhhhh!" Of course, he was totally unsuccessful in getting her to cooperate. That in itself was lesson enough and, luckily, he was a quick learner.

- Our family was very aware of the limitations of the deaf grandparents. Cocktail hour was always set in small seating areas where Grandma and Grandpa could easily read the lips of the other partygoers seated in the room. Over time, everyone learned that Grandma and Grandpa had favorite chairs that made speechreading easier for them. Those chairs became their "thrones," and we considered those chairs their territory.

- One patient who had a severe, and later profound, hearing loss from early adulthood, told us that dating was an interesting problem. She was never sure who was on the other end of the phone and was afraid she'd make a date with the wrong person. Then, when she was expecting someone, she would have to leave the door unlocked and ajar a bit, or sit within six feet of it, so she would know when the mystery person arrived.

- One wife stated, "I'm like an echo. I have to repeat everything."

- A patient came in and said he'd known he had a hearing loss for a while, but after church on Sunday he decided it was time for hearing aids. The pastor told his congregation, "For those of you in Wednesday night Bible study, I have good news! Starting next week, we are going to have Dolly Parton." The patient said, under his breath, "Wow—awesome!" His wife said, "Why do you care? You don't go to Bible study." And he replied, "I will now! They're going to have Dolly Parton!" She looked at him and said, "No, honey—he said they are going to have VALET PARKING!"

- One of our patients relayed this story. He and his wife were visiting a travel agent to arrange a trip. The travel agent asked if they wanted a queen bed, and he answered, "Of course we want a clean bed."

- A patient was in the cafeteria getting lunch and asked for a bread roll. The server asked if the patient wanted him to heat it for her. She answered, "No, I'll eat it myself."

- A patient said, "My wife is complaining that I don't listen to her. At least I think that's what she's saying."

- A patient, waiting to see the doctor, called a nurse into the room. "Will they shave my head before they do a hearing test?" The nurse responded, "No, why would you think that?" With eyes open wide, the patient said, "They're paging HEAD SHAVER!" "No, no," responded the nurse. "They paged ED SHAFER, the maintenance man."

The Least You Need to Know

- Hearing is important in keeping us in continuous contact with the world around us.

- Hearing loss can get in the way of effective communication and interfere with interpersonal relationships.

- Hearing loss negatively affects quality of life and can lead to social isolation, depression, fears for safety, and loss of earning power, among many other things.

- Hearing loss doesn't affect only the person with the loss but family and friends as well.

- When speaking to a hearing-impaired person, make sure he or she can see your face, speak with good enunciation at a normal rate, and don't raise your voice.

- Be patient; listening with a hearing impairment is hard work.

Glossary

acute otitis media   Condition in which fluid in the middle ear becomes infected.

air-bone gap   A hearing test term for the difference between the best possible hearing acuity as measured by sound conduction to the cochlea through bone and hearing acuity a person is actually getting as measured by sound conduction through air.

allergen   A substance that causes an individual's immune system to produce antibodies for protection from what it thinks is a harmful substance but which isn't actually harmful in most people.

amplification   Making sound louder.

anaphylaxis (anaphylactic shock)   A sudden allergic reaction that is severe and involves the whole body. Tissues in different parts of the body release histamine and other substances, causing difficulty in breathing and other symptoms.

anastomosis   A process whereby cut ends of a nerve are sutured together.

anotia   Congenital absence of the outer ear.

articulation   The act of giving utterance or expression; to give clear and effective utterance to; to utter distinctly; articulation is the process by which sounds, syllables, and words are formed.

assistive listening devices (ALDs)   Devices, other than hearing aids or cochlear implants, that help with telephone communication, listening in the home, and listening in large groups or public areas, including alerting or alarm devices; such devices may use sound amplification as well as visual and vibration alternative stimuli.

ataxia   An inability to coordinate muscle activity, causing jerkiness, incoordination, and inefficiency of voluntary movement; a rare complication of surgery near the brain.

attic   The part of the middle ear behind the eardrum and above the ear canal, containing part of the malleus and most of the incus.

audiogram   The record of an individual's pure-tone hearing thresholds shown in decibels for each frequency, usually from 250 Hz to 8000 Hz; it often is shown as a graph with frequency along the top and intensity or level of sound detection along the left side.

audiology   The branch of science that studies hearing, balance, and related disorders; its practitioners, who test and treat those with hearing loss, are audiologists.

auditory-verbal therapist   Usually a speech language pathologist, teacher of the deaf, or audiologist who has special training and certification to work with hearing-impaired children on listening skills for the development of spoken language.

aural atresia   Congenital absence or closure of the external ear canal.

barotrauma   Injury to certain organs, particularly the ear, caused by changes in atmospheric pressure.

basilar membrane   A stiff membrane within the cochlea that separates two liquid-filled tubes, the scala media and the scala tympani, that run along the coil of the cochlea.

behavioral observation audiometry   A method for testing a young infant's response to sound by simply observing signs that the baby hears sounds at different frequencies and intensities.

biopsy   A procedure for obtaining a tissue sample to be examined by a specially trained physician known as a pathologist.

Carhart notch   A dip in the bone conduction hearing test at 2000 Hz without a similar dip in the air conduction test; it is often seen in otosclerosis.

cerebellopontine angle (CPA)   An area between the brain and the skull that contains the hearing and balance nerves as well as the nerve that controls facial movement and sensation.

cerebral spinal fluid (CSF)   Fluid secreted by structures in the brain that fills the open spaces (ventricles) and other cavities of the brain and spinal cord.

cerumen   The medical term for earwax, which is secreted by glands in the external ear to lubricate the ear canal, repel water, and trap debris.

cholesteatoma   A collection of skin cells and connective tissue that forms a cyst in the middle ear, usually following chronic otitis media; cholesteatomas have the capacity for continued growth and can damage the ossicles, producing hearing loss.

chorda tympani   A branch of the facial nerve giving taste sensation that crosses the middle ear cavity to the front part of the tongue.

chronic otitis media (COM)   A long-lasting infection of the middle ear that often produces a hole in the eardrum and can lead to damage of the middle ear bones or tissue membrane of the middle ear, producing hearing loss.

cochlea   The hearing portion of the inner ear shaped like a snail shell or spiral that contains the three fluid-filled ducts and the organ of Corti with its sensory cells that are vital for hearing.

cochlear hydrops   The presence of excess fluid, called endolymph, in the cochlea that produces symptoms of hearing loss and tinnitus or ear fullness.

cochlear implant   A surgically implanted device that electrically stimulates the hearing nerve to provide sound to the severely and profoundly deaf—people who cannot benefit significantly from a hearing aid.

cochlear nerve   A part of the acoustic nerve that conducts sound stimuli from the cochlea to the brain, also known as the vestibulocochlear nerve or eighth cranial nerve.

cochleostomy   A surgical opening into the cochlea made to insert a cochlear implant device.

concha   The depressed "bowl" in the cartilage of the outer ear, containing the opening to the external auditory canal.

conductive hearing loss   Hearing loss due to problems with the ear canal, eardrum, middle ear space, or any of the three bones of hearing; this type of loss is usually correctable with surgery or may be treated with a hearing aid.

decibel (dB)   A measure of the intensity of a sound wave where zero indicates the softest sound the average normal-hearing person can detect and 130 dB a level at which the average person feels pain.

endolymph   The fluid contained in the scala media of the inner ear.

Eustachian tube   A canal extending from the middle ear to the throat, otherwise known as the auditory canal; it is involved in pressure regulation of the middle ear space.

exostoses   A bony outgrowth of the ear canal often caused by exposure to cold water and wind; sometimes called "surfer's ear."

external auditory canal   The canal leading from the opening of the external ear to the eardrum.

feedback   The squealing sound produced by a hearing aid whenever sound that has been amplified leaks out of the ear and is forced back into the microphone of the hearing aid a second time.

frequency   In hearing tests, frequency refers to the "pitch" of sound, measured in hertz.

hair cells   The sensory receptors of both the auditory (hearing) and vestibular, or balance, systems in the organ of Corti of the inner ear.

helix   The curved fold forming most of the rim of the external ear.

hertz (Hz)   The unit of measurement of the frequency, or pitch, of a sound; 1 hertz is one cycle per second; humans can hear frequencies from 20 Hz to 20,000 Hz.

hydrops   An excessive accumulation of fluid in any of the tissues or cavities of the body; in the inner ear, hydrops is thought to produce the symptoms of Ménière's disease.

idiopathic   Of, relating to, or designating a disease having no known cause.

incus   The middle of a chain of three small bones in the middle ear, shaped like an anvil.

internal auditory canal (IAC)   The bony channel connecting the region of the cerebellopontine angle to the structures of the temporal bone; the seventh (facial) and eighth (hearing and balance) cranial nerves travel through the IAC as they move from the inner ear to the brain.

International Phonetic Alphabet (IPA)   A system of phonetic notation based on the Latin alphabet; devised by the International Phonetic Association (beginning in 1886) as a standardized way to represent in writing the sounds of spoken language; provides one symbol for each distinctive sound; used to transcribe speech by foreign language students and teachers, linguists, speech pathologists and therapists, singers, actors, lexicographers, and translators.

jugular bulb   A small dilation where the blood enters the internal jugular vein in the neck.

mainstreaming   The practice of having differently abled children attend school or classes with their same-aged, normally abled peers.

malleus   The outermost of a chain of three small bones in the middle ear, shaped like a hammer.

mastoid   The part of the skull above and behind the middle ear cavity containing air-filled bony "cells" that can become infected in chronic otitis media or with cholesteatoma, requiring surgical treatment.

mastoidectomy   The procedure for removing diseased bone and tissue such as cholesteatoma from the mastoid air cells and bone.

Ménière's disease   A disease of the inner ear, thought to be caused by fluid and electrolyte imbalances, that produces episodes of severe spinning vertigo as well as sensorineural hearing loss and tinnitus or ear fullness.

meningitis   Inflammation of the meninges—the outer membranes of the brain—and the spinal cord, most often the result of a bacterial or viral infection and characterized by fever, vomiting, intense headache, and stiff neck; bacterial meningitis requires emergency treatment in a hospital and can lead to death; it can cause hearing loss, including deafness.

microtia   Congenital abnormally small external ear.

mixed hearing loss   Hearing loss due to a combination of conductive hearing loss and sensorineural hearing loss.

mucous membrane or **mucosa**   A membrane lining all body passages that have contact with the air (such as the respiratory tract or, in this case, the middle ear) and having cells and associated glands that secrete mucus.

myringoplasty   The procedure used to repair a hole in the eardrum.

myringotomy   A surgical incision made in the eardrum to drain fluid from the middle ear; this can be done for otitis media with effusion or acute otitis media.

neurotology   The medical specialty involved in the diagnosis and treatment of the hearing nerve, balance nerve, and facial nerve; an otologist who has special training in performing surgery for treatment of ear disease is a neurotologist.

nystagmus   An involuntary rhythmical or jittery oscillation of the eyeballs; the direction and type of eye movements can be used to diagnose the source of dizziness.

organ of Corti   The organ in the cochlea that contains the hair cells, which act as the sensory cells of hearing.

ossicles   The three bones of the middle ear: the malleus (hammer), incus (anvil) and stapes (stirrup).

otitis externa   An inflammation of the outer ear and ear canal, often with bacterial or fungal infection of the skin of the ear canal; use of cotton swabs is the most common event leading to acute otitis externa.

otitis media with effusion (OME)   Fluid in the middle ear space, often seen during or after acute otitis media or chronically with infection or allergy involving the middle ear space; OME is the most common cause of hearing loss in children today.

otolaryngology   Also referred to as ear, nose, and throat, or ENT, this is the field of medicine broadly concerned with the ear and other head and neck area structures.

otology   The science and medical specialty involved in diagnosis and management of disorders of the ear and balance system and related structures of the head and neck; an otologist is a board-certified otolaryngologist who has sub-specialized specifically in treating ear disease.

otosclerosis   A disease of the ear in which abnormal growth of bone interferes with movement of the stapes bone, leading to a progressive loss of hearing, usually conductive in nature but sometimes sensorineural as well.

otoscope   A special instrument used by doctors for examining the external ear canal and eardrum, consisting essentially of a magnifying lens and a light.

oval window   An oval opening in the cochlea connecting the middle and inner ear through which the sound vibrations of the stapes are transmitted to the cochlea.

perilymph   A sodium-rich fluid between the bony and membranous labyrinths of the inner ear; that is, in the scala tympani and scala vestibuli.

perilymphatic fistula   Leakage of inner ear fluid into the middle ear, which is normally filled with air, resulting in balance disturbances, hearing loss, or infection.

phoneme   The smallest segment of sound that forms a meaningful difference between utterances.

pinna   The part of the outer ear that protrudes from the head, also referred to as the auricle.

play audiometry   A method for testing sound thresholds in children $2\frac{1}{2}$ to 3 years old. The child is conditioned to perform a specific play task whenever he or she hears a sound.

politzerization   A way to blow air into the Eustachian tube using a special instrument called a middle ear inflator.

postlingual deafness   Profound hearing loss that occurs after the acquisition of speech and spoken language skills, usually considered to be at least three years of age.

prelingual deafness   Profound hearing loss that is present at birth (congenital) or occurs early enough to interfere with normal acquisition of speech and language, usually prior to three years of age.

presbycusis   Deterioration of hearing as a result of natural degenerative changes in the ear that occur mainly with aging.

radiology   Field that involves X-rays, computerized axial tomography (CT), magnetic resonance imaging (MRI), and other radiological tests.

Reissner's membrane   A membrane inside the cochlea of the inner ear that allows nutrients to travel from the perilymph to the endolymph of the membranous labyrinth; also known as the vestibular membrane or vestibular wall.

round window   A membrane-covered opening between the middle and inner ear that compensates for changes in pressure in the cochlea.

scala media   The spiral-shaped canal in the middle of the bony canal of the cochlea that contains the organ of Corti; also known as the ductus cochlearis, cochlear canal, or cochlear duct.

scala tympani   One of the cavities in the cochlea filled with a liquid called perilymph; separated from the scala media by the basilar membrane and connects to the round window.

scala vestibuli   One of the cavities in the cochlea filled with a liquid called perilymph; separated from the scala media by Reissner's membrane; connects to the oval window and receives vibrations from the stapes.

semicircular canals   Any of the three half-circular, tubelike canals in the labyrinth of the ear that help provide the sense of balance.

sensorineural hearing loss   Hearing loss due to problems with the cochlea or auditory nerve; this type of loss is most commonly treated with hearing aid(s) or cochlear implants.

speech language pathologist (speech pathologist or speech therapist)   An individual with a clinical license to assess, diagnose, treat, and help to prevent disorders related to speech, language, cognitive-communication (brain damage, stroke), voice, swallowing, and fluency (for example, stuttering).

speechreading   The use of visual clues from the lips, facial movements, and gestures of the speaker to understand speech; a speechreader makes use of all visual cues not just lip movements.

stapedectomy   The surgical procedure to remove all or part of the stapes bone of the middle ear and replace it with an artificial prosthesis; most commonly performed for otosclerosis.

stapedius muscle   The smallest muscle in the body, it attaches to the stapes bone to help stabilize the bone and to protect the ear from overly large, damaging vibrations caused by very loud sounds.

stapes   The innermost bone of a chain of three small bones in the middle ear, shaped like a stirrup; the smallest bone in the body.

tectorial membrane   A jelly-like membrane that covers the surface of the organ of Corti.

telecoil   A small coil of wire around a core that induces an electric current in the coil when it's in the presence of a changing magnetic field; telecoils are used in hearing aids to pick up directly the sounds from a telephone without any of the background noises.

temporal bone   A compound bone forming part of the sides and base of the skull with five main parts—the squamous, petrous, and tympanic portions, the mastoid process, and the styloid process; the structures of the ear are found in the temporal bone.

temporal lobe   A large lobe on each side of the brain that contains an area associated with the organ of hearing.

temporary threshold shift (TTS)   A temporary decrease in sensorineural hearing acuity that can occur after exposure to loud sound; with repeated TTS, permanent sensorineural hearing loss may result.

tensor tympani muscle   A muscle in the middle ear that attaches to the malleus.

tinnitus   A sound in one or both ears, such as buzzing, ringing, hissing, or whistling, that occurs even when there is no external sound present; often referred to as head noise; is a common symptom in many diseases of the ear but may occur on its own without apparent cause.

total communication   A method for communicating that uses both speech and signs at the same time. In fact, all means of communication may be used together, including sign language, voice, fingerspelling, lipreading, amplification, writing, gesture, and visual imagery (pictures); the majority of educational programs for the deaf use total communication.

tragus   The triangle-shaped skin-covered piece of cartilage at the front of the external opening of the ear canal.

TTY (teletypewriter, text telephone yoke)   Also called TDD (telecommunication device for the deaf), these are telephone communication devices that present a readable text message for those unable to hear adequately on a standard or amplified telephone.

tympanic membrane   Eardrum; the thin, semitransparent, oval-shaped membrane that separates the middle ear from the external ear.

tympanocentesis   A procedure for collecting middle ear fluid for diagnostic purposes that involves piercing the eardrum with a needle.

tympanogram An examination used to test the condition of the middle ear and mobility of the eardrum and three bones of hearing by varying the air pressure in the ear canal; helps differentiate between sensorinueural and conductive hearing loss and shows the presence of liquid in the middle ear to help diagnose otitis media.

tympanoplasty Surgically repairing or replacing the middle ear bones.

tympanosclerosis The formation of scarring and calcification in the eardrum and middle ear from chronic ear infections, often resulting in hearing loss when the ossicles are involved.

universal newborn hearing screening (UNHS) The completion of one or more objective, physiologic tests to determine hearing status in each ear for all newborn babies, regardless of risk factors, before they leave the hospital or birthing center.

valsalva maneuver A means for getting air from the back of the nose into the Eustachian tube, accomplished by carefully blowing air into the middle ear while holding the nose, often called "popping the ear."

ventilation tubes Small plastic or silicone tubes inserted through the eardrum to allow drainage of fluid and ventilation of the middle ear spaces; also called tympanostomy or PE (pressure equalization) tubes.

vestibular schwannoma The correct, technical name for most tumors arising in the cerebellopontine angle because these tumors arise from specialized cells known as Schwann cells and almost exclusively arise from the vestibular (balance) division of the hearing and balance nerve (the eighth cranial nerve); however, historically people have called these tumors acoustic tumors, as we do, because they affect primarily hearing.

visual reinforcement audiometry (VRA) A method for testing sound thresholds in an infant who is old enough to sit up; the child is given a reward of a toy that lights up or moves when he or she turns toward a sound.

Resources

Organizations

- **House Clinic**
  2100 West 3rd Street
  Los Angeles, CA 90057
  Tel: 213-483-9930
  TDD: 213-483-5706
  Web: www.houseearclinic.com

- **House Ear Institute**
  2100 West 3rd Street
  Los Angeles, CA 90057
  Tel: 213-483-4431
  TDD: 213-484-2642
  E-mail: info@hei.org
  Web: www.hei.org

- **House Ear Institute's Children's Auditory Research and Evaluation (CARE) Center**
  2100 West 3rd Street
  Los Angeles, CA 90057
  Tel: 213-353-7005
  TDD: 213-483-2226
  Web: www.hei.org/children/children

- **American Academy of Otolaryngology—Head and Neck Surgery**
  1650 Diagonal Road
  Alexandria, VA 22314-2857
  Tel: 703-836-4444
  Web: www.entnet.org

- **American Academy of Otolaryngic Allergy (AAOA)**
  1990 M Street, NW
  Suite 680
  Washington, DC 20036
  Tel: 202-955-5010
  Web: www.aaoaf.org

- **American Speech-Language-Hearing Association**
  2200 Research Boulevard
  Rockville, MD 20850-3289
  Tel: 1-800-638-8255
  TTY: 301-296-5650
  Web: www.asha.org

- **Better Hearing Institute**
  1444 I Street, NW
  Suite 700
  Washington, DC 20005
  Tel: 202-449-1100
  E-mail: mail@betterhearing.org
  Web: www.betterhearing.org/

- **Hearing Loss Association of America**
  (Formerly Self-Help for the Hard of Hearing)
  7910 Woodmont Avenue, Suite 1200
  Bethesda, MD 20814
  Tel: 301-657-2248
  Web: www.shhh.org or www.hearingloss.org

- **Deafness Research Foundation**
  641 Lexington Avenue, Fl 15
  New York, NY 10022-4503
  Tel: 1-866-454-3924
  TTY: 888-435-6104
  Web: www.drf.org

- **National Institute on Deafness and Other Communication Disorders**
  National Institutes of Health
  31 Center Drive, MSC 2320
  Bethesda, MD 20892-2320
  Tel: 1-800-241-1044
  TTY: 1-800-241-1055
  E-mail: nidcdinfo@nidcd.nih.gov
  Web: www.nidcd.nih.gov

Find numerous other organizations via the National Institute on Deafness and Other Communication Disorders Directory of Organizations, listed either alphabetically, by topic, or by keyword at www.nidcd.nih.gov/directory.

Print References

This is just a brief list of recently published books about hearing loss that you can find at online booksellers. We have not reviewed these books but simply list them as a sampling of what else is available.

Bauman, Neil G. *Help! I'm Losing My Hearing—What Do I Do Now?: A Basic Guide to Hearing Loss (and Other Ear Problems)*. Stewartstown, PA: Guidepost Publications, 2005.

———— *Keys to Successfully Living with Your Hearing Loss*. Stewartstown, PA: Guidepost Publications, 2009.

Burkey, John. *Baby Boomers and Hearing Loss: A Guide to Prevention and Care*. Piscataway, NJ: Rutgers University Press, 2006.

Carmen, Richard E. *The Consumer Handbook on Hearing Loss and Hearing Aids: A Bridge to Healing*, 3rd ed. Sedona, AZ: Auricle Ink Publishers, 2009.

Dalebout, Susan. *The Praeger Guide to Hearing and Hearing Loss: Assessment, Treatment, and Prevention*. Westport, CT: Praeger, 2009.

Morris, Rebecca A. *On the Job with Hearing Loss: Hidden Challenges. Successful Solutions*. Garden City, NY: Morgan James Publishing, 2007.

Assistive Listening Devices (ALDs)

The American Speech-Language-Hearing Association (ASHA) recommends these companies and organizations for ALDs.

- **Assistech Special Needs**
  Tucson, Arizona
  1-866-674-3549 (V/TTY)
  www.azhearing.com

- **AudioLink Services**
  New York, New York
  1-800-516-6955
  www.audiolinks.com

- **Audiology Products**
  Wenatchee, Washington
  1-888-851-1374
  www.audiologyproducts.com

- **Harc Mercantile**
  Portage, Michigan
  1-800-445-9968 (V)
  269-324-1615 (V/TTY)
  www.harcmercantile.com

- **Harris Communications**
  Eden Prairie, Minnesota
  1-800-825-6758 (V)
  1-800-825-9187 (TTY)
  www.harriscomm.com

- **Hear-More, Inc.**
  Farmingdale, New York
  1-800-881-4327 (V)
  1-800-281-3555 (TTY)
  www.hearmore.com

- **Hitec**
  Burr Ridge, Illinois
  1-800-288-8303 (V)
  1-800-536-8890 (TTY)
  www.hitec.com

- **Soundbytes**
  New York, New York
  1-888-816-8191 (V)
  516-937-3546 (TTY)
  www.soundbytes.com

- **United TTY Sales**
  Olney, Maryland
  1-866-889-4872
  www.unitedtty.com

- **Weitbrecht Communications**
  Santa Monica, California
  1-800-233-9130 (V/TTY)
  www.weitbrecht.com

There are also centers across the country where you can examine the types of assistive listening devices available to determine which products to purchase. To locate loaner devices and device demonstrations, visit the National Assistive Technology Technical Assistance Partnership (NATTAP) website (www.resna.org/content/index.php?pid=133) and select from their state contact list.

Hearing Dog Programs

Many service dog programs around the United States train and provide hearing dogs. We suggest that you perform an Internet search using the search terms "hearing dogs", "service dogs," "hearing ear dog," or "dogs for the deaf." Or ask your hearing health-care provider for contact information for a local hearing dog program.

Noise Levels of Common Sounds*

Appendix **C**

Maximum dB Level**	Sound/Noise	Recommended Exposure Limit***
180 dB	Rocket launch	No unprotected exposure
161–170 dB	Shotgun (12-gauge)	No unprotected exposure
	Handgun	
	Fireworks	
	Artillery fire	
	M1 rifle	
151–160 dB	Balloon pop	No unprotected exposure
141–150 dB	Firecracker (large)	No unprotected exposure
	Bicycle horn	
130–140 dB	Jet engine take-off	No unprotected exposure
	Engine backfire	
	Dynamite blast	
	Noisy squeeze toys	
	Auto racing	
	Pig squeal	
130 dB Immediate Pain Threshold		
121–129 dB	Oxygen torch	No unprotected exposure
	Personal stereo (MP3 player)	
120 dB Severe Irritation to the Ear		
118–120 dB	Thunder	No unprotected exposure
	Jet plane at ramp	
	Rock concert	
	Hammer on nail	
	Ambulance siren	

continues

continued

Maximum dB Level**	Sound/Noise	Recommended Exposure Limit***
115–117 dB	Stadium	No unprotected exposure
	Generator	
	Compactor	
115 dB Unprotected noise exposure of any duration poses serious health risk		
112–114 dB	Diesel truck accelerating	1 Min
109–111 dB	Jackhammer	< 2 Min
	Chainsaw	
	Crying baby	
	Firecracker (small)	
106–108 dB	Home theater (loud peaks)	< 4 Min
	Snowmobile	
103–105 dB	Motorcycle	7.5 Min
	CD player	
	Bulldozer	
100–102 dB	Impact wrench	15 Min
100 dB Extremely Loud		
97–99 dB	Hand drill	30 Min
94–96 dB	Industrial fire alarm	1 Hr
	Tractor	
91–93 dB	Table saw	2 Hrs
	Belt sander	
90 dB	Subway	4 Hrs
	Power lawnmower	
	Leaf blower	
90 dB Hearing Protection Required by OSHA		
88 dB	Cockpit of propeller airplane	4 Hrs
85 dB Ear Damage Possible		
85–87 dB	Forklift	8 Hrs
	Smoke alarm	
	Blender	
	Elevator	
	Handsaw	

Maximum dB Level**	Sound/Noise	Recommended Exposure Limit***
74–82 dB	Ringing telephone	Unlimited
	Lathe	
	Hair dryer	
	Garbage disposal	
	Alarm clock	
	Vacuum cleaner	
65 dB Nonhazardous		
55–60 dB	Normal conversation	Unlimited
	Sewing machine	
	Dishwasher	
	Microwave oven	
50 dB	Background music	Unlimited
	Flowing stream	
	Rainfall	
	Paper rustling	
	Transformer	
	Large office	
50 dB Comfortable		
40–45 dB	Refrigerator	Unlimited
	Quiet residential area	
	Quiet library	
	Quiet office	
30 dB	Audible whisper	Unlimited
20 dB Threshold of Audibility		
0–10 dB	Normal breathing	Unlimited

* *Sound levels of common sounds reaching the ear may vary depending on many factors, including the specific make and model of an item and the distance the listener is from the sound source. The dB levels in this table are an approximation, based on the ear of the listener being right next to the sound source. As distance of the ear from the sound source increases, the measured dB level lessens but could still be loud enough to be harmful.*

** *Sound energy doubles every 3 dB; for example, if an 85 dB noise is doubled, it measures 88 dB. For devices that produce variable levels of sound, the dB level listed is the possible maximum.*

*** *National Institute for Occupational Safety and Health (NIOSH) recommended exposure time limit to reduce the risk of developing permanent hearing loss as a result of occupational noise exposure. The decibel level is a time-weighted average (sound is rarely at exactly the same level for an extended period. It varies, getting louder and softer). Every 3 dB above 85 dB, recommended exposure time is halved.*

Low-Sodium, Low-Caffeine Diet

Appendix

D

High-Sodium Foods to Avoid

Food Group	Foods to Avoid
Beverages	Buttermilk
Bread	Salted crackers (low-sodium bread recommended)
Cereals	Instant cooked cereal
Dairy	All cheese except cottage, hoop, cream, and low-sodium cheddar
Desserts	Desserts made with salt, baking powder, soda, or cake mixes
Eggs	No restrictions
Fat	Bacon fat, salted butter and margarine, regular salad dressing, and mayonnaise
Fruit juices	Tomato juice
Meat, fish, poultry	Salted, smoked, or canned meat such as ham, bacon, cold cuts, and wieners
Potatoes and substitutes	Potato chips and corn chips
Soups	Canned soups and bouillon cubes
Vegetables	Sauerkraut
Miscellaneous	Salt, onion or garlic salt, monosodium glutamate, ketchup, chili sauce, olives, pickles, relish, seasoned salts, lemon pepper, soy sauce, meat tenderizers, and Worcestershire sauce

Sodium Content of Common Foods

Food	Sodium (mg)
Meat, Poultry, and Fish	
Sirloin steak (3 oz.)	53
Baked salmon (3 oz.)	55
Chicken breast, roasted (3 oz.)	64
Ground beef patty (4 oz.)	87
Chicken leg, fried (2.5 oz.)	194
Tuna, canned (3 oz.)	468
Hot dog (1)	504
Salami (2 slices)	607
Fast-food hamburger (4 oz.)	763
Corned beef (3 oz.)	802
Ham, canned (3 oz.)	908
Smoked salmon (3 oz.)	1,700
Soups, Vegetables, and Fruit	
Apple (1)	0
Banana (1)	1
Mixed vegetables, frozen (1 cup)	64
Mixed vegetables, canned (1 cup)	243
Chicken noodle soup, canned (1 cup)	1,106
Tomato sauce, canned (1 cup)	1,482
Sauerkraut (1 cup)	1,560
Bread and Grains	
Oatmeal, cooked without salt (1 cup)	2
Wheat bread (1 slice)	106
Italian bread (1 slice)	176
Bagel (1)	245
English muffin (1)	378
Dairy Products	
Butter, salted (1 tsp)	116
Milk (1 cup)	122
Sour cream (1 cup)	123
Margarine (1 Tbsp)	164
Buttermilk (1 cup)	257

continues

continued

Food	Sodium (mg)
Cheddar cheese (1 cup)	701
Cottage cheese (1 cup)	911
Parmesan cheese (1 cup)	1,861
Snacks, Drinks, Condiments, and Desserts	
Orange juice (1 cup)	2
Peanuts, unsalted (1 cup)	22
Chocolate fudge (1 oz.)	54
Diet cola, with saccharin (12 oz.)	75
Club soda (12 oz.)	78
Potato chips (10)	94
Mustard (1 Tbsp)	129
Ketchup (1 Tbsp)	156
Baked custard (1 cup)	209
Hard pretzel, Dutch style (1)	258
Shortbread cookies (2)	300
Chocolate pudding (1 cup)	880
Apple pie (1 slice)	476
Peanuts, salted (1 cup)	626
Vegetable juice cocktail (1 cup)	883
Dill pickle (1)	928
Pretzel twist (10)	966

Caffeine Content of Common Foods*

Product	Serving Size	Caffeine (mg)
Beverages		
Coffee, drip method	8 oz.	135
Java water	16.9 oz.	125
Coffee, instant	8 oz.	95
Jolt cola energy drink	12 oz.	71
Edge 20 bottled water	8 oz.	79
XTC energy drink	8 oz.	58

Product	Serving Size	Caffeine (mg)
Mountain Dew	12 oz.	54
Espresso	1 oz.	40
Coca-Cola Classic/Diet Coke	12 oz.	46
Sunkist orange soda	12 oz.	40
Pepsi and Diet Pepsi	12 oz.	36
Tea, black (3-min brew)	6 oz.	35
Tea, instant	5 oz.	25
Tea, green	5 oz.	25
Chocolate milk	8 oz.	8
Decaffeinated coffee, drip	8 oz.	3
Decaffeinated coffee, instant	8 oz.	3
Food		
Ben & Jerry's no-fat coffee fudge frozen yogurt	1 cup	85
Starbuck's low fat mocha mambo ice cream	1 cup	60
Häagen-Dazs coffee ice cream	1 cup	58
Dannon coffee yogurt	8 oz.	45
Hershey's special dark chocolate bar	1.5 oz.	31
Baking chocolate	1 oz.	25
Milky Way bar	2.1 oz.	11
Raisinets	1.58 oz.	11
Carnation chocolate crunch breakfast bar	1.34	7
Jell-O chocolate vanilla swirl pudding	5.5 oz.	7
Other		
NoDoz, maximum strength	1 tablet	200
Excedrin	2 tablets	130
Anacin	2 tablets	54

Caffeine intake may vary due to plant variety and brand.

From Lempert, P. "Watching Caffeine Intake? Look Beyond Coffee." Before You Bite column, *Los Angeles Times*, S.2 (Section: Health) Jan. 1, 2001. Sources cited by Lempert: Mayo Clinic, International Food Information Council, National Coffee Association, Center for Science in the Public Interest, National Soft Drink Association.

Hearing Loss and Learning Needs

(Adapted from Better Hearing Institute, www.betterhearing.org)

16–25 dB Hearing Loss

Possible Impact on the Understanding of Language and Speech

- Impact of a hearing loss of approximately 20 dB can be compared to the ability to hear when index fingers are placed in your ears.

- Child may have difficulty hearing faint or distant speech. A child with a 16 dB hearing loss can miss up to 10 percent of speech signal when the teacher is at a distance greater than 3 feet.

- A 20 dB or greater hearing loss in the better ear can result in absent, distorted, or inconsistent parts of speech, especially word endings (such as those represented by the letters *s* and *ed*) and unemphasized sounds.

- Percent of speech signal missed will be greater whenever there is background noise in the classroom, especially in the elementary grades when instruction is primarily verbal. Younger children have greater difficulty listening in noise.

- Young children have the tendency to watch and copy the movements of other students rather than to attend to auditorily fragmented teacher directions.

Possible Social Impact

- May be unaware of subtle conversational cues, which could cause child to be viewed as inappropriate or awkward.

- Child may miss portions of fast-paced peer interactions that could begin to have an impact on socialization and self-concept.

- Behavior may be mistaken as immaturity or inattention.

- Extra effort needed for understanding speech may cause child to be more fatigued.

Potential Educational Accommodations and Services

- Noise in typical classroom impedes child from having full access to teacher instruction. Will benefit from improved acoustic treatment of classroom and sound-field amplification.

- Favorable seating is necessary.

- Child may often have difficulty with sound/letter associations and subtle auditory discrimination skills necessary for reading.

- Child may need attention to vocabulary or speech, even if the loss is due only to a long history of middle ear fluid.

- Depending on loss pattern, child may benefit from low-power hearing aid and/or a personal FM system assistive listening device.

- Appropriate medical management is necessary for conductive losses.

- Requires teacher in-service on impact of "minimal" (16–25 dB) hearing loss on language development, listening in noise, and learning.

26–40 dB Hearing Loss

Possible Impact on the Understanding of Language and Speech

- A 26–40 dB hearing loss causes greater listening difficulties than a "plugged ear" loss.

- Child can hear but misses bits of speech, leading to misunderstanding.

- Degree of difficulty in school will depend upon noise level in the classroom, distance from the teacher, and configuration of the hearing loss, even with hearing aids.

- At 30 dB, child can miss 25 to 40 percent of the speech signal.

- At 40 dB, child may miss 50 percent of class discussions, especially when voices are faint or speaker is not in line of vision.

- Child will miss unemphasized words and consonants, especially if thresholds are poorer in the high frequencies.

- Language skills and speech production may be affected, depending on the degree and configuration of the loss.

- Child often experiences difficulty learning early reading skills such as letter/sound associations.

- Speaker distance and background noise will substantially diminish child's ability to understand and succeed in the classroom, especially in the elementary grades.

Possible Social Impact

- Barriers begin to build with negative impact on self-esteem as child is accused of: hearing when he/she wants to, daydreaming, or not paying attention.

- Child may believe he/she is less capable due to difficulties understanding in class.

- Child begins to lose ability for selective listening and has increasing difficulty suppressing background noise, causing the learning environment to be more stressful.

- Child is more fatigued due to effort needed to listen.

Potential Educational Accommodations and Services

- Noise in typical class will impede child from full access to teacher instruction.

- Child will benefit from hearing aid(s) and use of a desktop or ear-level FM system in the classroom.

- Needs favorable acoustics, seating, and lighting.

- Child may need attention to auditory skills, speech, language development, speechreading, and/or support in reading and self-esteem and may benefit from speech/language therapy.

- Amount of attention needed is typically related to the degree of success of intervention prior to six months of age to prevent language and early learning delays.

- Teacher in-service on impact of a 26–40 dB hearing loss on listening and learning is needed to convey that the impact is often greater than expected.

41–55 dB Hearing Loss

Possible Impact on the Understanding of Language and Speech

- Consistent use of amplification and language intervention prior to age six months increases the probability that the child's speech, language, and learning will develop at a normal rate.

- Without amplification, child may understand conversation at a distance of 3–5 feet if sentence structure and vocabulary are known.

- The amount of speech signal missed can be 50 percent or more with 40 dB loss and 80 percent or more with 50 dB loss.

- Without early amplification the child is likely to have delayed or disordered syntax, limited vocabulary, imperfect speech production, and flat voice quality.

- Even with hearing aids, child can "hear" but may miss much of what is said if classroom is noisy or reverberant.

- With personal hearing aids alone, ability to perceive speech and learn effectively in the classroom is at higher risk.

- A personal FM system to overcome classroom noise and distance is typically beneficial.

Possible Social Impact

- Even with hearing aids, barriers build with negative impact on self-esteem as child is accused of: hearing when he/she wants to, daydreaming, or not paying attention.

- Without hearing aids, communication will be significantly compromised with this degree of hearing loss.

- Socialization with peers can be difficult, especially in noisy settings such as cooperative learning situations, lunch, or recess.

- Child may be more fatigued than classmates due to effort needed to listen.

Potential Educational Accommodations and Services

- Consistent use of amplification (hearing aids plus FM system) is essential.

- Child needs favorable classroom acoustics, seating, and lighting.

- Consultation/program supervision by a specialist in childhood hearing impairment to coordinate services is important.

- Speech/language therapy will be essential to help the child attain and maintain age-appropriate speech and language goals.

- Depending on early intervention success in preventing language delays, special academic support will be necessary if language and educational delays are present.

- Attention to growth of oral communication, reading, written language skills, auditory skill development, and self-esteem likely.

- Teacher in-service required with attention to communication access and peer acceptance.

56–70 dB Hearing Loss

Possible Impact on the Understanding of Language and Speech

- Even with hearing aids, child will typically be aware of people talking around him/her but will miss parts of words said resulting in difficulty understanding in situations requiring verbal communication (both one-on-one and in groups).

- Without amplification, conversation must be very loud to be understood; a 55 dB loss can cause a child to miss up to 100 percent of speech information without functioning amplification.

- If hearing loss is not identified before age one year and appropriately managed, delayed spoken language, syntax, reduced speech intelligibility, and flat voice quality is likely.

- Age when first amplified, consistency of hearing aid use, and early language intervention are strongly tied to success of speech, language, and learning development.

- Addition of visual communication system may be indicated if severe language delays and/or additional disabilities are present.

- Use of a personal FM system will reduce the effects of noise and distance and allow increased auditory access to verbal instruction.

- With hearing aids alone, ability to understand in the classroom is greatly reduced by distance and noise.

Possible Social Impact

- If hearing loss was identified late and language delay was not prevented, communication interaction with peers will be significantly affected.

- Children will have greater difficulty socializing, especially in noisy settings such as lunch, cooperative learning situations, or recess.

- Tendency for poorer self-concept and social immaturity may contribute to a sense of rejection; peer in-service is helpful.

Potential Educational Accommodations and Services

- Full time, consistent use of amplification (hearing aids plus FM system) is essential.

- May require intense support in development of auditory, language, speech, reading, and writing skills.

- Consultation/supervision by a specialist in childhood hearing impairment to coordinate services is important.

- Use of sign language or a visual communication system by children with substantial language delays or additional learning needs may be useful to access linguistically complex instruction.

- Note-taking, captioned films, etc. often are beneficial accommodations.

- Teacher in-service is required.

71–90 dB & 91+ dB Hearing Loss

Possible Impact on the Understanding of Language and Speech

- The earlier the child wears amplification consistently, with concentrated efforts by parents and caregivers to provide rich language opportunities throughout everyday activities and/or intensive language intervention (sign or verbal), the greater the probability that speech, language, and learning will develop at a relatively normal rate.

- Without amplification, children with 71–90 dB hearing loss may only hear loud noises about one foot from ear.

- When amplified optimally, children with hearing ability of 90 dB or better should detect many sounds of speech if presented from close distance.

- Individual ability and intensive intervention will determine the degree that sounds detected will be discriminated and understood by the brain into meaningful input.

- Even with hearing aids, children with 71–90 dB loss may be unable to perceive all high-pitch speech sounds sufficiently to discriminate consonants.

- The child with hearing loss greater than 70 dB may or may not receive sufficient benefit from hearing aids alone to develop speech and oral language as their primary communication mode. To develop these skills, consistent use of appropriate hearing aids and continuing intensive therapy are essential.

- The child with greater than 90 dB hearing loss will be unable to perceive most speech sounds at normal conversational levels, even with hearing aids. Children with severe to profound hearing loss may be candidates for cochlear implantation.

- A visual communication system may be indicated, either as the sole or primary mode of communication or as an aid to development of oral language.

- For full access to language to be available visually through sign language or cued speech, family members must be involved in child's communication mode from a very young age.

Possible Social Impact

- Depending on success of intervention in infancy to address language development, the child's communication may be moderately or very significantly affected.

- Socialization with hearing peers may be difficult.

- Children in general education classrooms may develop greater dependence on adults due to difficulty perceiving or comprehending oral communication.

- Children may be more comfortable interacting with deaf or hard-of-hearing peers due to ease of communication.

- Relationships with peers and adults who have hearing loss can make positive contributions toward the development of a healthy self-concept and a sense of cultural identity.

Potential Educational Accommodations and Services

- No one communication system is right for all hard-of-hearing or deaf children and their families.

- Whether a visual communication approach or auditory/oral approach is used, extensive language intervention, full-time consistent amplification use, and constant integration of the communication practices into the family (whenever possible, by six months of age) will highly increase the probability that the child will become a successful learner.

- A delayed language gap is difficult to overcome. The educational program of children with hearing loss, especially those with language and learning delays secondary to hearing loss, requires the involvement of a therapist or teacher with expertise in teaching children with hearing loss.

- Depending on the configuration of the hearing loss and individual speech perception ability, frequency transposition aids (frequency compression), or cochlear implantation may be options for better access to speech.

- If an auditory/oral approach is used, early training is needed on auditory skills, spoken language, concept development, and speech.

- Educational placement with other signing deaf or hard-of-hearing students (special school or classes) may be a more appropriate option to access a language-rich environment and free-flowing communication.

- Support services and continual appraisal of access to communication and verbal instruction is required.

- Note-taking, captioning, captioned films, and other visual enhancement strategies are necessary. Training in pragmatic language use and communication repair strategies is helpful.

- In-service of general education teachers is essential.

Unilateral Hearing Loss

Possible Impact on the Understanding of Language and Speech

- Child can hear and understand speech using the better ear but can have difficulty understanding in certain situations, such as hearing faint or distant speech, especially if poor ear is aimed toward the person speaking.

- Child will typically have difficulty localizing sounds and voices using hearing alone.

- The unilateral listener will have greater difficulty understanding speech when environment is noisy and/or reverberant, especially when normal ear is toward the overhead projector or other competing sound source and poor hearing ear is toward the teacher.

- Exhibits difficulty detecting or understanding soft speech from the side of the poor hearing ear, especially in a group discussion.

Possible Social Impact

- Child may be accused of selective hearing due to discrepancies in speech understanding in quiet versus noise.

- Social problems may arise as child experiences difficulty understanding in noisy cooperative learning or recess situations.

- Child may misconstrue peer conversations and feel rejected or ridiculed.

- Child may be more fatigued in classroom due to greater effort needed to listen if class is noisy or has poor acoustics.

- Child may appear inattentive, distractible, or frustrated, with behavior or social problems sometimes evident.

Potential Educational Accommodations and Services

- Child should be preferentially seated to direct the normal hearing ear toward the primary speaker.

- Student is at 10 times the risk for educational difficulties as children with two normal hearing ears. One third to half of students with unilateral hearing loss experience significant learning problems.

- Children may have greater difficulty learning sound/letter associations in typically noisy kindergarten and first-grade settings.

- Educational and audiological monitoring is warranted.

- Teacher in-service is beneficial.

- The child will typically benefit from a personal FM system with low gain/power or a soundfield FM system in the classroom, especially in the lower grades.

- Depending on the hearing loss, the child may benefit from a hearing aid in the impaired ear.

Mid-Frequency or Reverse Slope Hearing Loss

Possible Impact on the Understanding of Language and Speech

- This configuration of loss can escape detection on certain newborn screening tests.

- Child can hear speech but, because the speech signal is not heard completely, will have difficulty understanding in certain situations.

- The child may have difficulty understanding faint or distant speech, such as a student with a quiet voice speaking from across the classroom.

- The "cookie bite," or reverse slope listener, will have greater difficulty understanding speech when the environment is noisy and/or reverberant, such as a typical classroom setting.

- A 25–40 dB degree of loss in the low- to mid-frequency range may cause the child to miss approximately 30 percent of speech information, if unamplified. Some consonant and vowel sounds may be heard inconsistently, especially when background noise is present.

- Speech production of these sounds may be affected.

Possible Social Impact

- Child may be accused of selective hearing or hearing when he wants to due to discrepancies in speech understanding in quiet versus noise.

- Social problems may arise as child experiences difficulty understanding in noisy cooperative learning situations, lunch, or recess.

- The child may misconstrue peer conversations.

- Child may be more fatigued in classroom setting due to greater effort needed to listen.

- Child may appear inattentive, distractible, or frustrated.

Potential Educational Accommodations and Services

- Personal hearing aids are important but must be precisely fit to hearing loss.

- Child likely to benefit from an FM system or assistive listening device in the classroom.

- Student is at risk for educational difficulties.

- Child may experience some difficulty learning sound/letter associations in kindergarten and first grade.

- Depending upon degree and configuration of loss, child may experience delayed language development and articulation problems.

- Educational monitoring and teacher in-service is warranted.

- Annual hearing evaluation to monitor for hearing loss progression is important.

High-Frequency Hearing Loss

Possible Impact on the Understanding of Language and Speech

- This configuration of loss can escape detection on certain newborn screening tests.

- Child can hear speech but can miss important components of speech.

- Even a 26–40 dB loss in high-frequency hearing may cause the child to miss 20 to 30 percent of vital speech information if unamplified.

- Consonant sounds represented by the letters *t, s, f, th, k, sh, ch* are likely heard inconsistently, especially in the presence of noise.

- Student may have difficulty understanding faint or distant speech, such as a student with a quiet voice speaking from across the classroom and will have much greater difficulty understanding speech when in low background noise and/or reverberation is present.

- Many of the critical sounds for understanding speech are high-pitched, quiet sounds, making them difficult to perceive. For example, the words *cat, cap, calf, cast* could be perceived as "ca," word endings, possessives, or plurals. Unstressed brief words are difficult to perceive and understand.

- Speech production may be affected.

- Use of amplification is often indicated to facilitate normal speech and language development.

Possible Social Impact

- Child may be accused of selective hearing due to discrepancies in speech understanding in quiet versus noise.

- Social problems may arise as child experiences difficulty understanding in noisy cooperative learning situations, lunch, or recess.

- Child may misinterpret peer conversations.

- Child may be fatigued in classroom due to greater listening effort.

- Child may appear inattentive or distractible.

- Loss could affect self-concept.

Potential Educational Accommodations and Services

- Student is at risk for educational difficulties.

- Depending upon onset, degree, and configuration of loss, child may experience delayed language and syntax development and articulation problems.

- Child may have difficulty learning some sound/letter associations in kindergarten and first grade.

- Early evaluation of speech and language skills is suggested.

- Educational monitoring and teacher in-service is warranted.

- Student will typically benefit from personal hearing aids and use of an FM system in the classroom.

- Use of ear protection in noisy situations is imperative to prevent damage to inner ear structures and the resulting progression of the hearing loss.

Fluctuating Hearing Loss

Possible Impact on the Understanding of Language and Speech

- Of greatest concern are children who have experienced hearing fluctuations over many months in early childhood (multiple episodes with fluid lasting three months or longer).

- Listening with a hearing loss that is approximately 20 dB can be compared to hearing when index fingers are placed in ears. This loss or worse is typical of listening with fluid or infection behind the eardrums.

- Degree of difficulty experienced in school will depend upon the classroom noise level, the distance from the teacher, and the degree of hearing loss on any given day.

- At 30 dB, child can miss 25 to 40 percent of the speech signal.

- A child with a 40 dB loss may miss 50 percent of class discussions, especially when voices are faint or speaker is not in line of vision.

- Child with this degree of hearing loss will frequently miss unstressed words, consonants, and word endings.

Possible Social Impact

- Barriers begin to build with negative impact on self-esteem as the child is accused of: hearing when he/she wants to, daydreaming, or not paying attention.

- Child may believe he or she is less capable due to understanding difficulties in class.

- Typically poor at identifying changes in own hearing ability, with inconsistent hearing, the child learns to "tune out" the speech signal.

- Children are judged to have greater attention problems, insecurity, distractibility, and lack self-esteem.

- Tend to be nonparticipative and distract themselves from classroom tasks; often socially immature.

Potential Educational Accommodations and Services

- Impact is primarily on acquisition of early reading skills and attention in class.

- Screening for language delays is suggested from a young age.

- Ongoing monitoring for hearing loss in school, communication between parent and teacher about listening difficulties, and aggressive medical management is needed.

- Child may benefit from amplification, soundfield FM, or an assistive listening device in class.

- Child may need attention to development of speech, reading, self-esteem, or listening skills.

- Teacher in-service is beneficial.

Comparison of Digital Hearing Aids

Keep in mind that hearing aid features are constantly being upgraded. Some of the features listed on this table are manufacturer specific. No one hearing aid is likely to possess all features.

Digital features are available in most styles of hearing aids (BTE, ITE, CIC, open fit).

Check with your hearing specialist to select the features that best suit you.

continues

Digital Hearing Aid Level of Technology*

Feature	Basic	Advanced	Premium
Multiple programs with automatic switching: Recognizes the type of listening situation and automatically switches to the best listening program. More programs with higher level of technology.	For limited noise exposure	For slightly more active person; reacts more rapidly	For very active person; reacts rapidly to multiple listening environments
Digital noise reduction: Improves hearing by reducing background noise. Degree of noise reduction varies with level of technology.	Limited noise reduction; designed for home use	More active noise reduction; noise reduction in multiple frequencies	Advanced noise reduction; multiple band frequency suppression and enhancement of speech in noise
Directional microphones: Microphones focus on the desired sound source. The microphones can automatically adapt their zoom pattern, allowing you to hear in noisy situations.	Basic broadband directionality; typically only "in front" pattern	Multi-frequency adaptive directionality; directional feature frequency dependent	Multi-frequency adaptive and "zoom" control; allows user to determine direction of hearing
Feedback reduction: Controls annoying shrieking sound caused by sound leaking out and getting reamplified.	Basic feedback reduction	Advanced feedback reduction	Advanced feedback reduction
Volume learning: The hearing aid remembers the manual volume changes you made depending on the situation. Over time, the hearing aid uses this information to adjust the volume automatically.	Not available	Yes	Yes
Data logging: Provides an electronic record of hearing aid use, such as number of hours worn and type of sounds to which you've been exposed. This helps a hearing specialist fine-tune your hearing aid for your needs.	Limited	Yes	Yes

continued

Feature	Digital Hearing Aid Level of Technology*		
	Basic	**Advanced**	**Premium**
Wireless coupling: For people who use two hearing aids, this feature allows the two hearing aids to "talk" to each other and work in unison.	Yes	Yes	Yes
Wind noise control: Reduces the effects of wind noise on microphones. Useful feature for those who spend a significant time outdoors.	No or very little	Yes	Yes
Echo control: Reduces the negative effects that echo has on speech perception.	No	No	Yes
Wireless Bluetooth Capability: Allows the hearing aid to be connected wirelessly to cell phones, MP3 players, and other audio devices.	On some models	Yes	Yes
Cost range per hearing aid	$1,250–$1,750	$1,750–$2,750	$2,750–$3,750

*Hearing aid level of technology:

Basic: User usually in quiet environments; needs help with TV; occasionally attends small gatherings; hearing needs to be improved for just a few types of situations.

Advanced: User frequently attends meetings but is rarely in busy restaurants or large groups; family gatherings tend to be two to four people; wants improved hearing in many situations.

Premium: User often goes to dinner in busy restaurants, frequently attends large family functions, is active in meetings and other social gatherings, leads a busy life—indoors and outdoors, wants the best technology available and the most improved hearing possible for all situations.

Index

F–G